Medical Information Extraction & Analysis

From Zero to Hero with a Bit of SQL and a Real-life Database

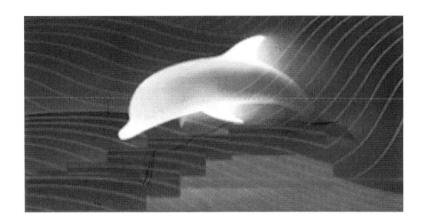

Alexander Scarlat MD, BSc Computer Sciences

Copyright © 2017 Alexander Scarlat
All rights reserved.
ISBN: 1544093373

ISBN-13: 978-1544093376

Dear Don,

I hope you'll find my second book useful.

Your friend,

[signature]

March 2018

Dedicated to my family

In loving memory of my father

Table of Contents

PREFACE	II
1. A BRIEF DATABASE PRIMER	1
DATABASES	2
TABLES, ROWS AND COLUMNS	3
KEYS	4
INDEXES	5
RELATIONSHIPS	6
STRUCTURED QUERY LANGUAGE (SQL)	8
2. MIMIC2 CLINICAL DATABASE	9
BACKGROUND	10
DE-IDENTIFICATION PROCESS	10
MIMIC2 - USER GUIDE & DOCUMENTATION	11
3. MYSQL WORKBENCH	12
INSTALL MYSQL WORKBENCH	13
HOSTNAME, USERNAME AND PASSWORD	14
IN CASE YOU FORGOT	15
CONNECT TO MIMIC2 WITH MYSQL WORKBENCH	16
DISCONNECT FROM MYSQL WORKBENCH	18
LOST CONNECTION TO SERVER	18
FAILED CONNECTION TO SERVER	19
WHEN TALKING WITH IT	19
4. INTRODUCTION TO THE MIGHTY SELECT	21
YOUR FIRST SQL COMMAND	22
RETRIEVE ALL COLUMNS AND ALL ROWS	24
RETRIEVE A SUBSET OF COLUMNS	26
ALIAS	28
RETRIEVE UNIQUE ROWS / REMOVE DUPLICATES	29
SORTING RESULTS	31
FILTERING RESULTS	34
OPERATORS	36
DATE AND TIME	41
THE SURPRISING NULL VALUE	44
SELECT WITHOUT A TABLE	46
PICKING THE RIGHT TABLES AND COLUMNS	47
A NOTE ON SQL FORMAT	47
5. AGGREGATE / SUMMARY FUNCTIONS	48

LET'S COUNT	49
MINIMUM & MAXIMUM	50
OTHER USEFUL SUMMARY / AGGREGATE FUNCTIONS	51
AVERAGE AND STANDARD DEVIATION	51
GROUP BY	52
HAVING	54
IDENTIFY OUTLIERS	57
SUBQUERIES	60

6. QUERYING MULTIPLE TABLES — 63

CONNECTING TABLES WITH JOINS	64
INNER JOIN	64
ALTERNATIVE TO THE INNER JOIN	66
LEFT JOIN	67
RIGHT JOIN	71
SELF-JOIN - COMPARING A TABLE TO ITSELF	71
RETRIEVING ROWS FROM 3 OR MORE TABLES	74
UNION – COMBINING MULTIPLE RESULTS SETS	75

7. ENTITY RELATIONSHIP DIAGRAM - ERD — 76

ERD - THE DATABASE BLUEPRINT	77
USING THE ERD	78
INFORMATION SCHEMA	86
FINDING RELEVANT TABLES AND COLUMNS	87
REVERSE ENGINEERING	90

8. SYSTEMATIC INFORMATION EXTRACTION — 91

CONCEPTUAL MODEL AND QUESTIONS OF INTEREST	92
CLINICAL QUERY DEVELOPMENT STRATEGY	95
MAP TABLE TO ENTITY AND COLUMN TO ATTRIBUTE	96
TEST SCENARIOS - 0, 1, N ROWS	99
ARE RESULTS CORRECT, RELEVANT, COMPLETE, CONSISTENT ?	99
QUERY BUILDING FLOWCHART	101

9. PATIENT — 102

PATIENT RELATIONSHIPS	103
PATIENT ATTRIBUTES	105
GENDER	109
DEMOGRAPHICS	110
AGE	111
GROUP ON DECADES	112
ADMISSIONS	113
WEIGHT, HEIGHT, BMI	117
ETHNICITY, RELIGION, INSURANCE	119
MIMIC2 PROFILE	122

10. MORTALITY — 125

MORTALITY RATE AND ITS MANY FLAVORS	126
MORTALITY BY GENDER	130

Mortality by age	**131**
Mortality by BMI	**134**
Mortality by admission type	**135**
Mortality over time	**136**

11. LENGTH OF STAY (LOS) — 139

LOS – stored vs. calculated	**140**
LOS by gender, age, BMI, admission type	**142**
LOS over time	**144**

12. READMISSIONS — 145

Readmissions calculation	**146**
Readmissions by gender, age	**147**
Readmissions over time	**152**

13. DIAGNOSIS — 153

Patients and admissions by diagnosis	**154**
Mortality by diagnosis	**157**
LOS by diagnosis	**162**
Readmissions by diagnosis	**164**
One patient - all diagnoses	**172**

14. SEPSIS PROFILE — 174

Profile structure	**175**
Sepsis related diagnosis	**177**
Volumes: with / without sepsis	**179**
Gender and age: with / without sepsis	**184**
Mortality: with / without sepsis	**190**
LOS: with / without sepsis	**195**
Readmissions: with / without sepsis	**196**

15. LAB — 200

Non-microbiology vs. microbiology	**201**
One patient – all labs	**202**
MRSA patients	**205**
Lab utilization	**206**
Hypoglycemia in diabetics	**208**
Hypoglycemia – time to next lab	**212**

16. DRUG — 217

IV vs. Non-IV	**218**
One patient – all drugs and medications	**220**
Drugs utilization: ordered vs. administered	**224**
Average time to execute an order	**225**
Nitroprusside toxicity	**226**

17. PROCEDURE — 230

One patient: all procedures	**231**

ONE PROCEDURE: ALL PATIENTS	232
VOLUMES BY PROCEDURE	233
MORTALITY BY PROCEDURE	234
LOS BY PROCEDURE	236
READMISSIONS BY PROCEDURE	237

18. CHART, NOTE AND MUCH MORE 239

PATIENT CHART: LABS, DRUGS, VITALS, ETC.	240
ONE PATIENT: ALL CHART INSTANCES	242
ONE ICU STAY: RESPIRATORY PARAMETERS	243
DISCHARGE, IMAGING REPORT AND MD NOTE	245
ONE PATIENT: ALL NOTES	246

19. PROVIDER AND CARE UNIT 248

CARE GIVER, CARE UNIT AND THEIR RELATIONSHIPS	249
ONE PATIENT: ALL CARE GIVERS	251
ONE PATIENT: ALL CARE UNITS	255
ONE CARE GIVER: ALL ICU STAYS RELATED	256
ONE CARE UNIT: ALL ICU STAYS RELATED	258

20. NURSING 259

ONE PATIENT: ALL NURSING EVENTS	260
ONE PATIENT: ALL NURSING NOTES	263
RESTRAINTS UTILIZATION	264
BRADEN SCORE	266

21. FLUID 267

FLUIDS ERD	268
ONE PATIENT: ALL FLUIDS	269
ONE PATIENT: ALL HOURLY FLUID BALANCES	270
HEMOGLOBIN LEVEL BEFORE BLOOD IS TRANSFUSED	271

22. SCORE AND SCALE 274

SCORE AND SCALE IN MIMIC2	275
ONE PATIENT: ALL SCORES AND SCALES	276
SOFA SCORE AND MORTALITY	278
SOFA SCORE AND LOS	281
SOFA SCORE AND READMISSIONS	282

APPENDIX A. ANSWERS TO QUESTIONS 287

ANSWER 1	288
ANSWER 2	289
ANSWER 3	290
ANSWER 4	291
ANSWER 5	292
ANSWER 6	293
ANSWER 7	294
ANSWER 8	295

ANSWER 9	**296**
ANSWER 10	**297**
ANSWER 11	**298**
ANSWER 12	**299**
ANSWER 13	**300**
ANSWER 14	**301**
ANSWER 15	**302**
ANSWER 16	**303**
ANSWER 17	**304**
ANSWER 18	**305**
ANSWER 19	**306**
ANSWER 20	**307**
ANSWER 21	**308**
ANSWER 22	**309**
ANSWER 23	**310**
ANSWER 24	**311**
ANSWER 25	**312**
ANSWER 26	**313**
ANSWER 27	**314**
ANSWER 28	**315**
ANSWER 29	**316**
ANSWER 30	**317**
ANSWER 31	**318**
ANSWER 32	**319**
ANSWER 33	**320**
ANSWER 34	**321**
ANSWER 35	**322**
ANSWER 36	**323**
ANSWER 37	**324**
ANSWER 38	**325**
ANSWER 39	**326**
ANSWER 40	**327**
ANSWER 41	**328**
ANSWER 42	**329**
ANSWER 43	**330**
ANSWER 44	**331**
ANSWER 45	**332**
ANSWER 46	**334**
ANSWER 47	**336**
ANSWER 48	**338**
ANSWER 49	**339**
ANSWER 50	**340**
ANSWER 51	**341**
ANSWER 52	**342**
ANSWER 53	**343**
ANSWER 54	**344**
ANSWER 55	**345**
ANSWER 56	**346**
ANSWER 57	**349**
ANSWER 58	**351**

ANSWER 59	352
ANSWER 60	353
ANSWER 61	354
ANSWER 62	356
ANSWER 63	357
ANSWER 64	358
ANSWER 65	359
ANSWER 66	360
ANSWER 67	361
ANSWER 68	362
ANSWER 69	363
ANSWER 70	365
ANSWER 71	367
ANSWER 72	368
ANSWER 73	370
ANSWER 74	371
ANSWER 75	373
ANSWER 76	374
ANSWER 77	375
ANSWER 78	377
ANSWER 79	379
ANSWER 80	380
INDEX	**381**
ABOUT THE AUTHOR	**385**

"Without data you're just another person with an opinion"

W. Edwards Deming

ACKNOWLEDGMENTS

I would like to express my sincere appreciation to all the individuals,
that have provided professional challenges in the clinical data extraction and analysis domain over the years.
Without these challenges I would have never improved my SQL skills.

All the dolphins in this book and on its cover are the logo and trademark of
MySQL - Oracle Corporation
Redwood City, CA, USA.

MIMIC2 Demo database used in this book, is a subset of the
ICU database from Beth Israel Deaconess Medical Center, Boston, MA, USA
MIMIC2 was developed in cooperation with
Physionet - MIT Lab for Computational Physiology, Cambridge, MA, USA

Preface

Why this book?
Electronic Health Records (EHR) as a technology, has been in use for more than two decades and as such, has accumulated vast amounts of clinical data.

This data, however, is not easily accessible.

Even with a reasonable reporting mechanism on top of your EHR, you'll quickly find a quality related question that your reporting infrastructure cannot answer. At least not without some tweaking on behalf of your beloved EHR vendor. These tweaks cost real money but what's worse, is the fact that by the time you'll get the report back, most probably you forgot what was the question at hand.
I was lucky, as I knew some SQL before I met my first EHR database many years ago. At that time there were no pre-canned reports, so I had to practically design my own SQL queries, based on what my colleagues were asking for, or just to satisfy my own curiosity. While developing queries on various EHR databases during the years, I've noticed a recurring pattern in terms of the process as well as the parameters involved:

- A question pops up, usually at a quality improvement / risk management meeting, that the existing EHR reporting system cannot answer in a timely manner.
- Information thus needs to be extracted from the EHR database and this information needs to be translated into a meaningful answer to the initial question.
- The questions asked are around volumes of patients or admissions involved, a specific diagnosis or procedure, utilization of resources, drugs, labs, providers, mortality, length of stay, readmission rates, costs, etc.

I believe that after the colossal effort invested in feeding data to EHR for years, the time has come for the machines to regurgitate back some useful information. Moreover, I think this extracted information should be translated into clinical insights: it should be cleaned and massaged into such a form and succinct format that a human being can swiftly come to a wise, evidence based conclusion about a clinical fact.
What if you could answer, by yourself, any of the questions you may have on the clinical information residing in your EHR?
In order to get some meaningful information out of an EHR, you'll need to know how to access the mysterious "back-end" of your EHR , "query the innards" of your EHR database and perform some "slicing-n-dicing". That may sound intimidating even if you are well versed with databases. Diving into a database and coming out with useful information, must seem like a mission-impossible for a clinical person with no knowledge of SQL.

This leads to the main reason for this book, as I believe that anyone should be able to:
- Easily learn the basic SQL necessary to query any clinical database, especially if one can experiment, hands-on, with the newly acquired skills, free from any fears of causing damage.
- Grasp the major healthcare quality metrics: mortality, length of stay (LOS), readmission rate, costs
- Understand the main interactions between the EHR entities: patient, provider, diagnosis, procedure, lab, drug, imaging, etc.
- Master the tricks and tips I have accumulated during the past years working in the healthcare domain, as they are distilled into a systematic, structured methodology in this book.

Whether you go by the adage "one cannot improve on what one cannot measure" or you are strict adept of the Six-Sigma DMAIC (Define, Measure, Analyze, Improve and Control) methodology, you'll agree that the crucial step in both cases is the data extraction.

Without the data, you can measure, analyze, improve and control absolutely nothing.

If you're curious enough, this book will teach you how to access and extract data from your EHR database and analyze this information so you can derive some wisdom and clinical insight from it, for your quality purposes.

What is in this book?
The book introduces the mighty SELECT command – the only command of the Structured Query Language (SQL) that you'll ever need for information extraction purposes.
As I believe in hands-on experience, I've uploaded to the proverbial cloud, a public, de-identified 4,000 ICU patients real-life database – MIMIC2 - for you to experiment with.
All you need is a computer with an internet connection in order to start interacting with a real-life clinical database. If on the other hand, you decide to read this book as is, without actually trying your SQL skills hands-on – that's Ok. All the SQL statements in this book are followed by the screens captured from my machine – so you can see how it would have looked, if you ran the SQL on your laptop.

Once you'll feel comfortable with counting patients and admissions and calculating averages on MIMIC2 tables, you'll get acquainted with a systematic approach and methodology to the slicing-n-dicing involved in clinical reporting for quality improvement initiatives.
Finally, the main concepts in MIMIC2: patient, diagnosis, procedure, lab, drug, fluid, provider, mortality, LOS, readmission, care-unit, etc. are systematically analyzed and explained.

Who should read this book?
You should consider reading this book if you see yourself in one of the following categories:
- You are involved with quality improvement and risk management initiatives and your current EHR reports doesn't satisfy your needs in this regard. Or, you are just curious to know what's in your EHR database, beyond what your EHR reports provide.
- Learning the lingua franca of databases – SQL – is very high on your bucket list. You've waited however, for a book using a real life database with clinical examples to come along.
- You need to extract information from an EHR database and prepare it for predictive analytics, machine learning and artificial intelligence algorithms – the next "big thing".

I hope you'll enjoy reading this book, learning SQL hands-on with the clinical database MIMIC2. When you're done - use your new skills to better understand your own EHR database, so you can help improve the quality provided at your healthcare organization.

Alexander Scarlat MD
Cupertino, California

1. A Brief Database Primer

- Databases
- Tables, rows and columns
- Keys
- Indexes
- Relationships
- Structured Query Language (SQL)

Databases

Databases are an integral part of most applications we use nowadays, since any decent app needs to store or "persist" the information it processes.

Databases are the conceptual and physical silos where data is at "at rest"

This is in contrast to the application input / output workflow which involves data being "in motion" - captured from the screen or another device or app and then stored in a database or conversely, data being retrieved from storage and then displayed to the user.

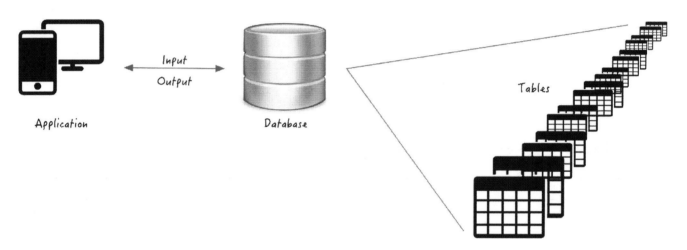

The majority of the databases currently supporting Electronic Health Records (EHR) are either Relational Database Management Systems (RDBMS) or hierarchical databases.
Both expose their databases to Structured Query Language (SQL) – the lingua franca of databases.

This book is based on one flavor of SQL - MySQL - an open source RDBMS. Once you've mastered the basics of SQL using MySQL, you'll find the transition and utilization of other SQL flavors to be very easy and intuitive.

Even if your organization uses a different than MySQL type of database, you will still be able to access it with the SQL you'll learn in this book.

A database can be as small as several kilobytes in one's cellular phone or it can store many terabytes over multiple servers dispersed geographically all over the world. A database may be installed locally on a cellular device / laptop / desktop or it may be stored in the cloud.

Cloud usually means that all the infrastructure (hardware, operating system, web and database server and all the other supporting software like anti-virus, backups, monitoring, as well as the physical security, electrical supply, air conditioning, etc.) – is being taken care of by somebody else and users pay for the cloud services like any other commodity.

For example, I have used Google Cloud to store a copy of the MIMIC2 database referenced in this book. Having the database secured, available anytime, anywhere, over the web, to multiple concurrent users – at very reasonable costs when compared to the alternatives of ownership or renting a machine – is an irresistible proposition, as many have realized during the last decade.

Still, the basic rules governing both the small and the large databases, the local or the cloud-based, are the same, and these databases can be manipulated with a simple, easy to learn, yet powerful language - SQL.

While most of the clinical database systems used nowadays can be accessed with SQL, other NoSQL technologies – Non-Relational databases – emerged during the last decade - MongoDB, Redis, HBase, etc. As currently, NoSQL technology has only a small presence in the EHR market, it is beyond the scope of this book to delve further into NoSQL databases.

Tables, rows and columns

A database is a collection of related tables, each table with its rows and columns.

A conceptual entity, such as Patients, Lab Orders or Lab Results, is usually implemented as one table in the database.

The attributes of an entity, such as Lab Unit or Lab Value, are represented by the table columns.
A column contains similar type of information (last name, date and time, numbers, etc.)
Each column in a database table can have only one type of data: integer, decimals, date and time, string of characters of variable length (varchar), binary (yes/no or true/false) and so on.
The data type for a column is set-up at the table creation time and usually will not change during the database life cycle.

An instance of an entity is usually represented by one row in a table.
A table row contains associated information related to one instance of the table entity – such as a single lab result with the patient identifier, date, time, numeric value and unit of measure, abnormality flag, etc. – all on the same row.

Columns contain similar data types

Rows are instances of associated data

itemid	test_name	fluid	category	loinc_code	loinc_description
50001	AADO2	BLOOD	BLOOD GAS	19991-9	Oxygen.alveolar - arterial [Partial pressure] Respiratory system
50002	BASE XS	BLOOD	BLOOD GAS	11555-0	Base excess in Blood
50003	CARBOXYHB	BLOOD	BLOOD GAS	20563-3	Carboxyhemoglobin/Hemoglobin.total in Blood
50004	CL-	BLOOD	BLOOD GAS	2069-3	Chloride [Moles/volume] in Blood
50006	GLUCOSE	BLOOD	BLOOD GAS	2339-0	Glucose [Mass/volume] in Blood
50007	HGB	BLOOD	BLOOD GAS	718-7	Hemoglobin [Mass/volume] in Blood

The intersection between a row and a column – a database table single cell - is used to store one (and only one) piece of information at a time.

Thus, one should not expect to find both the numeric value and the unit of measure of a lab result, reside in the same cell in a database table. In the above example, the **loinc_code** resides in a separate column than the **loinc_description**.

In a database table, columns contain similar data types, while rows are instances of associated data.

Keys

It is considered good database design to be able to uniquely identify each row in a database table. This is usually achieved by adding a column – Primary Key (PK) - to the table and storing in this column a unique value that identifies the row.

The value of the PK column can be automatically generated and increased by the RDBMS with each additional row added to the table. Usually the PK is not to be reused for identifying other instances in the future.

In the sample table below, the **iteimid** column is a PK column, uniquely identifying a row.

Primary Key (PK) ↘

itemid	test_name	fluid	category	loinc_code	loinc_description
50001	AADO2	BLOOD	BLOOD GAS	19991-9	Oxygen.alveolar - arterial [Partial pressure] Respiratory system
50002	BASE XS	BLOOD	BLOOD GAS	11555-0	Base excess in Blood
50003	CARBOXYHB	BLOOD	BLOOD GAS	20563-3	Carboxyhemoglobin/Hemoglobin.total in Blood
50004	CL-	BLOOD	BLOOD GAS	2069-3	Chloride [Moles/volume] in Blood
50006	GLUCOSE	BLOOD	BLOOD GAS	2339-0	Glucose [Mass/volume] in Blood
50007	HGB	BLOOD	BLOOD GAS	718-7	Hemoglobin [Mass/volume] in Blood

Indexes

In addition to PK a database table may have an Index defined on one or more of its columns. The use of an index can speed up the search and retrieval of a specific row significantly, since the RDBMS uses the index in the same way humans use the index of a book: instead of searching through all the pages to find the one term we are interested in, we use the book index to tell us the page(s) where the term appears.

Similarly, the RDBMS will use an existing database index in order to retrieve the relevant rows from a table, without the need to look through all the table rows. The time savings when retrieving data from an indexed column can be quite significant when compared to columns without an index and this effect is magnified the larger the table is.

So why not index all the columns in a table ? The downside of too many indexes, is that it increases the database size as it needs to store the indexes as well as the actual rows. In addition, too many indexes will slow-down the creation of a new row or the update of an existing row.
Usually a well-balanced database performance is achieved - both creation /update and retrieval of a row - when the columns that are most frequently used in retrieval queries are indexed.

Relationships

In addition to uniquely identifying a row in a table, the Primary Key (PK) mentioned above provides the mechanism to connect (or relate) the database tables. Tables are connected using the PK of one table being used as a Foreign Key (FK) in the relating table(s).

There are 3 types of database relationships:

1 to Many (1:M): where an instance (row) in one table is related to many instances (rows) in the other table.

For example: the relationship between the Patients and the Prescriptions entities (tables). Since a patient may have one or more prescriptions and a prescription belongs to one and only one patient – the relationship between the Patients table and the Prescriptions table is 1 to Many.

This 1:M relationship is achieved by using the PK of the patient (**PatientUID** column) as a FK in the Prescriptions table.

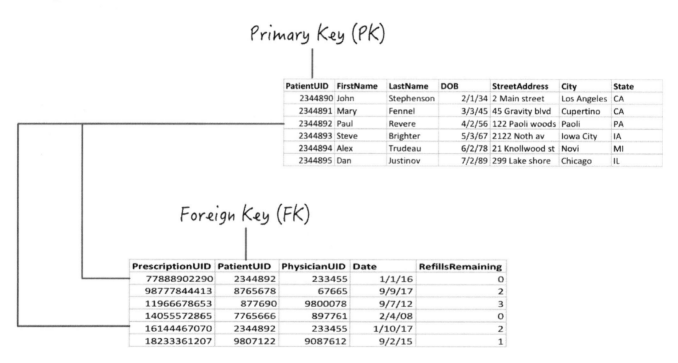

The patient named **Paul Revere** appears once in the Patients table, and its Unique Identifier (PK) **2344892** appears as FK, twice in the Prescriptions table.

While the Physicians table is not shown above, the **PhysicianUID** column in the Prescriptions table denotes a similar 1:M relationship between the Physicians and the Prescription tables. A physician may sign many prescriptions, but a prescription is signed by one and only one physician. Thus, the Physician entity is represented in the Prescriptions table by the **PhysicianUID** – the original Physicians table PK being used as a FK in the Prescriptions table.

The PK/FK mechanism of connecting tables minimizes redundancy, since one doesn't need to store the Patient (or Physician) details (name, address, phone, etc.) repeatedly in the Prescriptions table.

This in turn, improves the database consistency: if the patient's address changes, this change needs to be documented in one table only (the Patients table), while all the other tables that are related via PK/FK will remain correct and consistent without the need to modify the patient's address on each and every row in the Prescriptions table.

Finally, connecting tables with PK/FK minimizes the overall database size and this improves its performance.

Many to Many (M:N): where an instance (row) in one table is related to many instances (rows) in another table and vice-versa.

For example: the relationship between the Patients and the Physicians entities (tables). One patient may have one or more physicians treating him or her, while one physician usually treats many patients.
The M:N relationship necessitates further decomposition into an associative entity (table) that bridges between the two M:N tables.

Associative tables are known under many names, including: association table, bridge table, cross-reference table, crosswalk table, intermediary table, intersection table, join table, junction table, linking table, many-to-many resolver, mapping table, pairing table, etc.

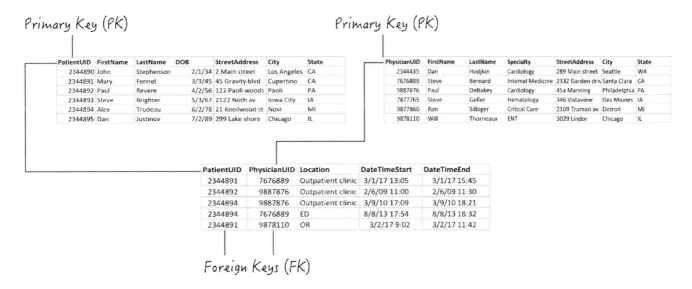

The associative table usually takes the name of the two related tables it intersects – Patients and Physicians - such as the associative table could be named PatientsPhysicians (or PhysiciansPatients) and will contain both the PK from the tables it connects, as FK in the associative table.

Usually an intersection table will have information specific to the associated instance, such as the date and time stamps for the start and the end of the patient visit, the location of the visit, etc.
The associative tables usually have a large number of rows in comparison to the tables that support these intersection tables.

One to one (1:1) relationship: where one instance (row) in one table is related to one and only one instance (row) in another table.

While the previous two relationships described above (1:M and M:N) are used extensively in modern database design, the 1:1 relationship is rarely employed, since the two 1:1 related tables could and most probably should be merged into one table, unless specific performance issues necessitate keeping these tables as separate entities.

Structured Query Language (SQL)

SQL is the programming language of the Relational Databases Management Systems. SQL was first standardized by the American National Standards Institute (ANSI) and the International Organization for Standardization (ISO) as ANSI/ISO SQL in 1986. There has since been a number of revisions – the last one being in 2011.

The various flavors of SQL are all compliant with these standards to various degrees of conformity. If you know one flavor of SQL (such as MySQL used in this book), you'd be efficient with any other SQL flavor (such as Microsoft T-SQL) in a short time, since they are all very similar.

While SQL is used in all aspects of a database life cycle, such as the creation of a new database or a new table, insert of new row(s) into an existing table, update or delete row(s) from a table or delete the table or database, etc. it is important to understand that for data extraction purposes, only one SQL command - the mighty SELECT statement - will cover all your needs.
Thus, this book will describe in depth the SELECT command, but it will not touch all the other SQL commands, since these commands are usually not used or needed in data extraction efforts.

Many newbies are concerned that their initial steps into SQL may cause damage to the underlying database they are using. These concerns are unfounded and you cannot cause any damage to a database - if you are going to use only the SELECT command.
The slight inconvenience a SELECT command could do, is to temporarily overload the RDBMS resources and thus may cause other SQL commands, from other concurrent users, to take longer than expected to complete. An example of a rogue SELECT command that may temporarily overload the RDBMS, can be a SELECT query that returns hundreds of millions of rows.

Rest assured, the MIMIC2 database we are going to use in this book (see next chapter), is configured so you can run only SELECT statements and none of the other, potentially more destructive SQL statements (such as CREATE, DELETE, INSERT, TRUNCATE, DROP, UPDATE, etc.). This book and the MIMIC2 database accompanying it are intended to help educate you on data extraction and analysis and thus the database is configured so it cannot be modified or damaged with well-intentioned SQL statements.

As for queries that may become a resource hog on the MIMIC2 database used for this book - any query that runs more than 60 seconds is being automatically discarded.

If you find SQL interesting, and you'd like to learn more about it, you are encouraged to read some of the many excellent books available on the subject.

2. MIMIC2 Clinical Database

- Background
- De-identification process
- MIMIC2 – User guide & documentation

Background

This book is based on the freely available MIMIC2 Demo clinical database from Physionet:
https://physionet.org/mimic2/demo/

MIMIC stands for Multiparameter Intelligent Monitoring in Intensive Care. The MIMIC2 Demo database contains de-identified information on approximately 4,000 patients hospitalized in one of the critical care units at Beth Israel Deaconess Medical Center in Boston, Massachusetts, USA.
MIMIC2 Demo database is an openly available dataset developed by the MIT Lab for Computational Physiology. It includes demographics, vital signs, lab results, medications, diagnoses, procedures, etc.
No living patients are included in MIMIC2 (although many of these patients lived for up to several years following their ICU admissions documented in this data set).

The MIMIC2 database was uploaded to Google Cloud Platform as a MySQL Community Server RDBMS, so it can be accessed anytime, anywhere and concurrently by multiple readers of this book.

Accessing MIMIC2 is free and you need to pay nothing in order to use this database, as the companion to the book. On the other hand, there is no guarantee, implied or otherwise, that the MIMIC2 database referenced in this book will always be available.

While one can read the book as it is, without accessing the MIMIC2 database – I recommend that you invest ten minutes in connecting to MIMIC2 database with the MySQL Workbench tool in the next chapter. If you believe in the old adage "practice makes perfect", you'll appreciate the opportunity to practice hands-on, executing SQL commands of your own design or solving the hundreds of quizzes and SQL challenges throughout the book. You can find the answers to all the questions in the book appendix.

De-identification process

The de-identification process, has removed any patient related HIPAA protected information from the MIMIC2 tables as well as any information related to the healthcare providers involved (physicians, nurses, etc.)
The de-identification process has also modified all the date and time stamps, so the time frames in MIMIC2 database are shifted to a time frame between March, 2501 and November, 3502.
Hopefully, the 1,000 years' future time span that the de-identified MIMIC2 covers, will not cause any undue cognitive dissonance while running queries on this database and examining the results.

MIMIC2 - User guide & documentation

An excellent guide to MIMIC2, which we'll refer to repeatedly in this book:

User Guide and Documentation for the MIMIC II Database
Gari D. Cliord, Daniel J. and Mauricio Villarroel
Harvard-MIT Division of Health Sciences & Technology

This free guide can be found at:
https://physionet.org/mimic2/UserGuide/UserGuide.pdf

3. MySQL Workbench

- Install MySQL Workbench
- Hostname, username and password
- In case you forgot
- Connect to MIMIC2 with MySQL Workbench
- Disconnect
- Lost connection to server
- Failed connection to server
- When talking with IT

Install MySQL Workbench

As mentioned, MIMIC2 database used in this book resides in the cloud – specifically on a server hosted at Google Cloud Platform. If you'd like to practice SQL hands-on with MIMIC2, you need a tool to access this database. In this chapter you are going to install such a tool, a client application - MySQL Workbench - on your computer / laptop and then you'll connect it to MIMIC2 database.

MySQL Workbench is the client we are going to use to connect to the MySQL server database.

Similar to MySQL Community Server, the database server used to store MIMIC2 for this book, MySQL Workbench is an open source client application and it is free of charge.
The name – MySQL - is a combination of the co-founder Michael Wildenius daughter's name and SQL – the abbreviation for Structured Query Language.
MySQL is owned by Oracle Corporation.

To install MySQL Workbench please follow the instructions at
https://dev.mysql.com/downloads/workbench/

On the download page, first select the operating system your computer uses (Windows, Mac, etc.) and then download and install MySQL Workbench.

Note that the Login or Sign Up offered are optional and you don't really need to login in order to download this app. On the lower part of the screen you'll find a "No thanks, just start my download" link you should click.

Once installed, open the MySQL Workbench application. On a Mac it should look similar to this:

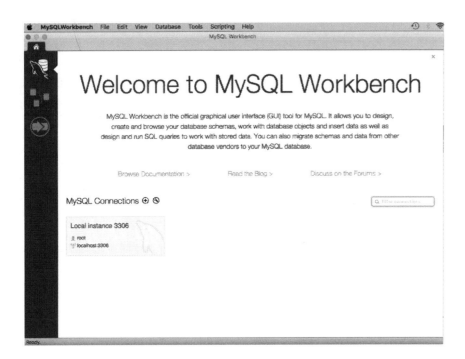

Hostname, username and password

In order to access the MIMIC2 database stored in the cloud, you'll need the hostname, username and password. BookGuests is a web application that will automatically provide you with these credentials for MIMIC2 database. BookGuests can be found at:

https://www.codixim.com/BookGuests/default/index

The BookGuests app is NOT the MIMIC2 database mentioned in the book.
BookGuests only provides the hostname, username and password to access MIMIC2.

How to use the BookGuests app in order to receive the username and password for MIMIC2:
1. First, you should sign-up ... Click on the "Log In", upper right corner
2. From the drop down menu pick "Sign Up"
3. Enter your details and provide a valid email for verification purposes
4. The password you provide is for this BookGuests web app only and it is not the password you'll use to access the book's MIMIC2 database
5. Prove you're not a robot
6. Once you submit this form, an email will be sent to you from text2codes@codixim.com
7. If you do not receive an email, check your spam folder

8. Click on the link in the email
9. Log into BookGuests app and you will be provided with a different set of username and password and the hostname.
10. The hostname, username and password provided by BookGuests app should be used to access the MIMIC2 database.
11. You cannot modify these parameters provided by BookGuests app.

Once you are logged in into BookGuests, you can retrieve the hostname, username and password for accessing the MIMIC2 database mentioned in this book:

BookGuests™   HOME

Welcome back Alexander Scarlat

Here are your credentials required to access the clinical database accompanying the book

Hostname ... 104.196.122.247
Username ... User3752120
Password ... 1:   9(

Please follow the instructions in the book in order to connect to the clinical database
Good luck and have fun !

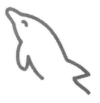

In case you forgot

If you forgot your username or password for MIMIC2, you can always retrieve them using the BookGuests application.

If you forgot the password to the BookGuests app, click on "Lost password?" under Log In – upper right corner of the screen - and an email will be sent to you, to reset your password.

Connect to MIMIC2 with MySQL Workbench

Assuming you have successfully installed the MySQL Workbench client application on your computer, as mentioned above:

On the upper menu of MySQL Workbench, click on **Database** and then select **Manage Connections**:

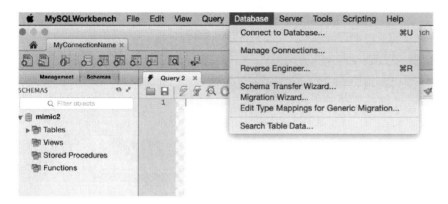

Next screen should look similar to this:

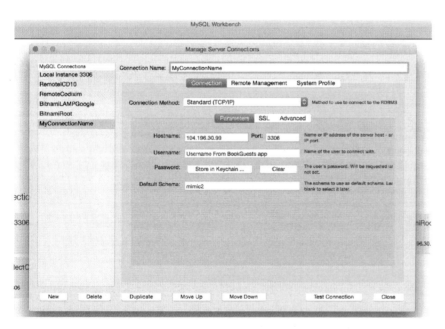

Fill out this form with the following parameters:

Connection Name: Enter a name for your connection to MIMIC2 (e.g. MyConnectionName)
Connection Method: Standard TCP/IP
Hostname: enter the Hostname as provided by the BookGuests app (e.g. 104.196.30.99)
Port: 3306
Username: enter your Username as provided by the BookGuests app (e.g. User4573227821)
Default schema: mimic2

Click **Test connection**

Password: enter your password as provided by the BookGuests app.
If you have the option to save the in your keychain, select it.

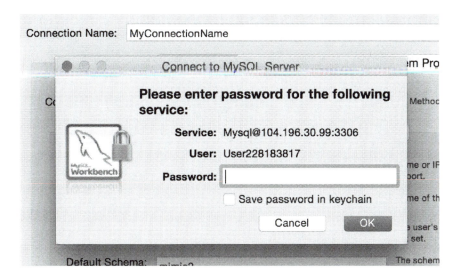

If connection is successful, you'll see the following notification:

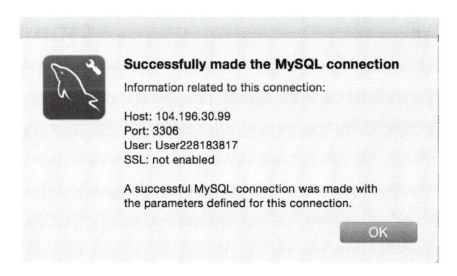

Once MySQL Workbench has connected successfully with the MIMIC2 database, the connection parameters are saved under the connection name you've given (e.g. MyConnectionName), so you can access the MIMIC2 in the future without entering the connection parameters again.

You can now connect to the MIMIC2 database:
On the upper menu bar of MySQL Workbench, click **Database**, then **Connect to database**, select your connection name and provide the password (if you haven't saved it in your keychain in the previous step).

Disconnect from MySQL Workbench

Disconnecting from the MIMIC2 database is simple: just close the tab with the connection name you've opened with MySQL Workbench (the small "X" on the right upper corner of the connection tab).

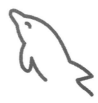

Lost connection to server

As mentioned above, queries attempting to retrieve tens of millions of rows may take a while to process. Since MIMIC2 resides on a modest machine in the cloud and it is planned to serve many users concurrently, a mechanism to prevent queries from draining this machine's resources was put in place:

- Queries that run over 60 seconds are discarded and you will get a message that the connection to the server was lost.

- You are limited to 2 concurrent connections at a time, with one connection used by the MySQL Workbench and the other by the queries you are actually running. Thus, it wouldn't be wise to share your username and password with others as they may block your access to MIMIC2, if they log-in before you do.

If you run a query that causes a "lost connection to the server", or if MySQL Workbench is idle for a long time - you may encounter the following error when trying to run a query:

Error Code: 1226 User 'User123456789' has exceeded the 'max_user_connections' resource (current value: 2)

Usually the server that hosts MIMIC2, cleans itself of stale or sleeping connections, queries running over 60 seconds and other potential resources hogs. It may take up to a minute for your MySQL Workbench connections to reset and the above error message to disappear so you can continue working with MySQL.

Failed connection to server

A failed connection to server is a completely different issue than a lost connection.
If you try to connect to MIMIC2 using MySQL Workbench and you receive the following error:

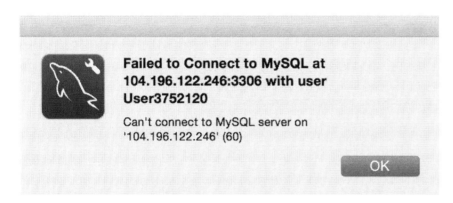

Then the problem may be with the actual machine hosting MIMIC2.
Rarely, the original IP address or Hostname of this machine may change and this will be reflected on BookGuests app at https://www.codixim.com/BookGuests/default/index
Please log-in to BookGuests app and review the Hostname published there:

- If the Hostname published on BookGuests is different than the one you currently have – you'll need to modify it accordingly on the MySQL Workbench – see above the steps required.
- If the Hostname published on BookGuests is the same one you have and you still cannot connect, please let me know.

When talking with IT

The following are important parameters in order to set up a connection between a client, such as your cellular device, laptop or desktop and a clinical database on a secured server, that your organization maintains. If you are not part of the IT department, most probably you're going to ask an IT person for help in setting up such a connection.
Remember, you are trying to establish a connection between a client and a server. For the handshake between the two to work nicely you'll need:

Client app: MySQL Workbench, Navicat or other SQL client tool ?
Connection name: Your pick
Connection method: Standard TCP/IP ? other ?
Hostname: 104.196.122.247… an IP address
Port: 3306 … usually the port reserved for MySQL, may be different for other SQL tools
Username / Password
Default schema: … usually optional, name of the default database
Select privileges only

This last point usually has a soothing effect on IT, since it shows your benevolent intentions: one cannot do much harm to the database structure or consistency with the SELECT command only.

If IT is still concerned with the potential resource-hogging queries you may run on the database, IT can limit your queries to a certain number of seconds, such as the 60 seconds limit employed in this book. Depending on the actual database used, putting such a limit in place may be quite easy to do.

4. Introduction to the Mighty SELECT

- Your first SQL command
- Retrieve all columns and all rows
- Retrieve a subset of columns
- Alias
- Retrieve unique rows / Remove duplicates
- Sorting results
- Filtering results
- Operators
- Date / Time parts and difference
- The surprising null value
- Select without a table
- Picking the right tables and columns
- A note on SQL format

Your first SQL command

If you've connected successfully to MIMIC2 database using MySQL Workbench, as detailed in the previous chapter, you should see something similar to this screen:

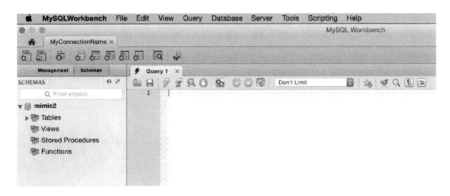

or

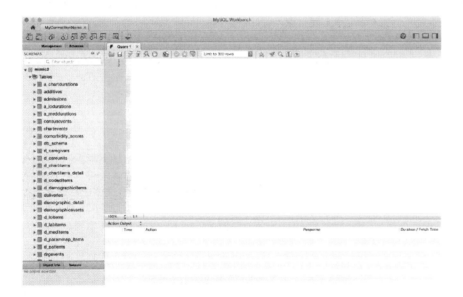

In order to see the tables in MIMIC2 database, either click on the small arrow, near **Tables** in the left panel, or type the following in the **Query 1** panel:

SHOW TABLES;

Then click on the third icon from the left – the lightning bolt - to run the query. The results will appear in the **Results Grid** below:

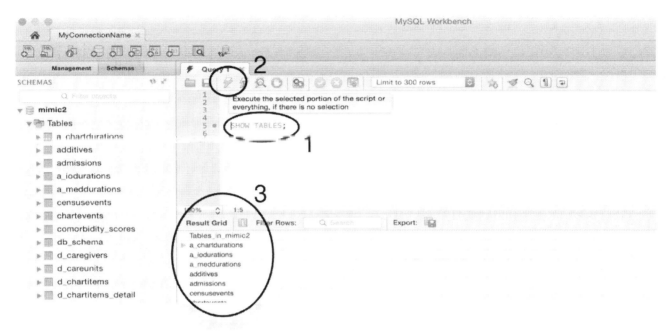

Congratulations! You've just run your first SQL command.

If you make a mistake or have an error in your SQL syntax, MySQL Workbench will underline the error in red and on the left side of the query panel, before you run it.

If you still run the erroneous query, there will be no **Result Grid** and on the bottom part of the screen, the **Action Output** panel will display the error:

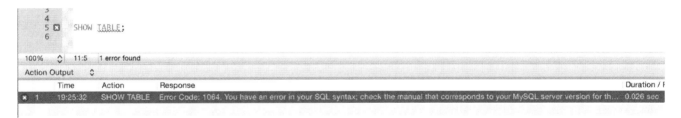

 Always check the left side of the panel where you write your SQL statements, before running a query:
If it shows a red x – you have an error, and this error may be specifically underlined in your SQL.
If it's a blue circle – you're Ok, at least from the basic SQL syntax perspective.

Retrieve all columns and all rows

The basic SELECT syntax is:

SELECT column(s)
FROM table(s)
WHERE condition(s);

The query to return all columns and all rows of a table, with no filters and no conditions:

SELECT *
FROM table_name;

The * symbol means "all columns" in SQL

Let's try it with one of the MIMIC2 tables. In the **Query 1** panel of MySQL Workbench, type:

SELECT *
FROM admissions;

Click the thunderbolt icon (third from the left, upper menu row) to run the query.

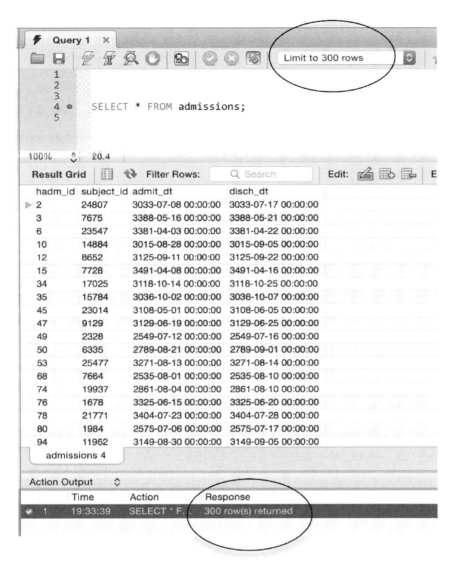

The resulting grid has 4 columns but only 300 rows. The reason we've received only 300 rows from the **admissions** table is that a limit has been set for MySQL Workbench to retrieve only 300 rows – see upper menu row.

Why would someone need to restrict the number of rows returned by a query ?
Since tables can be quite large, some having many millions of rows, and retrieving all these rows may take some time, you may consider limiting the number of rows while you develop your query statement, so you can see if the query runs Ok with a small subset of rows. If for example, a query takes forever to retrieve 300 rows, it wouldn't be any faster retrieving 3 million rows – you probably need to design a better query.

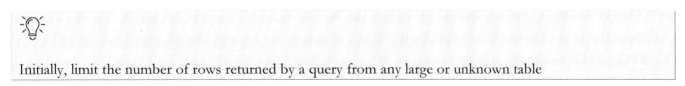

Initially, limit the number of rows returned by a query from any large or unknown table

You can easily modify this limit by changing the settings in the drop-down menu, for example: **Don't limit**.

Question 1

Remove the limit on the number of rows returned and run the above query again. How many rows are returned this time from the **admissions** table?

Retrieve a subset of columns

If we'd like to retrieve only a subset of the columns in a table, the SQL syntax is:

SELECT column1, column2, … columnX
FROM table_name;

Limiting the columns retrieved by a query is independent from any restrictions on the number of rows returned

Let's take a look at the **demographic_detail** table. First, since we don't know the names of the columns in this table, let's run a query to return all columns and all rows:

SELECT *
FROM demographic_detail;

Medical Information Extraction and Analysis

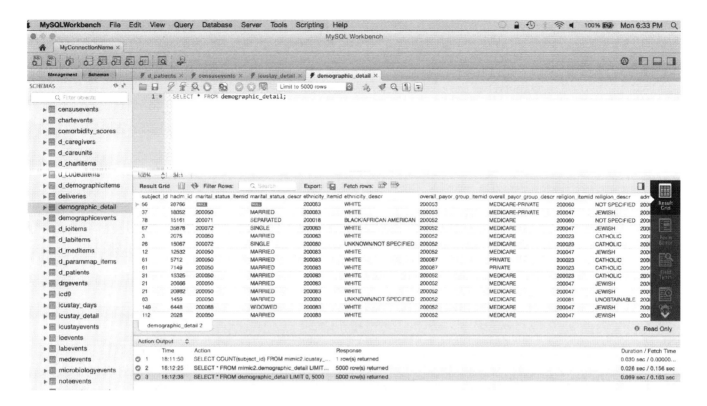

This table has several columns. If we are interested only in the marital status and the ethnicity of the patients:

SELECT marital_status_descr, ethnicity_descr
FROM demographic_detail;

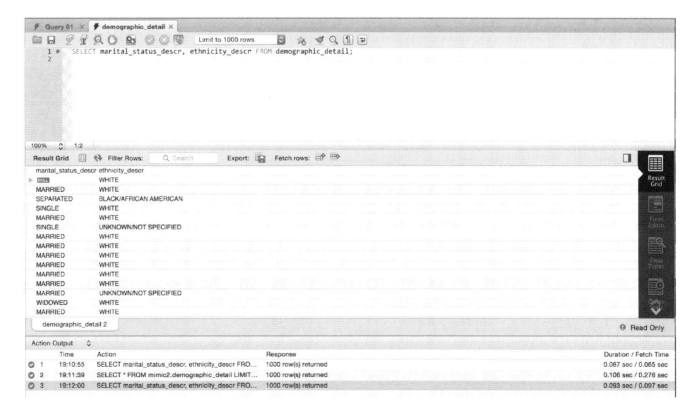

SELECT defines the columns or calculations you'd like the query to return
FROM defines the tables participating in the query

Alias

We can modify the names of the columns returned by the query to something more meaningful, so instead of **marital_status_descr** we can change it to the alias of **MaritalStatus** and instead of **ethnicity_descr** we can modify it to the alias of **Ethnicity** like this:

SELECT marital_status_descr AS MaritalStatus, ethnicity_descr AS Ethnicity
FROM demographic_detail;

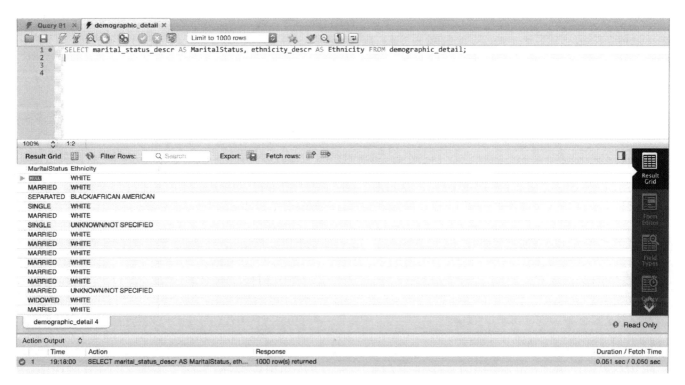

Later we'll use alias for table naming as well.

There is one caveat when using an alias – the new alias name cannot contain spaces such as **Marital Status**. The space between Marital and Status will cause a run-time SQL error. So either use an underline as in

Marital_Status or just concatenate the two with Camel case capitalization style (for readability purposes) as in MaritalStatus.

 Question 2

Using the table **icustay_detail**, retrieve only the gender, date of birth and date of death (and name these columns as PatientGender, BirthDate, DeathDate respectively).

Retrieve unique rows / Remove duplicates

If we run the following query:

SELECT drug_name, prod_strength
FROM poe_med;

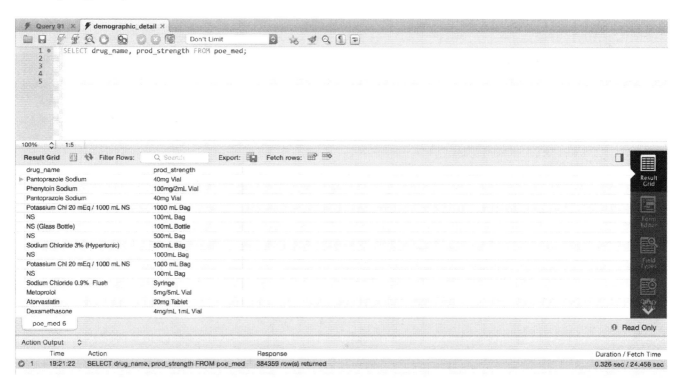

The results will contain 384,359 rows of all the combinations of drug names and their strengths, with a lot of duplicate values.

If we'd like the same list but only the unique combinations of drug name and strength - we'll use the following query:

```sql
SELECT DISTINCT drug_name, prod_strength
FROM poe_med;
```

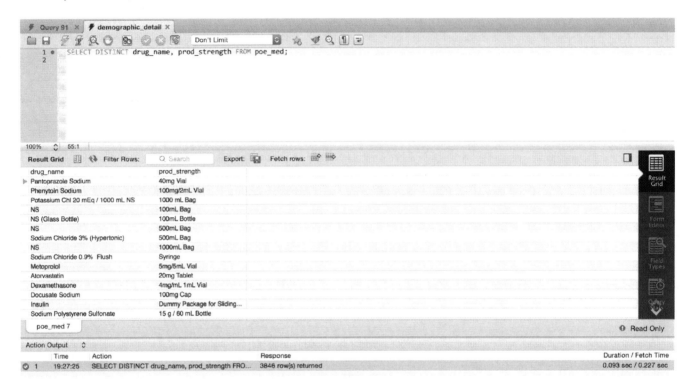

The results include only 3,846 rows, the unique combinations of **drug_name, prod_strength** as the **DISTINCT** SQL command has removed all duplicates.

DISTINCT defines the columns you'd like to retrieve only unique values, without repetitions

 Question 3

Using the table **noteevents**, find out the (unique) categories of these notes.

Sorting results

The previous list of drug names and their strengths is unsorted / unordered. We can sort the results by drug name alphabetically using the following command:

SELECT DISTINCT drug_name, prod_strength
FROM poe_med
ORDER BY drug_name;

Note the two rows related to "*NF* Micafungin":

NF Levocarnitine	200mg/ml-10ml vial
NF Lidocaine Patch 5%	5% PATCH
NF Micafungin	50 mg Vial
NF Micafungin	50mg Vial
NF Miralax	17gm Packet

"*NF* Micafungin" "50 mg Vial"
"*NF* Micafungin" "50mg Vial"

The above 2 rows seem like duplicates to us humans, but they are actually different from SQL perspective, due to the space between the "50" and "mg" on the first row – which doesn't appear on the second row. The lesson learned is simple: from a SQL standpoint, even one space within a string will make that string to be valued differently than the same string without the space.

We can sort results by more than one column, for example:

SELECT DISTINCT marital_status_descr, ethnicity_descr
FROM demographic_detail
ORDER BY marital_status_descr, ethnicity_descr;

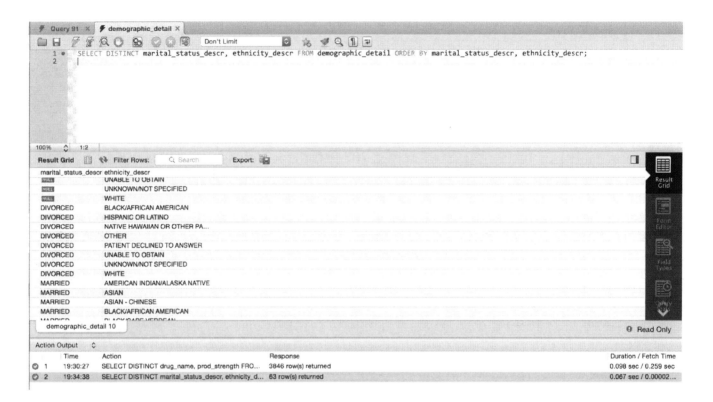

The above SQL command will sort alphabetically the (unique) rows first by **marital_status_descr** and then by **ethnicity_descr** columns. If we need the results sorted in reverse, descending alphabetical order, we add **DESC** at the end of the **ORDER BY**:

SELECT DISTINCT drug_name, prod_strength
FROM poe_med
ORDER BY drug_name DESC;

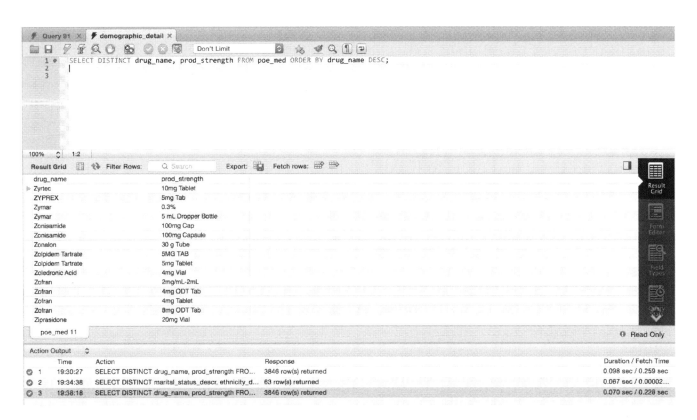

We can sort results on numeric or date / time columns as well as character strings.

ORDER BY defines the columns you'd like to sort on

Question 4

Using the table **poe_order**, retrieve the (unique) medications and the number of doses for 24 hours and sort them in ascending order of the medication name (alphabetically) and the number of doses (numerical order from the smallest to the largest number).

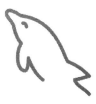

Filtering results

The WHERE clause is used to filter the results returned by a query, to extract only the rows that fulfill a specific condition:

SELECT column1, column2, ...
FROM table_name
WHERE condition;

If we are interested in retrieving from the **poe_med** table only the rows that are related to the drug "Metoprolol", the SQL syntax should be:

SELECT *
FROM poe_med
WHERE drug_name = 'Metoprolol';

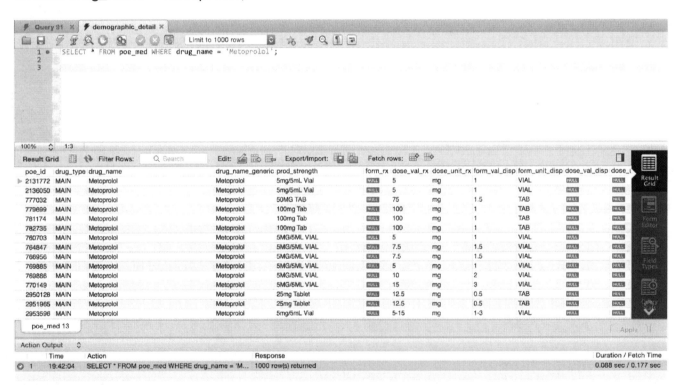

Note that since "Metoprolol" is a string, it is enclosed within single quotes. MySQL (and other RDBMS) allows text strings to be enclosed within double quotes as well, so the following is considered a correct SQL statement and it is identical to the single quotes command above:

SELECT *
FROM poe_med
WHERE drug_name = "Metoprolol";

The string used for comparison is case-insensitive, so "Metoprolol" is the same as "mEtoProlol"

When filtering results with the WHERE clause on a numerical column, you don't need any quotes around the condition considered, though MySQL would allow quotes on numerical values as well. Retrieving from **poe_med** all the rows related to "Metoprolol" and **dose_val_disp** = 50, has two conditions and the logical "AND" operator connecting them:

SELECT *
FROM poe_med
WHERE drug_name = "Metoprolol" AND dose_val_disp = 50;

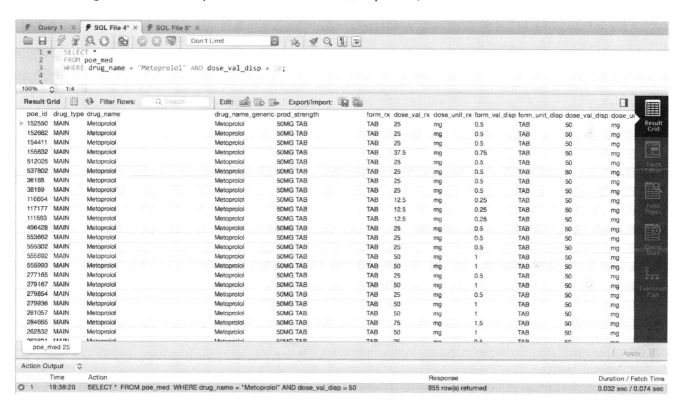

WHERE defines the conditions that restrict the number of rows considered by a query

Operators

The following operators can be used with the WHERE clause:

AND | OR | NOT	Logical operators
=	Equal
<>	Not equal (MySQL allows the != notation for Not equal as well)
>	Greater than
>=	Greater than or equal
<	Less than
<=	Less than or equal
BETWEEN	Between an inclusive range (equivalent to >= …AND… <=)
LIKE	Fits a specific pattern (with wildcards)
IN	List of multiple values, instead of using multiple "OR" operators
+ - * /	Arithmetic operators (addition, subtraction, multiplication, division)
CONCAT	String concatenation

Question 5

Using the table **poe_order**, retrieve all the rows where the Diazepam medication was not administered by mouth (route is not "PO")

Question 6

Retrieve all the patients that have been admitted between Jan 1st, 3000 and Dec 31st, 3100 and order them by the admission date (Remember all the dates are skewed by the de-identification process of the real-life MIMIC2 clinical database)

The **LIKE** operator is used with the **WHERE** clause to search for a specific pattern. There are two wildcards commonly used with the **LIKE** operator:

The **%** percent sign is used to represent between zero and many characters in a pattern
The **_** underscore sign represents one and only one character placeholder in the pattern

If we need to retrieve all the unique drug names that begin with the characters "Mo":

```
SELECT DISTINCT drug_name
FROM poe_med
WHERE drug_name LIKE 'Mo%';
```

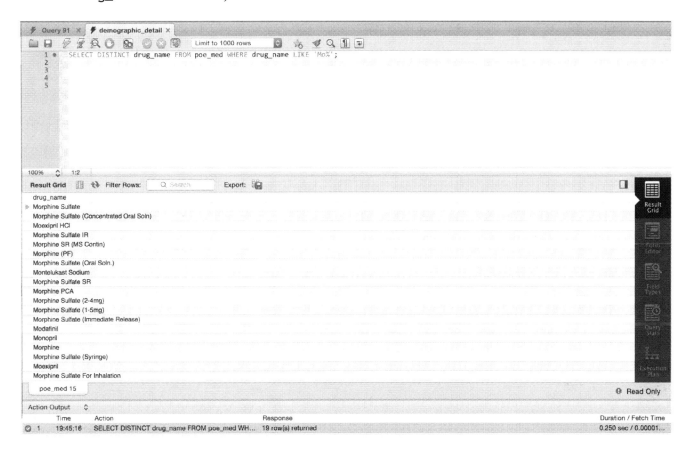

This query will return "Morphine", "Morphine Sulphate", "Morphine PCA", "Moexipril HCL", "Monopril", "Modafinil", etc.

LIKE used together with the % place holder is useful for finding a piece of string within other larger strings

 Question 7

Retrieve all the (unique) drug names that end with "azolam" from the **poe_med** table

The IN operator can be used instead of multiple OR conditions. So instead of this query:

SELECT DISTINCT drug_name
FROM poe_med
WHERE drug_name = 'norepinephrine'
OR drug_name = 'epinephrine'
OR drug_name = 'neo-synephrine' ;

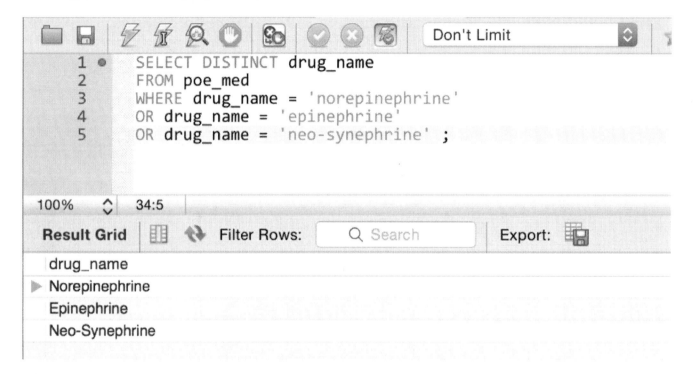

For the same results, we can use the equivalent and succinct IN operator:

SELECT DISTINCT drug_name
FROM poe_med
WHERE drug_name IN ('norepinephrine' , 'epinephrine' , 'neo-synephrine');

IN (list of parameters) is useful when you have to compare something to a large list of parameters and you find yourself using many OR in your SQL

The negation operator NOT can be used with the other operators:
NOT IN
NOT BETWEEN
NOT LIKE

Question 8

Retrieve all the rows from the **poe_order** table, that contain the characters "ephrine" in the medication name, the route is not IV, IV Drip, IM or SC and the start date is within the time frame of Jan 1st, 3000 and Jan 1st, 3500

If we'd like the dose of the drug imipenem to be displayed in grams in addition to the dose in mg, we can use the division operator:

SELECT drug_name, dose_val_rx AS DoseInMg, dose_val_rx / 1000 AS DoseInGrams
FROM poe_med
WHERE drug_name LIKE '%imipenem%';

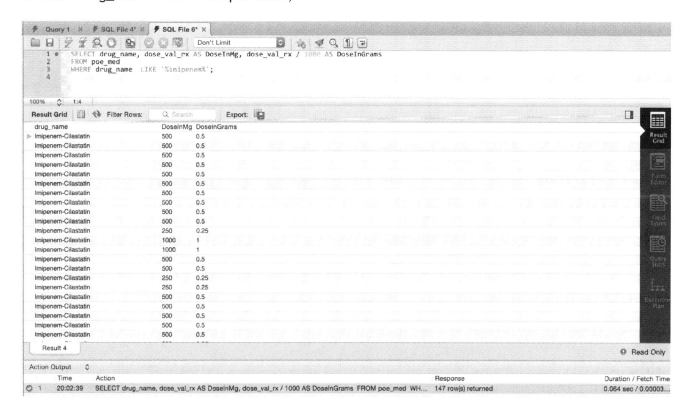

SQL can concatenate two or more columns with the CONCAT operator. These columns are being evaluated as strings even if originally they were numerical. If we need the **expiration_val** and **expiration_unit** from the **poe_order** table to be concatenated with the "-" character in between, the query would be:

SELECT DISTINCT expiration_val, expiration_unit,
CONCAT(expiration_val, "-", expiration_unit) as ExpValUnit
FROM poe_order;

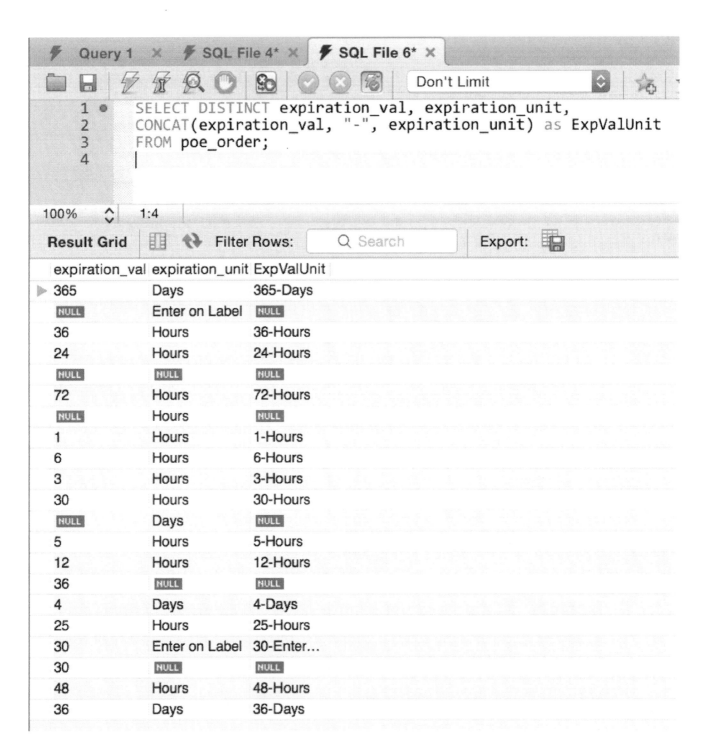

Date and Time

We can extract a part from a date and time column - year, month, day, etc. with the simple syntax:

SELECT Unit(DateTimeColumn)
FROM table_name;

Where **Unit** can be **DAY, HOUR, MINUTE, WEEK, MONTH, YEAR**, etc.
If we'd like only the year and month of the admission date and time stamp from the **admissions** table:

SELECT YEAR(admit_dt), MONTH(admit_dt)
FROM admissions;

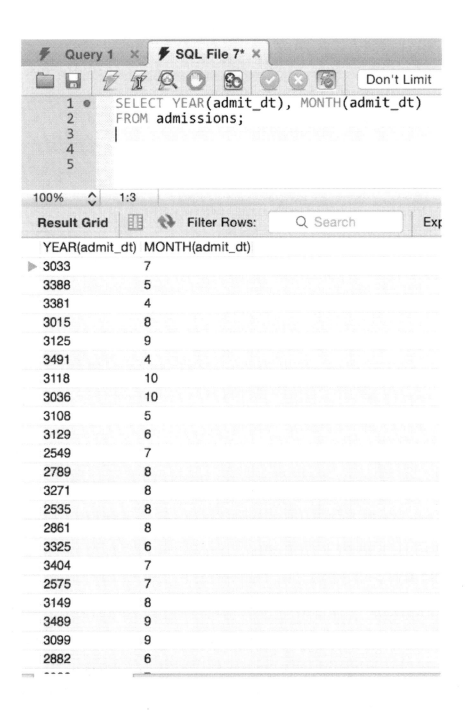

Date / Time difference follows the syntax:

```
SELECT TIMESTAMPDIFF(Unit, FirstDateTime, SecondDateTime)
FROM table_name;
```

Where **Unit** can be **DAY, HOUR, MINUTE, WEEK, MONTH, YEAR**, etc.
In order to calculate the number of days between admission and discharge, we can use:

```
SELECT *, TIMESTAMPDIFF(DAY, admit_dt, disch_dt) AS DTdifference
FROM admissions;
```

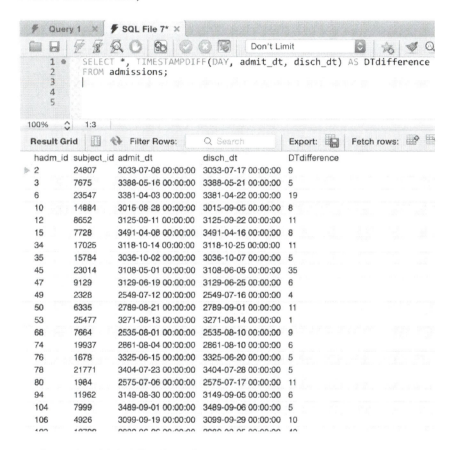

When comparing two columns that contain date and time data, and the time is set as 00:00:00 in one column, make sure that the other column is in the same format and it doesn't have any time values as 02:32:45 for example.

In case one of the two date and time columns that need comparison has the time defined other than **00:00:00**, say **02:32:45** – then we'd need employ a comparison that extracts the date part from both fields for the equate clause, such as **DATE(datefield) = DATE(admit_dt)**. This eliminates the TIME part from being considered by the query. Without specifying which part of the column we are interested in, these columns – one with the time values of 00:00:00 and the other with time values other than 00:00:00 - can never be equal, only because of the time differences, which we may or may not have cared about.

Question 9

Using the **poe_order** table, retrieve the medication name, start and stop date / time stamps and calculate the number of hours patients have been on the "Propofol" medication (IV anesthetic). Limit the results to those that have been on Propofol for more than 24 hours.

The surprising null value

To quote the MySQL tutorial:

"The NULL value can be surprising until you get used to it"

- The NULL value means a missing or unknown value .
- Conceptually it is different than the zero "0" value or an empty space string " " value.
- Actually you may have seen the NULL value in some of the queries results we've discussed above.
- Comparing a NULL with a non-null value will return a NULL
- An arithmetic operator using a NULL value will return a NULL.
- To make it more intriguing, comparing between two nulls will return a NULL as well.
- When ordering / sorting results, the NULL values will appear first (if ascending order).
- Any expression that contains a NULL will return a NULL.

With such a finicky value, one needs a way to find the NULL values or conversely, those that are not null, and SQL provides the operators that can evaluate whether there is a null value involved:

IS NULL
IS NOT NULL

If we'd like to retrieve all the patients that have both their min. and max. Sequential Organ Failure Assessment (SOFA) scores defined in the **icustay_detail** table:

```
SELECT *
FROM icustay_detail
WHERE sofa_min IS NOT NULL AND sofa_max IS NOT NULL;
```

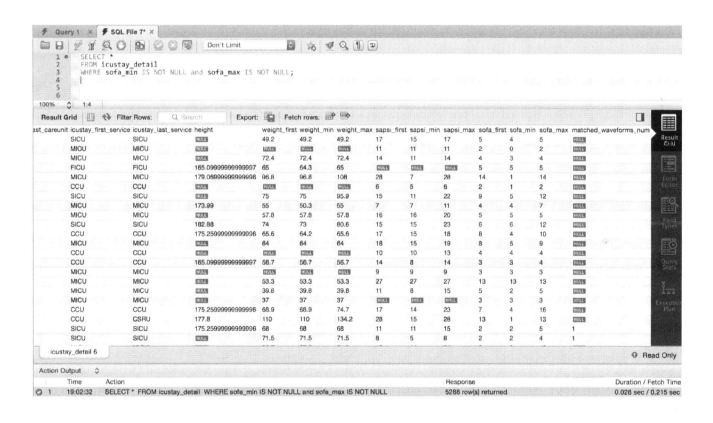

Another useful function is **IFNULL(expression, value)**.
If an **expression** is **NULL**, this function will replace the **NULL** with the **value**.
This becomes handy when we'd like to replace NULLs with zeroes:

IFNULL(expression, 0)

 ## Question 10

Using the **icustay_detail** table, retrieve all the rows with non-null values in the height and weight_max columns.

Select without a table

We can use the SELECT statement without a table:

Arithmetic:
SELECT 3 * 4;
SELECT 3 * 4 + (5 *6);

Current date and time:
SELECT NOW();

Current logged-in user:
SELECT USER();

Current database used:
SELECT DATABASE();

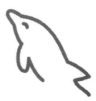

Picking the right tables and columns

Until this point and for the next couple of chapters, the tables and columns used in the examples may seem as randomly picked from MIMIC2 database. One may wonder, how did I choose the specific tables and columns used in the examples so far.

There's nothing mysterious or magical about it.

Starting with the chapter on ERD, the book will introduce a more structured approach to the subject of navigating a database map and some methods to find specific information about patients, labs, meds, outcomes, etc. in *any* haystack of tables and columns – not only MIMIC2 database - but any other database with a SQL interface.

By the end of this book, you will be able to apply the principles discussed in order to pick the right tables and columns from *any* database and execute SQL queries for your specific needs.

A note on SQL format

Throughout the book, the SQL commands are capitalized for clarity, but you don't have to capitalize your SQL commands.

The semicolon ";" at the end of a SQL statement is optional when you execute only one query at a time. If you'd like to execute several statements, you must separate them with ";"

Also for clarity, I've separated the SQL statements with line breaks, so 'SELECT' is on the first line, 'FROM' is on a separate line, 'WHERE' on a third line, etc. – but you don't need to separate your SQL statements in the same fashion.

While correct SQL statements will run with or without capitalization or separation of clauses on different lines, I found the above helps with the readability and maintainability of a query.

5. Aggregate / Summary Functions

- Let's count
- Minimum & Maximum
- Other useful summary / aggregate functions
- Average & Standard deviation
- Group by
- Having
- Identify outliers
- Subqueries

Let's count

The most basic summary function is COUNT().
If we'd like to know how many rows are in the **admissions** table:

SELECT COUNT(*)
FROM admissions;

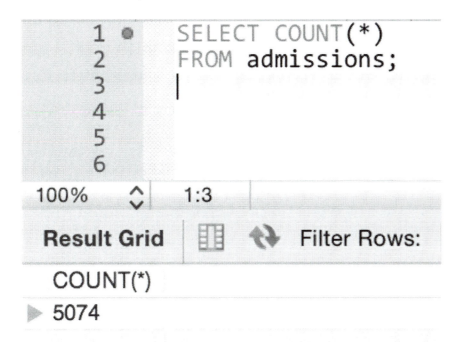

Note the parenthesis () following the function name is characteristic of SQL functions.

If we need to know the number of unique patients in this table, as some patients may have been admitted more than once, then we'll use the DISTINCT operator and the specific column inside the parenthesis:

SELECT COUNT(DISTINCT subject_id)
FROM admissions;

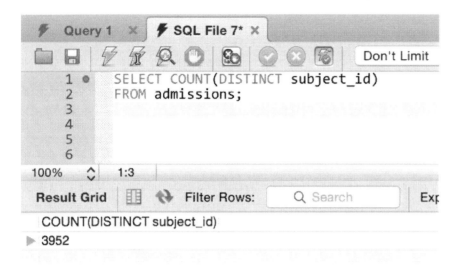

Question 11

How many unique drug names are in the **poe_med** table?

Minimum & maximum

Similar to COUNT, we have the MIN and MAX aggregate functions, that will find the minimum and maximum values. For the minimum and maximum doses of Morphine in the **poe_med** table:

SELECT MIN(dose_val_disp), MAX(dose_val_disp)
FROM poe_med
WHERE drug_name LIKE '%morphine%';

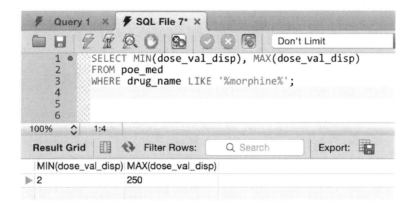

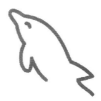

Other useful summary / aggregate functions

SUM()   Total
AVG()   Average
STD()   Standard deviation (population)
STDDEV_SAMP()   Standard deviation (sample)
VARIANCE()   Variance (population)
VAR_SAMP()   Variance (sample)

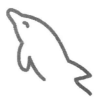

Average and standard deviation

The length of stay (LOS) in the **censusevents** table is displayed in minutes in the **los** column.
To calculate the average and standard deviation of LOS in hours we divide the number of minutes by 60:

```
SELECT AVG(los/60), STD(los/60)
FROM censusevents;
```

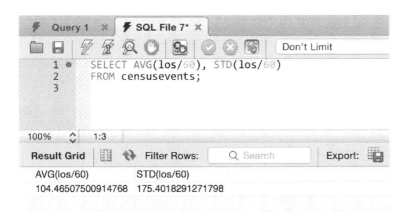

Question 12

Using the **poe_med** table, find the average and standard deviation (population) of the **dose_val_disp** for the drug Morphine

Group by

The aggregate functions become more useful when used in conjunction with the GROUP BY clause using the syntax:

SELECT NameOfColumn, AggregateFunction1, AggregateFunction2
FROM table_name
WHERE conditions
GROUP BY NameOfColumn

GROUP BY will split the table into groups of rows, according to the unique values in the **NameOfColumn** and then will calculate the aggregate function(s) on each group.
We can apply the aggregate functions on each group of rows created by the GROUP BY clause.
To calculate the average **dose_val_disp** for all the drugs in **poe_med**:

SELECT drug_name, AVG(dose_val_disp) AS Average
FROM poe_med
GROUP BY drug_name;

Medical Information Extraction and Analysis

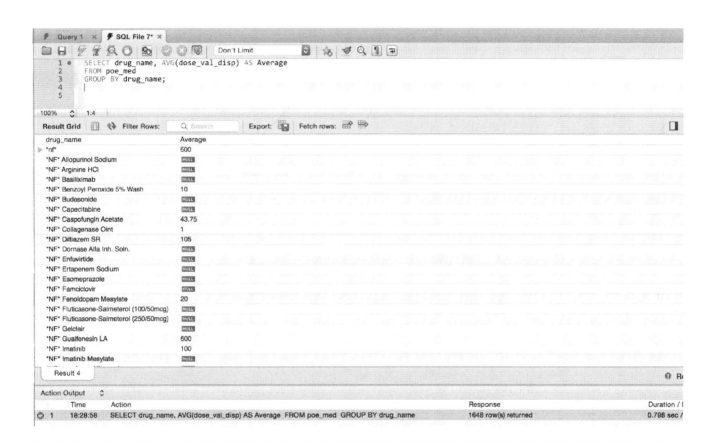

GROUP BY defines the columns you'd like to aggregate, in order to calculate a metric on each group

The above query will return 1648 unique rows, but many have the NULL values as average, which is not very useful.

 Question 13

Modify the above query, so it will return the non-null averages of all the drugs in **poe_med** table

Having

While WHERE operates on rows, HAVING operates in a similar fashion on the aggregate functions used in a GROUP BY clause.

Consider the following:

```
SELECT drug_name, COUNT(dose_val_disp) AS Counter, AVG(dose_val_disp) AS Average
FROM poe_med
WHERE dose_val_disp IS NOT NULL
GROUP BY drug_name;
```

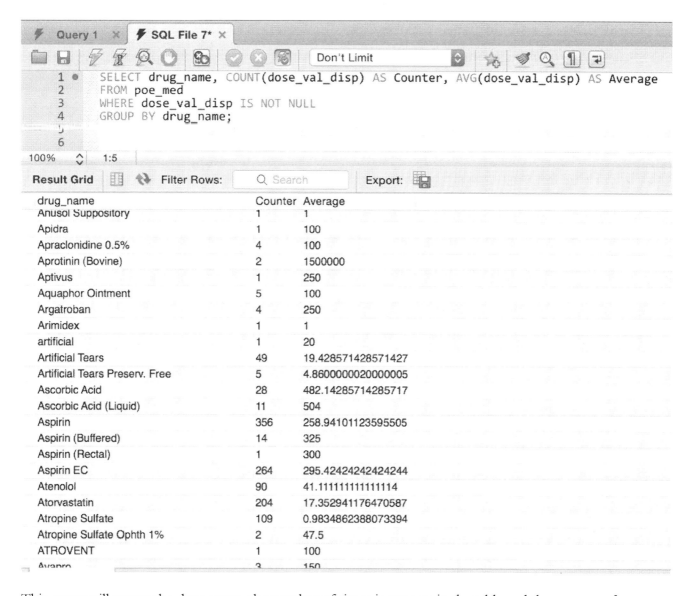

This query will return the drug name, the number of times it appears in the table and the average of **dose_val_disp** for non-null values.

Suppose we are interested in retrieving only those drugs that have been prescribed more than 1000 times in the **poe_med** table.
We need apply a condition on an aggregate function – COUNT - but after this aggregate function was evaluated.
Such a condition will not work if it is applied before the aggregate function was evaluated, in a WHERE clause. If we apply the condition in the WHERE clause, it will only restrict the rows to be evaluated later by the aggregate function.

Hence the HAVING clause, that restricts a query results based on conditions applied after the WHERE and GROUP BY clauses and all the aggregate functions have been evaluated:

```sql
SELECT drug_name, COUNT(dose_val_disp) AS Counter, AVG(dose_val_disp) AS AvgDose
FROM poe_med
WHERE dose_val_disp IS NOT NULL
GROUP BY drug_name
HAVING Counter > 1000
ORDER BY Counter DESC;
```

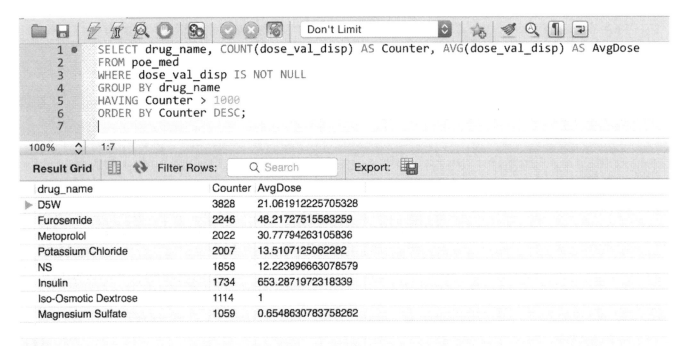

These results list all the drugs ordered more than 1000 times in the **poe_med** table, from the most common drug to the least one used, each with the number of times it was ordered and the average dose on vial.

The ordering was achieved with the **ORDER BY Counter DESC.** ORDER BY is not mandatory within a GROUP BY or a HAVING clause, but if you decide to use it, please note its location at the end of the statement.

Similarly, the HAVING clause is optional within a GROUP BY clause, but if you use it, note the proper location within the SQL syntax.

HAVING defines the condition(s) to be applied to the results of an aggregate function, after the function was calculated

Identify outliers

Using the GROUP BY and HAVING clauses introduced above, one can retrieve specific rows from tables, group them based on the columns' unique values, calculate aggregate functions on these groups and then further filter the query based on the evaluation of these aggregate functions' results.

We can employ the above technique to identify outliers – values that are at a more than a certain distance from a metric, such as their group average.

For example, retrieve the drugs, that their **dose_val_disp** is two times or more than their group average:

SELECT drug_name, dose_val_disp, AVG(dose_val_disp) AS Average
FROM poe_med
WHERE dose_val_disp IS NOT NULL
GROUP BY drug_name
HAVING dose_val_disp >= 2 * Average;

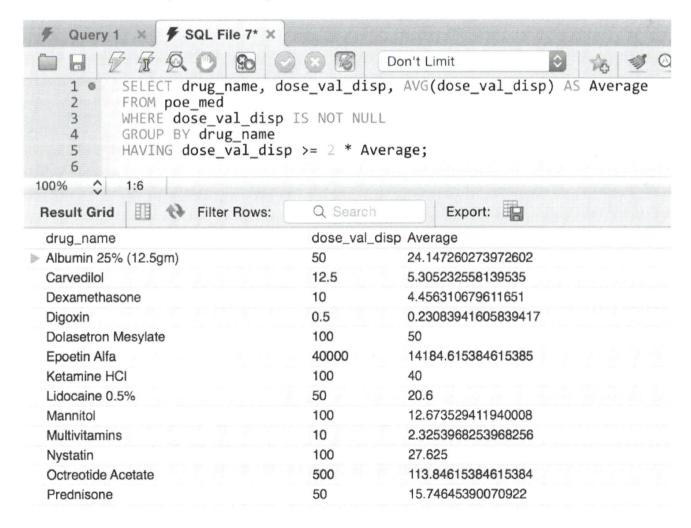

- The query retrieves the columns **drug_name, dose_val_disp, AVG(dose_val_disp)** from the **poe_med** table, while eliminating the rows where **dose_val_disp** has NULL values.

- Next the query groups the rows according to their unique **drug_name** values.
- It proceeds to calculate the average of **dose_val_disp** for each **drug_name** group.
- Lastly, the query filters the final results to display only those HAVING their **dose_val_disp** as twice or more than the average for their group, calculated in the previous step.

Using the **poe_order** table, let's find out the patients that have had more than 100 drug orders :

```
SELECT subject_id, COUNT(medication) AS Counter
FROM poe_order
GROUP BY subject_id
HAVING Counter > 100
ORDER BY COUNTER DESC;
```

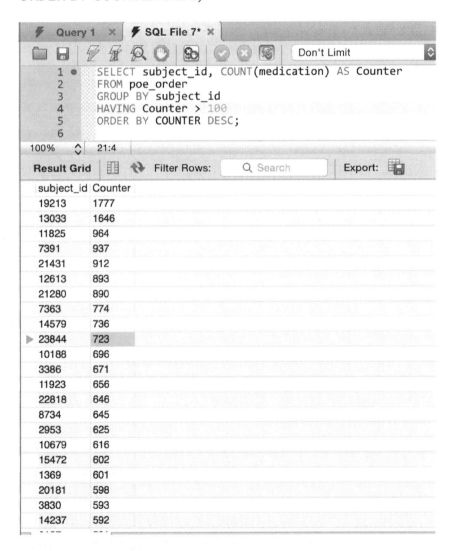

Note the above query GROUP BY is on the **subject_id** column (patient), while the HAVING clause is on the number of medications ordered for that patient.

We can **GROUP BY** on more than one column, so if we'd like to identify the patients with more than 30 drug orders per patient, per day, we add the **start_dt** column to the GROUP BY clause in the above query:

```sql
SELECT subject_id, COUNT(medication) AS Counter
FROM poe_order
GROUP BY subject_id, start_dt
HAVING Counter > 30
ORDER BY Counter DESC;
```

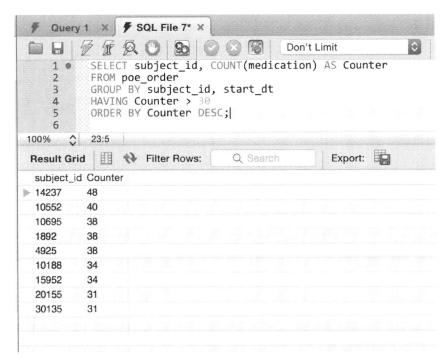

HAVING is useful in identifying outliers

🯄 Question 14

Modify the above query, so it will return those patients (subject_id) with more than 20 different, unique drug orders per day.

While 100 medication orders per patient may seem impressive, it is just an arbitrary number and not a useful threshold for identifying outliers, as we do not know the average number of medication orders per patient.

We need to find first the average number of medication orders per patient in order to be able to identify outliers.

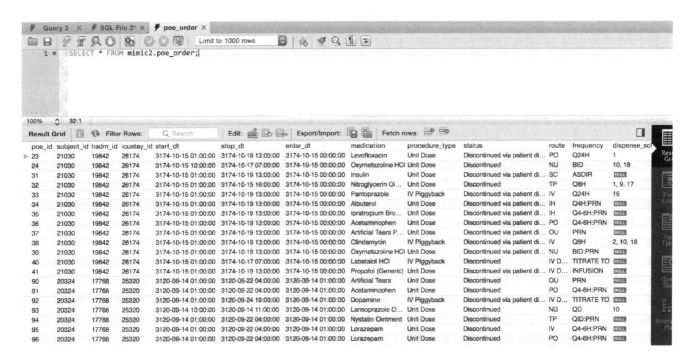

The initial obstacle is that the **medication** column in the **poe_order** table contains the actual name of the medication (e.g.: Levofloxacin, Insulin, Tylenol, etc.) – and we cannot calculate an average on this column as it is a text column. The average function has to run on numbers, not text.

The query plan is to first count the number of (text) meds for each patient and then calculate the average over these (numeric) values.

For this purpose, let's introduce the concept of subqueries: running a query on the results of another query.

Subqueries

The general syntactic template for running a query on the results of another, nested subquery:

SELECT ... FROM
(
SELECT ... FROM
) AS X;

The first SELECT is the outer query.
The second SELECT, within the parenthesis, is the inner query or subquery – and it will be executed by the SQL engine before the outer query.
The structure must have an alias **AS X**, otherwise SQL will throw an error: **Every derived table must have its own alias.** As the result of the inner query is a derived table, it must have a name or an alias.

Returning to the previous question, what is the average number of medication orders per patient in the **poe_order** table:

First we create the inner, subquery – counting the number of medication orders each patient has:

SELECT subject_id, COUNT(medication) AS MedCounter
FROM poe_order
GROUP BY subject_id

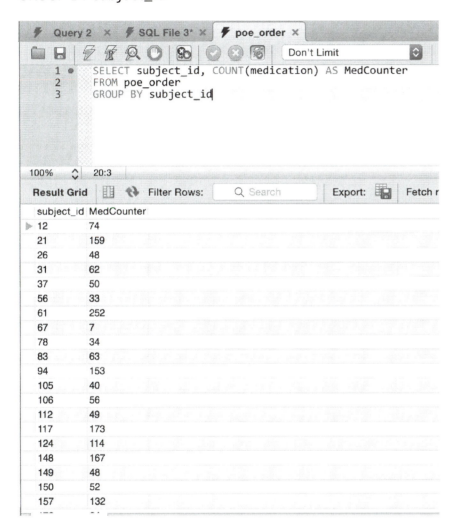

On the above results, we run the outer / final query, calculating the overall average:

SELECT AVG(MedCounter) FROM
(
SELECT subject_id, COUNT(medication) AS MedCounter
FROM poe_order
GROUP BY subject_id
) AS MyTable;

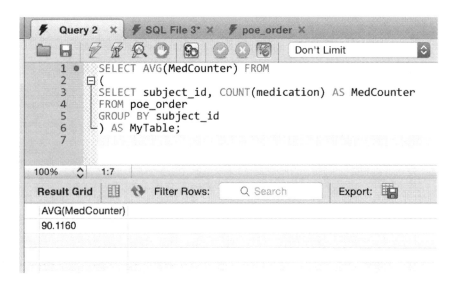

Note the mandatory, **MyTable** alias for the derived table and the unrelated, optional **MedCounter** alias for the **Count(medication)** column.

On average, each patient has 90 medication orders in the **poe_order** table.

Now we can set the threshold for identifying outliers at a more informed level - in terms of the average or a or a combination of the average and the standard deviation.

 ## Question 15

Retrieve the subject_id, start_dt and number of daily medication orders per day of the patients that had more than 5 times the average of med orders per patient, per day. Arrange results in a descending order of the number of daily meds per patient.

6. Querying Multiple Tables

- Connecting tables with joins
- Inner join
- Alternative to inner join
- Left join
- Right join
- Self-join - Comparing a table to itself
- Retrieving rows from 3 or more tables

Connecting tables with joins

All the query examples till now, have used a single table. In real life though, we usually need to query multiple tables, especially with the 1:M and M:M relationships between tables that have been introduced in the first chapter.

When we're querying two tables, it is beneficial to know initially what we'd like to retrieve:
- Only the rows that have matching values in both tables (Inner Join)
- All the rows from one table and only the rows that have matching values in the other table (Left / Right Outer Join)

Inner Join

The syntax to retrieve rows that have matching values in two tables:

SELECT table1.columnX, table2.columnY
FROM table1 INNER JOIN table2
ON table1.column_name = table2.column_name;

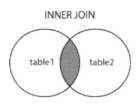

Note the notation **table1.column_name** which defines the table name explicitly in the column specification. Since the **column_name** is exactly the same in both tables, the INNER JOIN clause has the table1 and table2 qualifiers in the specifics of the columns. If **columnX** or **columnY** appear in only one table, then there is no need to explicitly specify the table name within the definition of the column, and the above can be simplified as:

SELECT columnX, columnY
FROM table1 INNER JOIN table2
ON table1.column_name = table2.column_name;

If you forget to explicitly define a column with the table qualifier when needed, such as when the name of the column is the same in both tables, SQL will throw an error, complaining about ambiguity it cannot resolve.

If two columns have the same name, you must specify their respective tables

Consider the **d_labitems** (table 1) - it is a dictionary table, with the lab test names, descriptions, fluid, category, etc.
Similarly **d_meditems** (table 2) has the names of the medications items.

Are there any lab tests with the same name as a medication ?

In the Venn diagram above, we'd like to retrieve the rows from table 1 and table 2 that equate on **test_name = label**. Since these columns' names are not the same, we don't need specify their tables.

```
SELECT *
FROM d_labitems INNER JOIN d_meditems
ON  test_name = label;
```

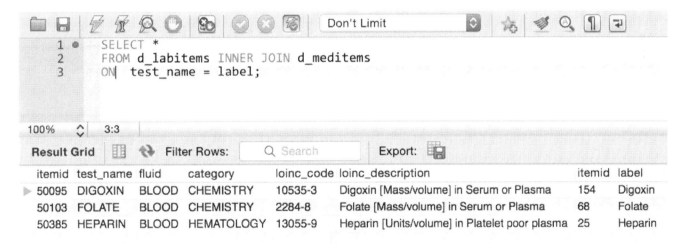

Alternative to the Inner Join

SQL allows an alternative mechanism to retrieve rows from two or more tables, based on common value(s) that match in both tables, using the following syntax:

SELECT columnX, columnY
FROM table1, table2
WHERE table1.column_name = table2.column_name;

Note the comma between **table1, table2** and the familiar WHERE clause that links the two tables.

 Question 16

Using the second mechanism to retrieve rows with matching values mentioned above, retrieve the information on meds and labs with the same name from the **d_meditems** and **d_labitems** tables.

For clarity purposes, the rest of the book will employ the Alternative to Inner Join approach when linking tables

Left Join

Left Join (or Left Outer Join) will retrieve all the rows from the left (table1) and the rows that have a match in the right (table2).

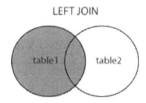

In order to understand when to use a left join, let's run the following query, which summarizes the number of admissions by year and month:

```
SELECT YEAR(admit_dt) AS YearAdmit, MONTH(admit_dt) AS MonthAdmit, COUNT(admit_dt)
AS MonthlyAdmissions
FROM admissions
WHERE admit_dt BETWEEN '2501-01-01' AND '2700-01-01'
GROUP BY YearAdmit, MonthAdmit
ORDER BY YearAdmit, MonthAdmit;
```

The time frame limit was added so the query will not run over 60 seconds.

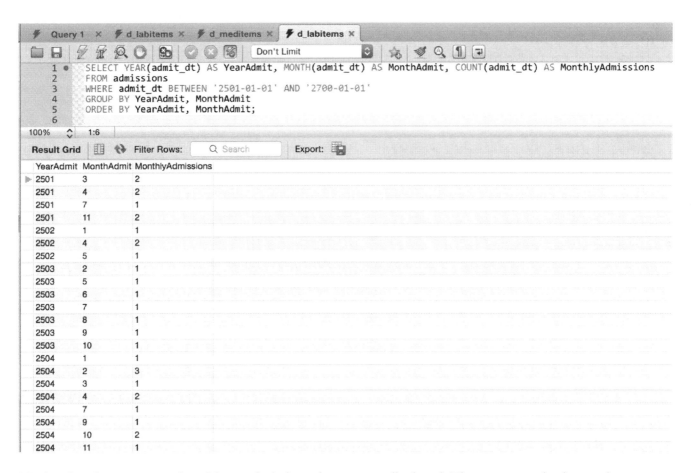

Notice that there are months with no admissions that are not displayed. There are gaps in the results. Gaps in time series usually induce cognitive errors when trying to interpret a table or chart.

This peculiar fact, which I've exploited in this example - months with no patients in ICU ? – originates from the de-identification process used on the MIMIC2 database, which spreads the admissions over a thousand years.

Still, you may encounter situations where a gap appears in a time series. For example when reviewing mortality by month, as there are departments / units with zero monthly mortality and most probably, you'd like to see those departments in your mortality report.

We'd like the query results to display the months without admissions (or mortality), as zero.

That's where a Left Join can help, with the general syntax:

```
SELECT columnX, columnY
FROM table1 LEFT JOIN table2
ON table1.column_name = table2.column_name;
```

I've added to the original MIMIC2 database, a table named **calendar**, with the daily dates between the years 2501 and 3502. We are going to use this **calendar** table as the Left table (the one to always show its rows) in the Left Join query:

```
SELECT YEAR(datefield) AS YearAdmit, MONTH(datefield) AS MonthAdmit, COUNT(admit_dt) AS MonthlyAdmissions
FROM calendar LEFT JOIN admissions
ON datefield = admit_dt
WHERE datefield BETWEEN '2501-01-01' AND '2511-01-01'
GROUP BY YEAR(datefield), MONTH(datefield)
ORDER BY YEAR(datefield), MONTH(datefield);
```

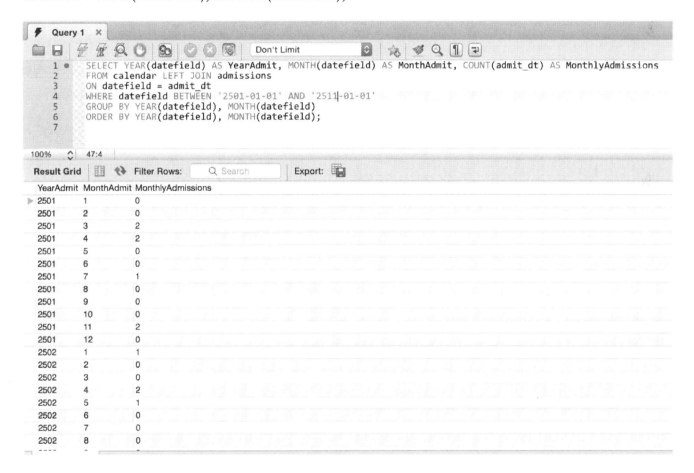

The results above display all the year and month fields (between the dates in the WHERE clause) from the **calendar** (Left) table.

The months that have a counterpart (on the same month and year) with a row from the **admissions** (Right) table are summarized, while those months that do not have any admissions, appear as zero.

- The Left Join query has the **datefield** from the (Left) **calendar** table in the select statement – and not the **admit_dt** from the (Right) **admissions** table. Remember, we'd like to see the Year and Month of the **datefield,** even if there are no admissions for that time frame.
- The order of the tables within the ON clause is important, it should be the Left Join **calendar** table ON the (Right) **admissions** table.
- The ON clause is evaluating **datefield = admit_dt** and it works only because in this specific case, both fields / columns have the time set as **00:00:00.**
- If one of the fields had the time defined other than **00:00:00**, say **02:32:45** – then we'd need employ a comparison that extracts the date part from both fields for the equate clause, such as **DATE(datefield) = DATE(admit_dt)** for these two fields to be possibly equal.
- The aggregate Count function is on **admit_dt** – and not the **datefield** - since the **admit_dt** is the field we'd like to aggregate / summarize.
- Grouping is on the **datefield** and not the **admit_dt** for the same reasons as the first point above.
- Last but not least – the use of the Where clause within the Left Join query is optional, but necessary in this case, limiting the query to 10 years. Without it – the query may run for more than a minute and will most probably cause a "lost connection to server" error, as detailed in chapter 3.

Use a different, complete table of values and the Left Join when you need the NULL values in your results to appear as 0

 Question 17

Retrieve all the years and months between 2501-01-01 and 2601-01-01 and the number of discharges per month, using the **calendar** and **censusevents** tables. If there are no discharges in a specific month, query should return a zero.

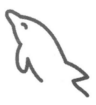

Right Join

Right Join (or Right Outer Join) will retrieve all rows from the right (table2) and the rows that have a match in the left (table1). Since it is exactly the opposite of the Left Join discussed above, there's nothing more to add on this type of join.

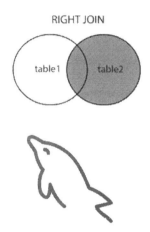

Self-Join - Comparing a table to itself

Consider the following task: retrieve from the **poe_order** table the patients that have received both the opiate (pain killer) Morphine and the reversal antidote Naloxone.
If we run a query such as:

SELECT *
FROM poe_order
WHERE medication LIKE 'Morphine%';

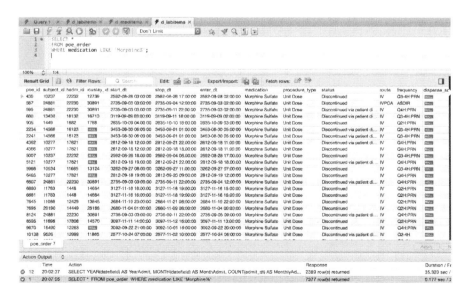

The results will include the patients that have received Morphine.
Running a similar query on Naloxone:

```
SELECT *
FROM poe_order
WHERE medication LIKE 'Naloxone%';
```

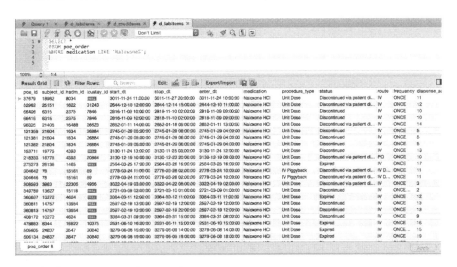

Will undoubtedly return the patients that have received Naloxone.
But running the following query:

```
SELECT *
FROM poe_order
WHERE medication LIKE 'Morphine%'
AND medication LIKE 'Naloxone%';
```

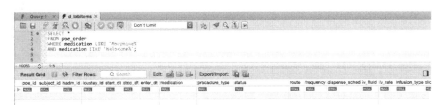

There are no results – an empty set.
The reason is simple: the query evaluates one row at a time and since there is no drug that has both Morphine and Naloxone in its name – the query finds absolutely nothing.

We need to compare the **poe_order** to itself and query it once for "Morphine" and once for "Naloxone", while checking that it is the same patient.

This is where a Self-Join becomes useful:

```
SELECT A.columnX, B.columnX
FROM table_name A, table_name B
WHERE A.columnX = B.columnX;
```

- The table name needs to appear twice in the FROM clause: once as A and once as B, so SQL can distinguish between them. You can pick any other letters or synonyms for the tables, as long as they do not contain spaces.
- The columns used in the SELECT clause, need to be defined as either A.column or B.column, otherwise there is an ambiguity about the table, which SQL will complain about by throwing an error.
- We have to define in the WHERE clause what is equal (and what is not if we'd like) - when comparing the table to itself.

The query on patients that have received both Morphine and Naloxone:

SELECT DISTINCT A.subject_id, A.medication, B.medication
FROM poe_order A, poe_order B
WHERE A.subject_id = B.subject_id
AND A.medication LIKE 'Morphine%'
AND B.medication LIKE 'Naloxone%';

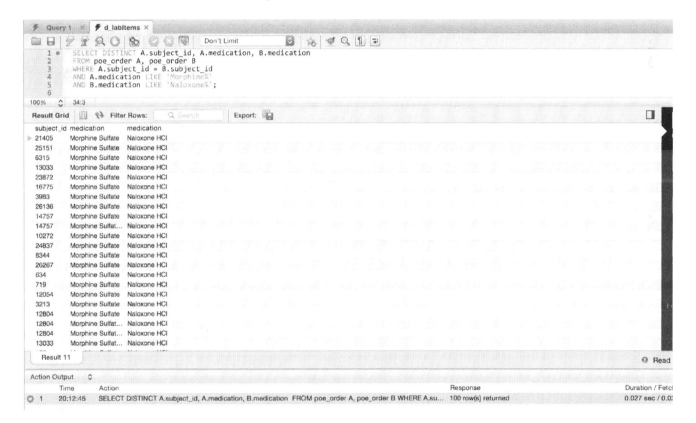

- The table we are comparing to itself appears twice in the FROM clause, once as A and once as B: **poe_order A, poe_order B**
- We are making sure it is the same patient being compared, with the **A.subject_id = B.subject_id** equate in the WHERE clause
- The DISTINCT in the SELECT prevents similar rows to appear more than once.

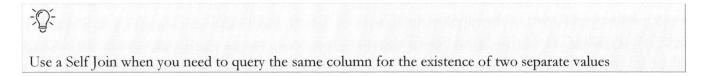

Use a Self Join when you need to query the same column for the existence of two separate values

Question 18

Retrieve all the patients from the **poe_order** table that have received Morphine and Naloxone within 24 hours, the time of administration for both these drugs and the number of hours that have passed between these drugs administration.

Retrieving rows from 3 or more tables

There are situations where we need to connect more than two tables in the same query. The general syntax for relating 3 or more tables in the same query:

SELECT table1.columnX, table2.columnY, table3.columnZ
FROM table1, table2, table3
WHERE table1.columnA = table2.columnB
AND table2.columnC = table3.columnD
AND Other Conditions;

- The need to identify unambiguously the columns we are interested in, using the table names qualifiers. This is especially important if a column name from one table is similar to the column name from another table.
- Tables are separated by commas in the FROM clause.
- We must connect all the tables used in the query with several conditions in the WHERE clause of the query. These conditions are usually around the unique identifiers and the PK / FK mechanism previously explained.
- Without these necessary conditions, SQL will return the result of the tables multiplication: a huge Cartesian product of the two tables' rows.
- Connecting the tables within the WHERE clause is mandatory and in addition to any other conditions we may have in the query statement.

When linking N (3) tables in a query, there should be at least N-1 (2) conditions in the WHERE clause for the linking to work properly

UNION – combining multiple results sets

If you need to consolidate several query results into one set and these queries have the same number and type of columns, use the SQL **UNION**:

(SELECT ...)
UNION
(SELECT ...)
UNION
(SELECT ...)

UNION is used to combine similar results from multiple SELECT statements into a single set

From the MySQL tutorial:
*"The column names from the first **SELECT** statement are used as the column names for all the results returned.*
*Selected columns listed in the corresponding positions of each **SELECT** statement should have the same data type.*
For example, the first column selected by the first statement should have the same type as the first column selected by the other statements."

7. Entity Relationship Diagram - ERD

- ERD - the database blueprint
- Using the ERD
- Information schema
- Find relevant tables and columns
- Reverse engineering

ERD - the database blueprint

The Entity Relationship model or Diagram (ERD) is basically the database blueprint. It displays the entities (tables) and the relationships between instances (rows) of these entities.
Think of the ERD as a map, the same map used by the database developers many years ago, when the database was conceived. The ERD assures one doesn't literally get lost in the myriad pathways and relationships that may exist between hundreds and thousands of tables, columns and the relationships between them.

The ERD can help when designing a query on a database, as it helps to visually grasp the various tables and their relationships.

We are going to use the MIMIC2 ERD as published in:

User Guide and Documentation for the MIMIC II Database
Gari D. Cliord, Daniel J. and Mauricio Villarroel
Harvard-MIT Division of Health Sciences & Technology

The guide can be found at:
https://physionet.org/mimic2/UserGuide/UserGuide.pdf

Even with its inherent succinct format, an ERD can become huge in size and complexity and thus may become less readable.

The MIMIC2 ERD in the above mentioned document, is presented in several parts and we are going to gradually introduce and use these ERD parts as we progress through the book.

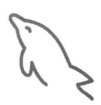

Using the ERD

Below is one part of the MIMIC2 ERD, the one that details the Patients, Diagnoses and DRG (Diagnoses Related Group) – the relevant entities (tables), columns and their types and the relationships between their instances (rows):

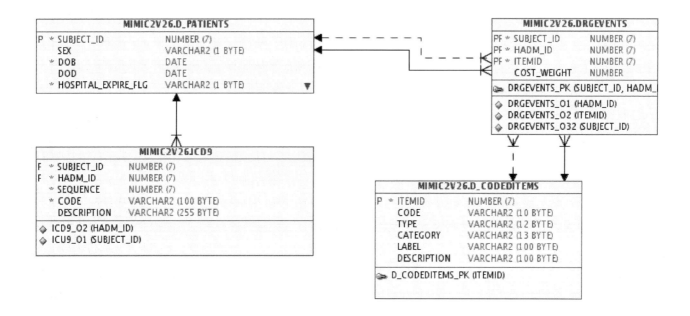

- The boxes are entities or tables.
- The name of the table is on the top line of each box.
- An entity / table name has two parts separated by a period: First part is the database name **MIMIC2V26**.
- The second part of the table title is the actual table name.
- In the above ERD, you should be able by now to identify and access with MySQL Workbench the following tables: **D_PATIENTS, ICD9, DRGEVENTS** and **D_CODEDITEMS** in the MIMIC2 database.

 Question 19

Using the **D_CODEDITEMS** table, find what are the types of coded items in this table.

 Question 20

Modify the previous query and retrieve the types of coded items and the number of instances in the table for each.

Within the box, there are the column names of that table.
In the table **D_PATIENTS,** there are **SUBJECT_ID, SEX, DOB, DOD, HOSPITAL_EXPIRE_FLG** columns.

The letter "P" on the left side of the column name denotes a Primary Key (PK). In the **D_PATIENTS** table, **SUBJECT_ID** is the PK.

The table **ICD9** has the same column **SUBJECT_ID** as **D_PATIENTS** denoted as "F", meaning Foreign Key (FK).

The "crow feet" end of the relationship line between the two tables and the arrow ending on the other side, define the relationship between these tables:

- The crow feet ending means that one instance (row) of **D_PATIENTS** may have one or more related instances in the **ICD9** table. Basically, one patient may have one more ICD9 diagnoses.
- The arrow ending means that one instance in the **ICD9** table must be related to one and only one instance in the **D_PATIENTS** table.

It is important to conceptually navigate the relationship lines in an ERD in both directions, as from **D_PATIENTS** towards **ICD9** and vice versa, in the example above.

Sometimes there is an additional relationship dotted line, as the relationships between **D_PATIENTS** and **DRGEVENTS** tables or between **DRGEVENTS** and **D_CODEDITEMS** tables. A dotted line, depending on the specific ERD symbols and nomenclature used, may be interpreted as either:

- A "weak" type of relationship – where the relationship is not based on PK but on other columns
- An optional relationship (as opposed to mandatory), so it may or may not exist between the entities

There are tables where there is no single column tagged with a "P". Instead there are several "PF" columns, such as **DRGEVENTS** table where **SUBJECT_ID, HADM_ID** and **ITEMID columns** are all defined as "PF". It means that all three column together are a composite PK. A combination of these three columns must be unique and it will uniquely identify a row (instance).

Sometimes there is no PK defined for a table, only FK – such as the **ICD9** table.

We've previously mentioned intersection entities / tables a.k.a. junction or association tables, that resolve M:M relationships. These tables can be identified in an ERD by having at least two M:1 relationships with other tables (so each of these other tables in turn, will have a 1:M relationship with this junction table).

The **DRGEVENTS** table in the above ERD is an intersection / junction table, between the **D_PATIENTS** and **D_CODEDITEMS** tables. It resolves the M:M relationship between these two tables: one patient may have many coded items and one coded item may be assigned to many patients.

Why is the relationship between patients and coded items M:M requiring an intersection table, while a quite similar situation with the ICD9 diagnosis codes - was solved with a different design approach, with a simple 1:M relationship ? We'll never know, but I can only guess that the coded items table is a bit more complex than the ICD9 table and thus the database designers, chose many years ago to represent these entities in this specific fashion in the ERD.

For our querying purposes, it's good enough to know the tables, their relationships and the column names participating in these relationships.

By reviewing the partial ERD above, we can better understand the relationship between the tables **d_patients** and **ICD9**:

- The **d_patients** table has the patient unique identifier **subject_id**. How do we know **subject_id** is the column with the unique identifiers ? Since it is the only column defined in this table in the ERD as **P** – Primary Key.
- The **ICD9** table has the same **subject_id** as **F** – Foreign key.
- The arrow and crow feet complete the picture: one instance of **d_patients** may have many instances of **ICD9** while one **ICD9** instance must have one and only one instance of **d_patients**.
- Basically, one patient may have many diagnoses and one diagnosis must be related to one patient only.
- In addition to the relationships, we can see all the columns' names and types that exist in these tables.

In a database with patient names, addresses, phones and etc., we would have to first search in a table similar to the **d_patients** table, using the patient name, SSN, phone or email, etc. as search parameters and eventually would have found the patient unique identifier – the **subject_id**.
As MIMIC2 is de-identified and there are no patient names or other patient identifying details, we'll need to skip this initial search. Let's assume we've found the patient we're interested in, and the patient unique identifier is **subject_id** = 16994.

What are the ICD9 diagnosis codes assigned to this specific patient ?
The table that holds the Many side of the 1:M relationship between patients and ICD9 diagnosis is the **ICD9** table:

SELECT *
FROM icd9
WHERE subject_id = '16994';

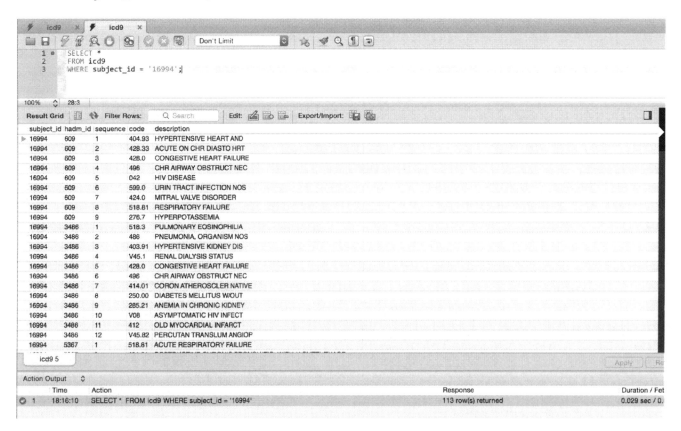

There are several hospital admissions related to this patient, identified by the **hadm_id** column.

Each admission has a related series of ICD9 codes, their descriptions and these diagnoses in turn, have been sequenced according to their clinical importance during that episode of care.

Question 21

Find all the ICD9 diagnosis used in MIMIC2 and the number of patients each diagnosis was assigned to. Arrange the results from the most common diagnosis to the rarest one. What is the most common diagnosis in MIMIC2 ?

If we try a similar query on the **drgevents** table:

```
SELECT *
FROM DRGEVENTS
WHERE subject_id = '16994';
```

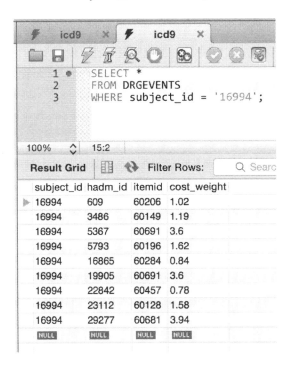

- In the results, **itemid** is not the DRG code, but a unique identifier.
- The results display **itemid** and their **cost_weight**, but we don't know what these **itemid** actually represent in terms of DRG.
- The reason for the lack of DRG details in the query results, is that **drgevents** table is a junction / intersection entity and the details on the **itemid** resides in the table **d_codeditems**.
- Note that **d_codeditems** is considered a dictionary table – a table that holds the details of an entity, but not the actual transactions this entity has participated in.
- While **d_codeditems** has the details on the DRG codes, **drgevents** has the information about the patients with these DRG codes.

When reviewing an ERD, try to identify and differentiate between dictionary tables that detail the attributes of an entity and the tables that contain the actual, transactional information about these entities' interactions. Usually a dictionary is much smaller than the transactions table it relates to.

The query to retrieve all the **drgevents** and their meaning for a specific patient:

SELECT *
FROM drgevents, d_codeditems
WHERE subject_id = '16994'
AND drgevents.itemid = d_codeditems. Itemid;

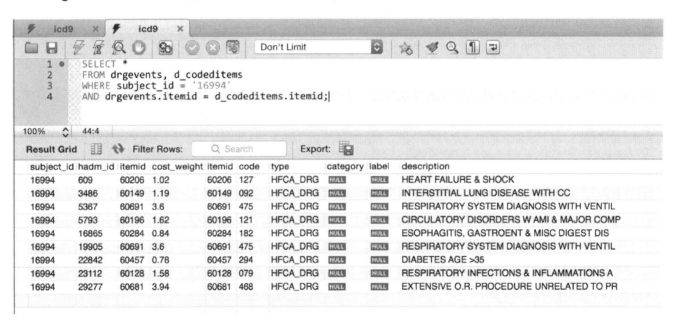

Note that each hospital admission has one and only one DRG (with its cost weight and description attached) summarizing the care episode. This is to be expected, as only one DRG is used to summarize one hospital episode.

As in your own queries you will probably have access to tables with detailed patient identification information, you may ask yourself:
How would a similar to the above query look, if **d_patients** wasn't de-identified, if it actually had patients' names and etc. and we were looking for a specific patient named "John Doe" and his DRG codes ?
Assuming the first and last name were in separate (imaginary, as currently non-existent in MIMC2) columns in this hypothetical **d_patients** table, then a tentative query may look like:

SELECT *
FROM d_patients, drgevents, d_codeditems
WHERE d_patients.FirstName = 'John' AND d_patients.LastName = 'Doe'
AND d_patients.subject_id = drgevents.subject_id

AND drgevents.itemid = d_codeditems.itemid;

Note: the above italicized query will cause an error if you try to run it, as there are no first and last names columns in MIMIC2.

Still, for educational purposes this imaginary query would relate the three tables mentioned in the FROM clause: **d_patients, drgevents, d_codeditems** - by employing two conditions. (Remember, f there are N=3 tables, you'll need at least N-1=2 conditions to be dedicated to connecting these table):

d_patients.subject_id = drgevents.subject_id
AND drgevents.itemid = d_codeditems.itemid

Without these restricting conditions the query will return a Cartesian product of all the rows from these 3 tables in an astonishing display of a very large and useless combinatorics results set.

The first condition in the WHERE clause
d_patients.FirstName = 'John' AND d_patients.LastName = 'Doe'
identifies the patient in the **d_patients** table by searching the first "John" and last "Doe" names against the respective (imaginary in the case of MIMIC2) columns.

Then, using the **subject_id** satisfying the previous condition, the second condition in the WHERE clause
d_patients.subject_id = drgevents.subject_id
would retrieve the rows from the **drgevents** table with the specific **subject_id** previously found in the **d_patients** table.

Finally, using the **itemid**, the last condition in the WHERE clause
drgevents.itemid = d_codeditems.itemid
would filter the descriptions and other details from the **d_codeditems** table, for the rows that have the same **itemid** as the ones found in the **drgevents** table. These rows in turn have the same **subject_id** as John Doe in the **d_patients** table. The 3 tables would be correctly related for this query.

Usually the name of a PK column will be the same when representing a FK in another table. Use these PK / FK columns to link tables in the WHERE clause

 ## Question 22

Find all the DRG used in MIMIC2 and the number of patients each DRG was assigned to. Arrange the results from the most common DRG to the rarest one. What is the most common DRG in MIMIC2 ?

As previously mentioned, DRG is a measure used to summarize one episode of care with many diagnoses, procedures, complications and comorbidities into one parameter, for billing purposes.

Suppose we'd like to know the most common diagnosis for a specific DRG, such as **Septicemia Age > 17**.

Using the ERD introduced above, the query plan may have the following steps:

1. In the SELECT clause – we'd like to have the ICD9 diagnosis and the number of times each diagnosis was counted for a specific DRG – the relevant column names are picked from the ERD
2. Find the unique identifier of the DRG whose description is **Septicemia Age > 17** in the dictionary table **d_codeditmes** (the letter **d**, conveniently denoting a dictionary table in MIMIC2, is not guaranteed to be part of the naming convention of your database ERD)
3. Using this DRG unique identifier, find the patients' unique identifiers that have been assigned this DRG in the intersection / junction table **drgevents**. Correlate the two tables with an equality condition in the WHERE clause using the ERD arrow and crowfeet notation and the columns defined as PK / FK.
4. Using these patients' unique identifiers, GROUP BY and COUNT their ICD9 diagnoses from the **ICD9** table.
5. Order results so the most common diagnosis would be on top

SELECT ICD9.Description AS ICD9Diagnosis, COUNT(ICD9.subject_id)
FROM drgevents, d_codeditems, ICD9
WHERE d_codeditems.Description = 'SEPTICEMIA AGE >17'
AND drgevents.itemid = d_codeditems.itemid
AND drgevents.subject_id = ICD9.subject_id
GROUP BY ICD9.Description
ORDER BY COUNT(ICD9.subject_id) DESC;

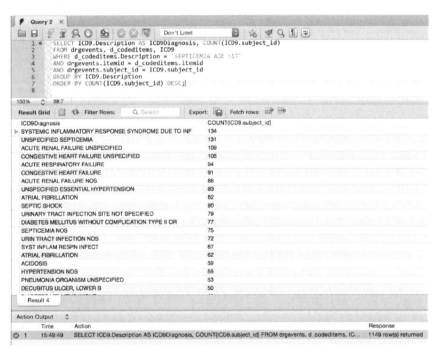

- The SELECT clause has the **ICD9.Description** and the count of the patients from the **ICD9** table.
- All the other tables used in the FROM clause are for restricting results and nothing from these tables will be included in the final results.
- Since **subject_id** appears in all tables, we must have the table specified in order to avoid ambiguity. Ditto for **description**, as it appears in two tables.
- **d_patients** table is not required for this query. The 3 tables used in the query are the only ones needed.

- The first restriction of the query plan is achieved with: **d_codeditems.Description = 'SEPTICEMIA AGE >17'**
- The tables used in the query are connected with the following equality conditions on columns derived from the ERD above: **AND drgevents.itemid = d_codeditems.itemid AND drgevents.subject_id = ICD9.subject_id**
- The grouping of the results is on the diagnosis **GROUP BY ICD9.Description** while the aggregate function, the counting **COUNT(ICD9.subject_id)** is performed on the **subject_id** - as the SQL translation of the question: how many patients have this diagnosis ?
- Lastly, ordering from most to least common with **ORDER BY COUNT(ICD9.subject_id) DESC;**

Information Schema

From MySQL tutorial:
"**INFORMATION_SCHEMA** *is a database within each MySQL instance, the place that stores information about all the other databases that the MySQL server maintains.*"

We can query this **INFORMATION_SCHEMA** when we are searching for tables or columns that may contain information we are interested in.
The initial syntax for querying this database of databases, on tables' names:

SELECT *
FROM INFORMATION_SCHEMA.TABLES;

The above query will return many rows and columns, and if we browse the results we can identify the **TABLE_SCHEMA** related to MIMIC2 database.
Note that the results include other system, MySQL own engine tables, which are not particularly useful when searching for tables or columns that may contain "Diagnosis", "Procedures", "Medications", etc. We can limit the results to MIMIC2 database with the following SQL statement:

SELECT *
FROM INFORMATION_SCHEMA.TABLES
WHERE TABLE_SCHEMA = 'mimic2';

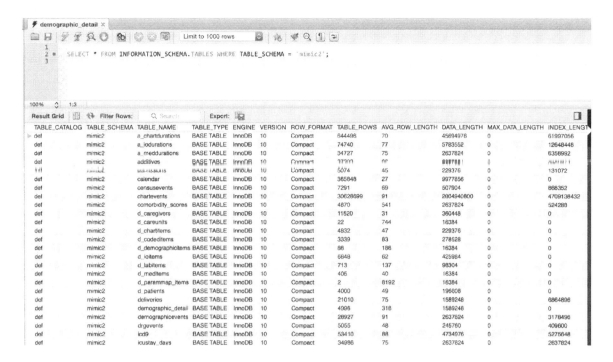

The results include the 37 tables from MIMIC2 database.

Finding relevant tables and columns

If we'd like to find the tables in MIMIC2 that have **lab** in their names, the query becomes:

SELECT *
FROM INFORMATION_SCHEMA.TABLES
WHERE TABLE_SCHEMA = 'mimic2'
AND TABLE_NAME LIKE '%lab%';

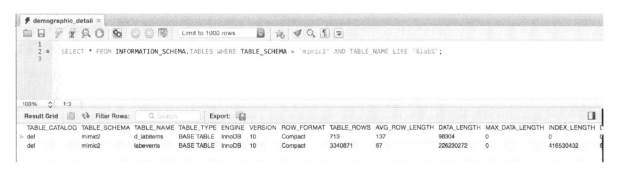

Browsing only the first thousand rows of these two tables, we can guess that one is a dictionary table and the other holds the actual lab results.

When executing a SELECT * on a new or unknown table, it is best to limit the number of rows returned as the results may have many millions of rows.

As we count the rows in the d_labitems (713 rows) and labevents (3,740,682 rows) – it becomes clear that the first one is a dictionary table (small) while the second table is the one actually holding the information on lab results (large).

SELECT * (with limits on) and COUNT(*) - on a new or unkown table, will get you familiar with the table and it can help differentiate between dictionary tables and the transactional ones

Question 23

The **labevents** table has other columns that end with **id**, besides the **itemid** - such as **subject_id**, **hadm_id**, **icustay_id**. What is the purpose of these **id** columns in **labevents** ? What kind of table is **labevents** ?

If we are searching for all the columns (not tables) in the MIMIC2 information schema:

```
SELECT *
FROM INFORMATION_SCHEMA.COLUMNS
WHERE TABLE_SCHEMA = 'mimic2';
```

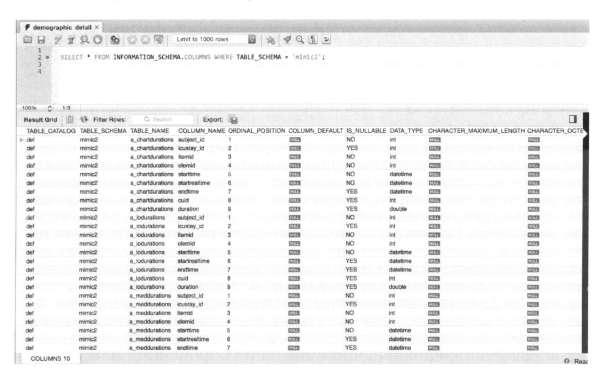

But if we try to find the columns related to lab :

```
SELECT *
FROM INFORMATION_SCHEMA.COLUMNS
WHERE TABLE_SCHEMA = 'mimic2'
AND COLUMN_NAME LIKE '%lab%';
```

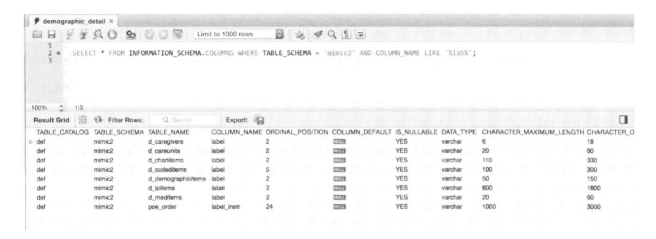

The results are unrelated to labs, since the column names retrieved form the schema are related to "labels".

 Querying the INFORMATION SCHEMA is one of the methods to quickly find tables and columns of interest

ERD and Information Schema are two complementary tools:

ERD

Pros	Cons
Visual map of the whole database	ERD can be quite large and is best digested in small bites
Clearly depicts the relationships	Not good for search

Information Schema

Pros	Cons
Finds tables and columns quickly	Doesn't display results graphically
Usually doesn't require admin credentials	Not easy to retrieve relationships

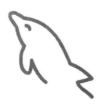

Reverse engineering

If you don't have a database ERD, you may try to reverse engineer it. While engineering a database for an ERD requires the knowledge of design and engineering principles, you definitely don't need an engineering degree to reverse engineer a database.

Most of the modern RDBMS have a mechanism in place to automatically review all the PK / FK constraints and create an ERD out of it.

Depending on the type of database you may have, it may be as easy as going to the **Database** on the top menu and click on **Reverse engineer**, point the engine to the right table and MySQL will create the ERD. If you try do it yourself on MIMIC2, MySQL will throw an exception error as you do not have the right access level and privileges to reverse engineer a database.

Best is to ask the database administrator for the ERD.
If the admin doesn't have one, ask the admin to reverse engineer the database with the RDBMS.
It is not a lot of work but it may require the admin credentials to do it.

8. Systematic information extraction

- Conceptual model and questions of interest
- Clinical query development strategy
- Map table to entity and column to attribute
- Test scenarios – 0, 1, N rows
- Are results correct, relevant, complete, consistent ?
- Query building flowchart

Conceptual model and questions of interest

When first approaching an information extraction project, a good starting point is the conceptual model of the domain you intend to query. From Wikipedia:

*"A **conceptual model** is a representation of a system, made of the composition of concepts which are used to help people know, understand, or simulate a subject the model represents. It is also a set of concepts ...The term conceptual model may be used to refer to models which are formed after a conceptualization or generalization process. Conceptual models are often abstractions of things in the real world whether physical or social."*

This conceptual model is initially unrelated to the database at hand.
It depicts hypothetical entities that:

- Help you define domain boundaries – what is in and what is out
- Help you conceptualize your initial queries around the possible interactions between entities you expect to find represented as tables in the database

A tentative conceptual model of an EHR:

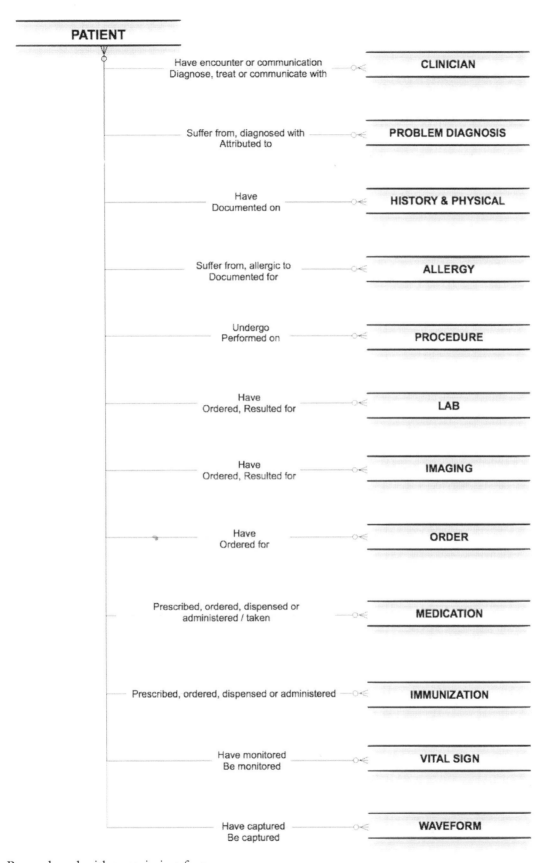

Reproduced with permission from:
Electronic Health Record: A Systems Analysis of the Medications Domain - A. Scarlat MD (CRC Press, 2012)

In the tentative conceptual model above:

- Patient is the center of the model
- Patient has M:N relationships with other entities (labs, meds, etc.)
- This M:N relationship means that the entities depicted are dictionary entities
- The transactional tables - the intersection / junction tables that are resolving this M:N relationship and hold the actual information about the entities interactions - are not displayed in a conceptual model

Use the above conceptual model as a starting point. Add to or remove from it, as you fit it to your needs.

Once you have defined the boundaries of the domain you intend to search with a conceptual model, the next step is to formulate the question of interest.

At this stage, try to focus on the entities involved and the interactions of interest to you – and write down the question(s) in plain English.

Do not attempt to write SQL before you have a clear question formulated in plain language.

While not knowing yet what exactly the entity Patient may contain, we can expect this entity to hold the data for simple queries on the subject of patients. For example:

Questions on a single entity - Patient:
- How many patients
- How many admissions
- Female / Male
- Minimum, Maximum, Average age, weight, height and BMI
- Ethnicity groups

Questions involving multiple entities:
- The most common diagnosis for a specific DRG or vice-versa
- Mortality rate for a specific diagnosis / procedure
- Monthly LOS by department
- Medications taken by patients with a specific diagnosis / procedure
- Lab results of patients taking a specific med / undergoing a procedure / having a diagnosis
- Calculating time intervals between specific events such as a med administered and a lab result or vice-versa
- Distribution over time of the above in order to detect trends

These examples are high-level questions that encompass the interactions between entities.
Some of the terms used in these questions are related to entities (e.g., Patient) and some are related to attributes of the entities (e.g., the Date / Time stamp of an event).

Clinical query development strategy

As we'll work thru the mentioned conceptual entities, a recurring theme of a query strategy emerges: For many of the conceptual entities (diagnosis, procedure, drug, fluid), we'd like to know:

- **Volumes** of patients / admissions – which instance is the most common or most frequent (e.g.: most common procedure, most common vital sign abnormality)
- **Mortality** e.g.: mortality for all diagnosis
- **LOS** e.g.: LOS for all procedures
- **Readmissions** rate e.g.: Readmissions for all the DRG codes
- **Profile of one patient** – all the instances of an entity, related to one patient (e.g.: all the lab results for one patient with their time stamps)
- **Profile of one instance** of an entity (e.g.: a diagnosis, a procedure or one lab abnormality) – with comparison to the population without that instance:
    - Volumes, Mortality, LOS, Readmission – current (last month), average, distribution over time.
    - Comparison between 2 situations: when the instance is present vs. when the instance is not present (e.g. mortality rate of admissions with sepsis vs. mortality without sepsis)
    - Age of population when profile instance is present vs. missing (e.g.: average age of the population with atrial fibrillation diagnosis vs. average age of the population without the diagnosis of atrial fibrillation)
    - Gender distribution when profile instance is present vs. absent (similar to age parameter above)
    - Other instances of the same entity that commonly accompany the profile instance (e.g.: other lab abnormalities that usually accompany high creatinine)

Starting with the chapter on Diagnosis, we're going to follow the above strategy while developing interesting queries around the MIMIC2 patients.

If you have access to the financial database of your organization, you can add to the above list of queries – the costs, revenue, etc. as related to the clinical concepts.
Basically, you'll be able to attach $ values to specific procedures, DRG codes, labs, imaging, etc.

Map table to entity and column to attribute

Once you have formulated your question in plain language, the next step is to map between the conceptual model and the ERD:
- Entities – Tables
- Attributes – Columns

Entities in the conceptual model map to tables in the database
Attributes in the conceptual model map to columns in the database

For example, a partial ERD of MIMIC2, that you can use as an exercise to map concepts from the conceptual model above, may look like this:

Medical Information Extraction and Analysis

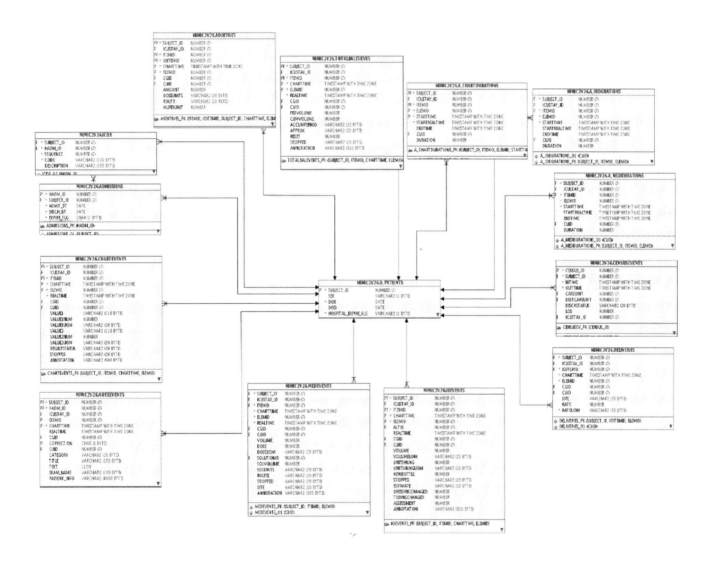

Start writing down the tables, you may discover as relevant to your query by:
- Reviewing the ERD
- Reviewing the tables names
- Querying the Information Schema

With a list of tentative tables, and for each candidate table:
- Count the number of rows in the table
- Retrieve all the columns of the table (while limiting the number of rows returned, if the table is large)
- If table is relevant, identify its relationships with other tables by noting down the PK / FK involved
- Try to differentiate between dictionary (usually small) tables and transactional tables (much larger than the dictionary table)

Entities that are logically related to your question, need to be identified and mapped to the database tables, with their PK / FK and columns.
Also note any other relationship a table of interest may have with other tables, especially dictionary tables.

During the above exercise, you'll start discovering the columns a.k.a. attributes you'll need for your queries. When you review column candidates and for each column of interest:
- Note the type of column – text, numeric, binary, date / time, etc.
- Check how many NULL values are in the column. If most of the column values are NULL, the column is worthless
- Arrange with ORDER BY (ascending and descending) to quickly identify outliers
- If you need to eliminate NULL values or other outliers, make a note of it to add later to your query
- Use DISTINCT in order to grasp the unique values in a column
- Use a GROUP BY and COUNT to grasp the values distribution in a column
- When two or more tables hold the same attribute, try to understand the fine nuances between them. Most probably only one of these tables holds the correct, complete, relevant and consistent information that you need.

Test scenarios - 0, 1, N rows

As you review tables and columns, and as practice towards the big query you intend to design, run a few queries with the specific goals of returning:

- **0 rows** – an empty set. Run some queries that you plan to return no rows. If results are not an empty set, you'll learn something about the database.
- **1 row only** – Test your knowledge of the database and SQL skills and run a query that will return a single row as a result. Again, if you receive anything else, no rows or more than one row – something needs to be improved: your SQL skills or your understanding of the database ERD
- **N rows** – Run a query that you know approximately the number of rows to be returned. Does the result make sense ?

Start small initially: limit the number of rows returned.
For example, limit the time frame of your query to a couple of years (instead of the 1,000 years in MIMIC2)

Are results correct, relevant, complete, consistent ?

Both newbies and SQL masters would like to know the answer to this question, each time they run a query.

Sometimes the answers are obvious (such as the 15 feet patient's height or a negative blood pressure measurement), but occasionally it requires additional work to construct and test various querying techniques – just to validate previous results in terms of correctness, completeness, relevancy and consistency.

Correct and complete query results will have the following characteristics:
- Low false-positives: Ideally the query retrieves no rows it should not have
- Low false-negatives: Ideally the query misses no rows that should have been retrieved

Relevance measures:
- High precision (a.k.a. positive predictive value): Ideally the fraction of relevant instances among the retrieved rows is high
- High recall (a.k.a. sensitivity): Ideally the fraction of relevant instances retrieved among all the relevant rows is high

Consistent query results are expected to have the following characteristics:
- No intrinsic logical inconsistencies are identified, such as an overlap or a gap between two mutually exclusive groups. For example: there should be no overlap between the patients that lived and those that died and there should be no patients that are missing from both these groups
- High degree of agreement internally with other tables in the same database
- High degree of agreement externally with other data sources (e.g., clinical vs. financial databases)

In addition to the above, don't forget to use your common sense when reviewing the results of a query. If something doesn't make sense, you have to identify the anomaly / inconsistency that may exist at the database level.

Query building flowchart

Start with a conceptual model of the entities involved — Use the ERD and / or Information Schema

Formulate questions around interactions between entities

Identify the tables representing the entities of interest

Identify the columns representing the attributes of interest

More than one entity / table needed ? — N

Y

Identify the PK / FK of the tables involved

Check results:

Identify the dictionary vs. transactional tables

- Correct ?
- Complete ?
- Relevant ?
- Consistent ?

Unique values important ? — Y — Use DISTINCT

- Count the number of rows
- Arrange from most common to least common
- Min, Max, Avg

Test - 0, 1 and Many situations

Group results on unique values ? — Y — Use GROUP BY

- Overlapping mutually exclusive groups?
- Gap between mutually exclusive groups?
- Are the results compatible with human life?

- Start with small subsets
- Limit time frame to several months or years

Identify outliers?
Filter on the results of an aggregate function ? — Y — Use HAVING

Need Count, Average, Sum, etc. ? — Y — Use aggregate function

Need different values from the same column ? — Y — Use Self Join

Need NULL values to appear as 0 ? — Y — Use a complementary table and Left Join

9. Patient

- Patient relationships
- Patient attributes
- Gender
- Demographics
- Age
- Group on decades
- Admissions
- Weight, height, BMI
- Ethnicity, religion, insurance
- MIMIC2 profile

Patient relationships

Let's start with the high level view of the table **D_PATIENTS** and its relationships with other tables. MIMIC2 guide offers only a partial ERD related to **D_PATIENTS**:

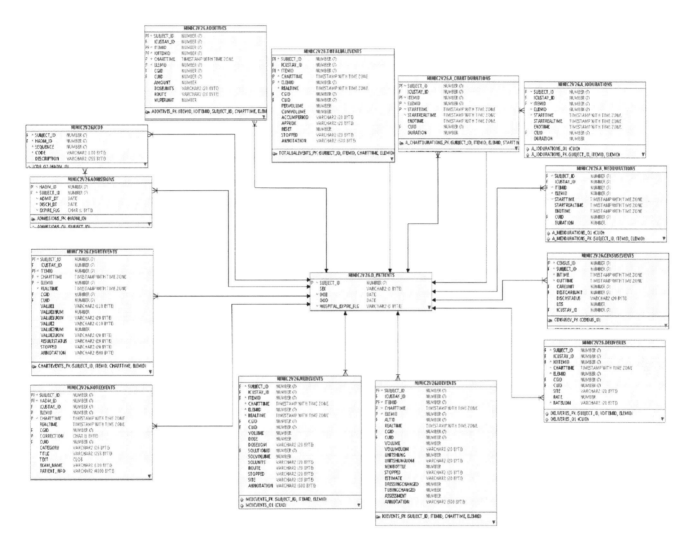

As the **D_PATIENTS** table is such a central concept in MIMIC2 database and the above ERD is only partial, we must identify all the tables that relate to **D_PATIENTS** by using other means.

If you have only a partial ERD or no ERD at all, use the Information Schema to quickly find relevant tables or columns

Using the Information Schema introduced earlier and realizing from the partial ERD above, that the **subject_id** is the PK in **D_PATIENTS** and the same **subject_id** is used to connect to other tables as FK:

```sql
SELECT * FROM INFORMATION_SCHEMA.COLUMNS
WHERE TABLE_SCHEMA = 'mimic2'
AND COLUMN_NAME = 'subject_id'
ORDER BY TABLE_NAME;
```

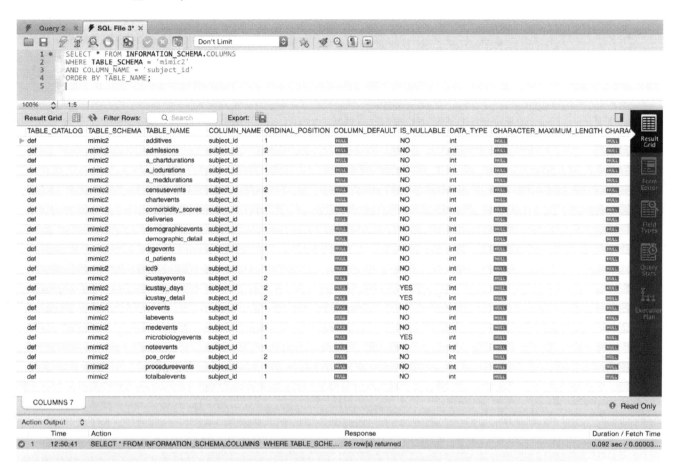

The query retrieved 25 (out of 37) tables containing a column **subject_id**.

Try to map the EHR conceptual entities from the previous chapter to the tables found in the Information Schema related to **d_patients**

Order in the conceptual model most probably will map to **poe_order** table in MIMIC2.
A quick **SELECT * FROM poe_order** (with a prudent limit of say 1,000 rows) will tell you if you're right about your initial hunch. While you browse the columns of **poe_order**, try to get familiar with its PK / FK, their types, examples of their content, if there are many null values, etc.

Repeat this process for each table of interest and you'll quickly become familiar with the MIMIC2 tables, columns and relationships.

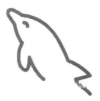

Patient attributes

As you approach an unknown table, first step is to do a COUNT(*):

SELECT COUNT(*)
FROM d_patients;

Counting the number of rows will let you know whether this table can be queried in the next step to retrieve all the rows and columns or only a subset of the rows. If the count is in the millions, you'll need to limit the number of rows to retrieve, for the query to run in less than the allowed 60 seconds.

There are 4,000 rows in this table, but does it mean 4,000 unique patients?
As we know the unique identifier of this table is **subject_id**, we should query whether there are 4,000 unique **subject_id**:

SELECT COUNT(DISTINCT subject_id)
FROM d_patients;

Indeed, there are 4,000 unique patients in **d_patients.**

If you need identify the number of unique rows in a table, pick the identifier of interest and run a COUNT(DISTINCT IdentifierName) on the table. Compare the results with the total number of rows.

As **d_patients** doesn't have millions of rows, we can safely run:

SELECT *
FROM d_patients;

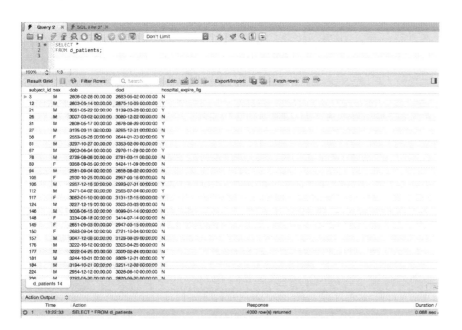

On top of the PK (**subject_id**), the table **d_patients** has the patient gender, date of birth, date of death and whether the patient has died in the hospital. Mortality will be discussed in a separate chapter.

SELECT *
FROM d_patients
ORDER BY sex;

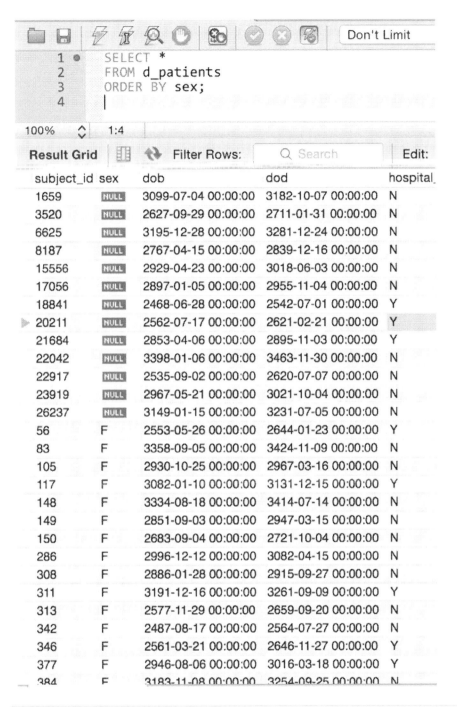

ORDER BY on a column can quickly identify NULL values by arranging them on top of the list

You could get the same result if you count the null values:

SELECT COUNT(*)
FROM d_patients
WHERE sex IS NULL;

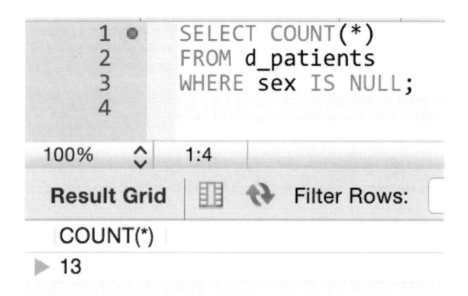

There are 13 patients with no information on gender as the **sex** column has 13 NULL values. 13 out of 4,000 rows missing on gender - 0.325% - seems reasonable.

Counting the NULL values in a column will tell you how much information is missing from that column. If most of the column has NULL values, then obviously it doesn't hold much information and you should search for a more complete data set, in other column(s).

Gender

From **d_patients** we can retrieve the patients' gender distribution:

SELECT sex, COUNT(subject_id)
FROM d_patients
GROUP BY sex;

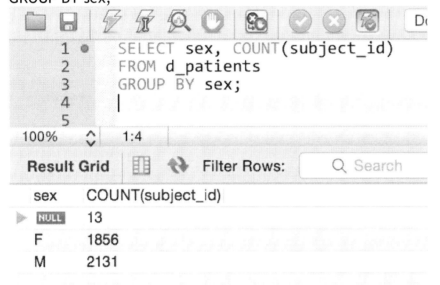

When you execute a COUNT together with a GROUP BY, SQL will first group the rows on the unique values of the column and then it will count the number of instances each group may have.
This method provides the values distribution of a column.

Demographics

The demographics part of MIMIC2 ERD (slightly modified from the original):

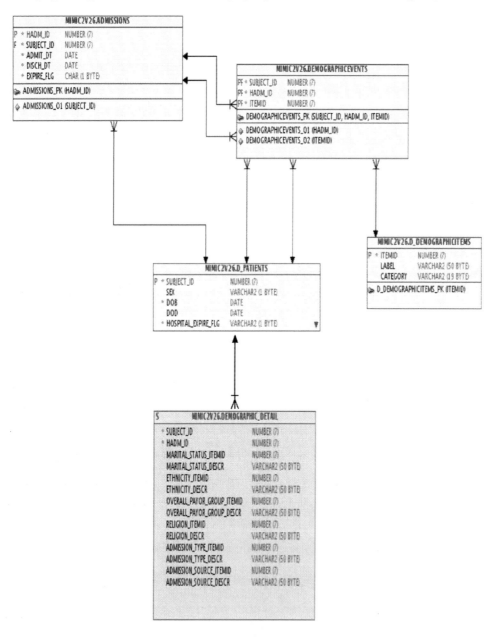

Age

In order to calculate the patients' age at admission, we need two parameters: date of birth and admission date.

 ## Question 24

Using the previous demographics ERD, calculate and retrieve:
1. All the patients: id, date of birth, admission date, age at admission - ordered by id
2. Minimum, maximum and average age at admission

If you search the Information Schema for columns with the characters "age" in their name:

```
SELECT * FROM INFORMATION_SCHEMA.COLUMNS
WHERE TABLE_SCHEMA = 'mimic2'
AND COLUMN_NAME LIKE '%age%'
ORDER BY TABLE_NAME;
```

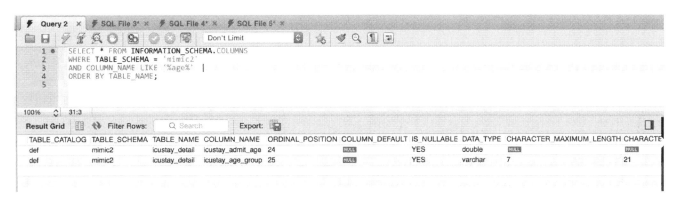

Usually information that can be calculated, should not be stored in a database. However, most probably for reasons of simplifying future frequent calculations, there is a column which needs further elaboration - **icustay_admit_age**.

Comparing simple statistics between 2 tables that contain similar information, can lead to interesting insights

 ## Question 25

Calculate the minimum, maximum and average age at admission from **icustay_admit_age** column and compare the results of this stored value with the statistics you've calculated in the previous question. Explain the slight differences between these results sets.

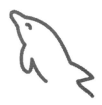

Group on decades

Sometimes in order to simplify a visualization, we may be interested in grouping the rows on larger units than the individual values. For example, when viewing the age distribution we'd likely group patients on decades instead of yearly values.

The goal is to group the patients by their age, measured by decades: 0-9 first decade, 10-19 second decade, etc. In order to achieve this type of grouping let's introduce two aggregate functions:

ROUND() - Rounds the argument
ROUND(X,D) function returns D decimal places of X
29.9 will **ROUND** to 30

FLOOR() – Floors the argument
FLOOR(X) function returns the largest integer value not greater than X
29.9 will **FLOOR** to 29

If we'd like the age distribution of the patients at admission, grouped by decades, **FLOOR()** function works best. Grouping patients by the decades of their age and then counting the patients in each group:

SELECT FLOOR(icustay_admit_age/10) AS Decade, COUNT(subject_id)
FROM icustay_detail
GROUP BY Decade;

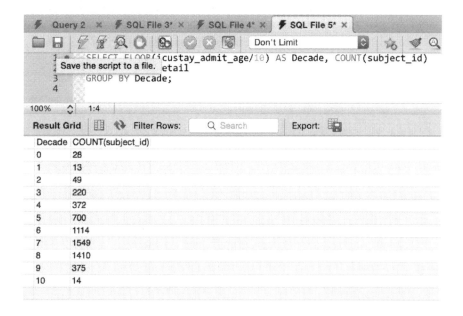

Decade	COUNT(subject_id)
0	28
1	13
2	49
3	220
4	372
5	700
6	1114
7	1549
8	1410
9	375
10	14

Question 26

In the previous query results, the age in decades begins with the first decade (age 0-10) as 0. Modify the query so the decades extracted will begin with 1 instead of 0.

Admissions

As we review the demographics part of the ERD, it is clear from the crow-feet / arrow line connecting the two tables **admissions** and **d_patients**, that one patient may have one or more admissions.

Question 27

Retrieve all admission and discharge dates of one patient: subject_id = 25030

Let's see how many admissions each patient had:

```
SELECT d_patients.subject_id, COUNT(hadm_id)
FROM admissions, d_patients
WHERE d_patients.subject_id = admissions.subject_id
GROUP BY d_patients.subject_id
ORDER BY COUNT(hadm_id) DESC;
```

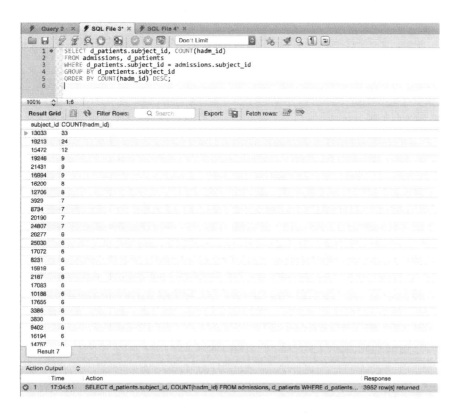

There are two suspected anomalies in the above results (and it is not the 33 admissions **subject_id** 13033 had)...

- There are only 3,952 patients in the admissions table – instead of the 4,000 expected. 48 patients (1.2%) are missing from the admissions table.
- There are no patients with 0 admissions.

Are these two anomalies connected ?

Identifying the source of even minor differences or anomalies between the expected and actual results of a query, can help you achieve a better understanding of the database structure as well as your query design.

Question 28

Retrieve all the patients' **subject_id** and the number of admissions, even if patients have 0 admissions.
Hint: review the chapter on Left-Join

Question 29

Identify all the patients **subject_id** that had no admissions

As you may have noticed in the ERD, the table **demographic_detail** has two interesting columns: **admission_type_descr** and **admission_source_descr**.

Let's retrieve the admission types and the number of patients in each group.

SELECT admission_type_descr, COUNT(DISTINCT subject_id) AS Counter
FROM demographic_detail
GROUP BY admission_type_descr
ORDER BY COUNT(DISTINCT subject_id) DESC;

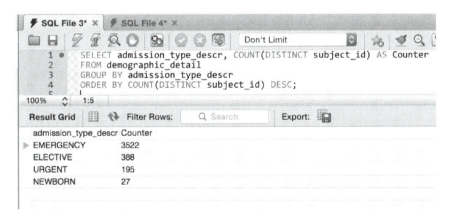

If we'd like to see the number of patients and admissions over time, grouped by century:

Volumes	Total	Average month	Oct 2018
Patients	4,000	382	388
Admissions	5,074	492	504

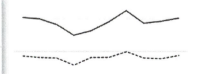

Patients over time:

```
SELECT FLOOR(YEAR(hospital_admit_dt)/100) AS CenturyAdmit,
COUNT(DISTINCT subject_id) AS NumPatients
FROM icustay_detail
GROUP BY CenturyAdmit;
```

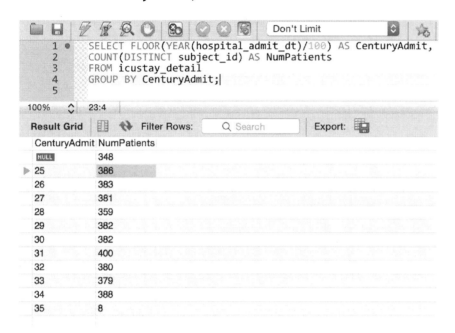

Admissions over time:

```
SELECT FLOOR(YEAR(hospital_admit_dt)/100) AS CenturyAdmit,
COUNT(DISTINCT hadm_id) AS NumAdmissions
FROM icustay_detail
GROUP BY CenturyAdmit;
```

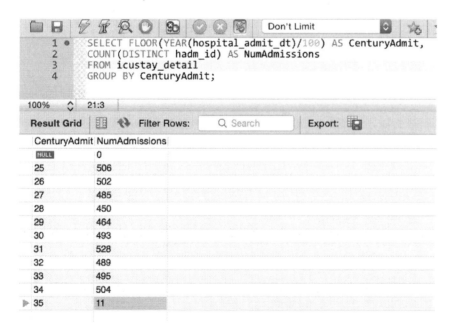

Weight, Height, BMI

Using the Information Schema, let's find the columns that may contain data related to weight:

SELECT * FROM INFORMATION_SCHEMA.COLUMNS
WHERE TABLE_SCHEMA = 'mimic2'
AND COLUMN_NAME LIKE '%weight%'
ORDER BY TABLE_NAME;

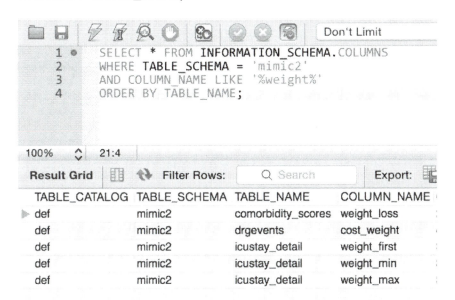

 ## Question 30

Using **weight_first**, calculate the minimum, maximum, average and standard deviation of the patients' weight at admission. Round the results to one decimal.

 ## Question 31

Calculate the minimum, maximum, average and standard deviation of the patients' height. Round the results to one decimal.

Note that the results of the previous question, include at least one very tall patient with a height of 457 centimeters (almost 15 feet).

This is a computer anomaly – hopefully not a biological one.

In order to check how skewed / incorrect is the information in the **height** column, we can simply arrange all patients in a decreasing order of their height. This way we can easily identify outliers:

```
SELECT height
FROM icustay_detail
ORDER BY height DESC;
```

There are 5 height values that are just incompatible with humans, most probably errors in data entry, no validation performed during data entry, a bug, etc. These incorrect measurements, don't seem like a significant issue as there are only 5 extremely high values and this is only 0.125% of the 4,000 patients.

 ## Question 32

Assuming the tallest (human) patient in the **icustay_detail** table is 208.28 centimeters tall, modify the previous query so it will disregard any heights above this limit.

BMI = Weight (kg) / Height (meters) ^{2}

X^2 translates in MySQL to **POWER(X , 2)**

 ## Question 33

Using the BMI formula, calculate the average BMI in MIMIC2. Disregard any BMI over 100 or under 10. Round the results to 2 decimals.

 ## Question 34

Retrieve the admission sources and the number of patients in each group.

Ethnicity, religion, insurance

Let's retrieve the patients ethnicities' distribution:

SELECT ethnicity_descr, COUNT(DISTINCT subject_id) AS Counter
FROM demographic_detail
GROUP BY ethnicity_descr
ORDER BY COUNT(DISTINCT subject_id) DESC;

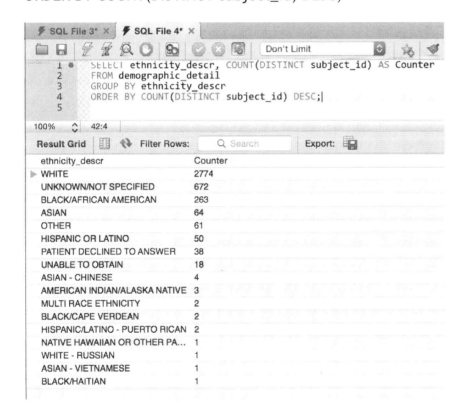

 Question 35

Similar to the above, retrieve the patients religions' distribution. Order from highest to lowest number of patients in a group.

If we'd like to know the patients' type of insurance (a.k.a. payor):

```sql
SELECT overall_payor_group_descr, COUNT(DISTINCT subject_id) AS Counter
FROM demographic_detail
GROUP BY overall_payor_group_descr
ORDER BY COUNT(DISTINCT subject_id) DESC;
```

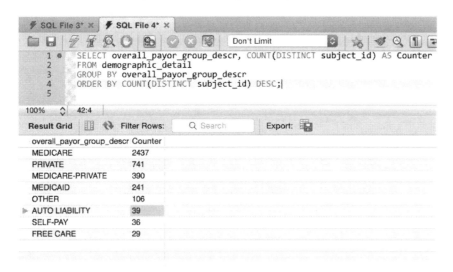

Now suppose you'd like to know the ethnicities' distribution for each insurance type, arranged so the most common ethnicity for each insurance group would appear on top:

```sql
SELECT overall_payor_group_descr, ethnicity_descr, COUNT(subject_id) AS Counter
FROM demographic_detail
GROUP BY overall_payor_group_descr, ethnicity_descr
ORDER BY overall_payor_group_descr, Counter DESC;
```

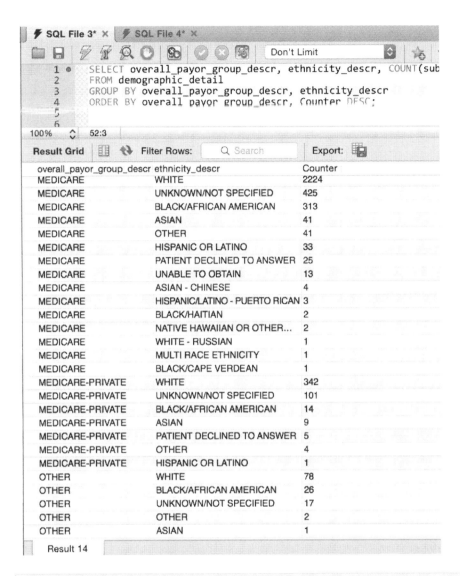

Always try to think bi-directionally.
If previously we've checked the distribution of ethnicities for each insurance type, let's check the insurance types for each ethnic group.

 ## Question 36

Similar to the above, retrieve the insurance types' distribution for each ethnic group. Arrange results so the insurance types that are used most would appear on top.

MIMIC2 profile

The number of patients / admissions, mortality, LOS and readmission rate, gender and age distributions are parameters we'd like to monitor in relation to diagnosis, procedure, drug, lab, etc.

Before we dive into the details of how to create a specific profile, related to one of the parameters above, here's how a tentative MIMIC2 profile may look, while the centuries have been modified to hypothetical months:

Medical Information Extraction and Analysis

MIMIC2 Profile . October 2018

printed Nov 15, 2018 by Alex Scarlat MD

Volumes	Total	Average month	Oct 2018
Patients	4,000	382	388
Admissions	5,074	492	504

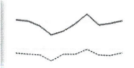

	Average	Oct 2018
Mortality	37.7%	36.0%
LOS	13.9 days	13.7 days
Readmissions	8.0%	9.2%

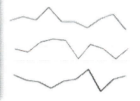

Top ICD9 Codes

code	description	NumPts	NumAdmis
428	CONGESTIVE HEART FAILURE UNSPECIFIED	1490	1845
401.9	UNSPECIFIED ESSENTIAL HYPERTENSION	1570	1777
427.3	ATRIAL FIBRILLATION	1292	1553
584.9	ACUTE RENAL FAILURE UNSPECIFIED	1013	1132
518.8	RESPIRATORY FAILURE	1051	1123
414	CORONARY ATHEROSCLEROSIS OF NATIVE CORONARY ARTERY	900	1030
250	DIABETES MELLITUS WITHOUT COMPLICATION TYPE II OR	749	884
599	URINARY TRACT INFECTION SITE NOT SPECIFIED	733	817
486	PNEUMONIA ORGANISM UNSPECIFIED	599	630
496	CHRONIC AIRWAY OBSTRUCTION NOT ELSEWHERE CLASSIFIE	535	625
507	PNEUMONITIS DUE TO INHALATION OF FOOD OR VOMITUS	550	589
38.9	UNSPECIFIED SEPTICEMIA	561	584
276.2	ACIDOSIS	484	513
995.9	SYST INFLAM RESPN INFECT	483	509
272	PURE HYPERCHOLESTEROLEMIA	466	501
403.9	UNSPECIFIED HYPERTENSIVE RENAL DISEASE WITH RENAL	350	471
410.7	SUBENDOCARDIAL INFARCTION INITIAL EPISODE OF CARE	444	459
244.9	UNSPECIFIED ACQUIRED HYPOTHYROIDISM	361	434

Top DRG Codes

code	description	NumPts	NumAdmis
428	CONGESTIVE HEART FAILURE UNSPECIFIED	1490	1845
401.9	UNSPECIFIED ESSENTIAL HYPERTENSION	1570	1777
427.31	ATRIAL FIBRILLATION	1292	1553
584.9	ACUTE RENAL FAILURE UNSPECIFIED	1013	1132
518.81	RESPIRATORY FAILURE	1051	1123
414.01	CORONARY ATHEROSCLEROSIS OF NATIVE CORONARY ARTERY	900	1030
250	DIABETES MELLITUS WITHOUT COMPLICATION TYPE II OR	749	884
599	URINARY TRACT INFECTION SITE NOT SPECIFIED	733	817
486	PNEUMONIA ORGANISM UNSPECIFIED	599	630
496	CHRONIC AIRWAY OBSTRUCTION NOT ELSEWHERE CLASSIFIE	535	625
507	PNEUMONITIS DUE TO INHALATION OF FOOD OR VOMITUS	550	589
38.9	UNSPECIFIED SEPTICEMIA	561	584

Insurance

Payor	Pts
MEDICARE	2437
PRIVATE	741
MEDICARE-PRIVATE	390
MEDICAID	241
OTHER	106
AUTO LIABILITY	39
SELF-PAY	36
FREE CARE	29

Average age 70.2 years

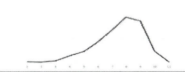

Female : Male   1 : 1.15

Admission types

Admission Type	NumPts	NumAdmit
EMERGENCY	3522	4438
ELECTIVE	388	408
URGENT	195	201
NEWBORN	27	27

Top Procedures

Procedure	NumPts	NumAdmit
VENOUS CATHETER NEC	1825	1825
INSERT ENDOTRACHEAL TUBE	1486	1486
PACKED CELL TRANSFUSION	1268	1268
EXT INFUS CONC NUTRITION	1134	1134
CONTINUOUS INVASIVE MECH	1081	1082
CONTINUOUS INVASIVE MECH	915	915
ARTERIAL CATHETERIZATION	683	683
PARENTERAL INFUS CONC NU	524	524
CORONAR ARTERIOGR-2 CATH	511	511
HEMODIALYSIS	491	491
SERUM TRANSFUSION NEC	413	413
SM BOWEL ENDOSCOPY NEC	358	358
ENDOSCOPIC BRONCHIAL BR-	357	357
RT/LEFT HEART CARD CATH	355	355
DX ULTRASOUND-HEART	339	339
EXTRACORPOREAL CIRCULAT	329	329
THORACENTESIS	273	273
TEMPORARY TRACHEOSTOMY	271	271
PERCUTANEOUS ABDOM DRAIN	250	250
LEFT HEART CARDIAC CATH	246	246
INFUSION OF VASOPRESSOR	246	246
PLATELET TRANSFUSION	246	246

As MIMIC2 is dispersed over 1,000 years – the charts depict centuries as months, in order to minimize any cognitive dissonance that may be caused by a millennium of data.
The following chapters will explain how to derive the numbers and charts used for this and other profiles.

10. Mortality

- Mortality rate and its many flavors
- Mortality by gender
- Mortality by age
- Mortality by BMI
- Mortality by admission type
- Mortality over time

Mortality rate and its many flavors

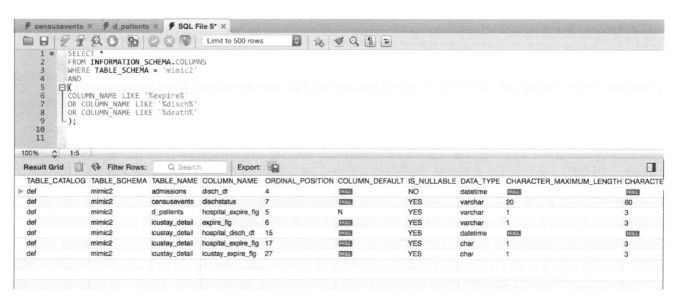

Using the Information Schema, let's find first the columns in MIMIC2 tables that are related to the terms discharge, expired or death:

```
SELECT *
FROM INFORMATION_SCHEMA.COLUMNS
WHERE TABLE_SCHEMA = 'mimic2'
AND
(
COLUMN_NAME LIKE '%expire%'
OR COLUMN_NAME LIKE '%disch%'
OR COLUMN_NAME LIKE '%death%'
);
```

There are 5 columns we need to further explore in search of the mortality rate in MIMIC2:
1. dischstatus in censusevents table
2. hospital_expire_flg in d_patients table
3. expire_flg in icustay_detail table
4. hospital_expire_flg in icustay_detail table
5. icustay_expire_flg in icustay_detail table

For each column above, we are grouping the data on the unique values and then count the number of patients in each group.

1.
SELECT dischstatus, COUNT(DISTINCT subject_id)
FROM censusevents
GROUP BY dischstatus;

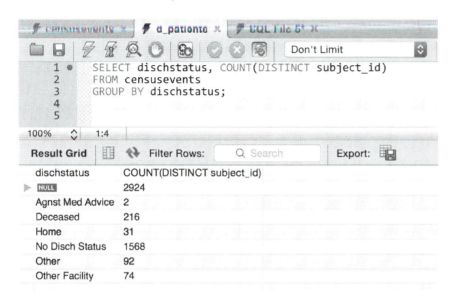

Out of 4,907 instances, there are 4,492 instances with no information (2,924 **NULL** values and another 1,568 **No Disch Status**). Even with a name like **dischstatus** - 91.5% of this column has no useful information on discharge status – thus, we eliminate it from the list of tentative sources for mortality.

2.
SELECT hospital_expire_flg, COUNT(DISTINCT subject_id)
FROM d_patients
GROUP BY hospital_expire_flg;

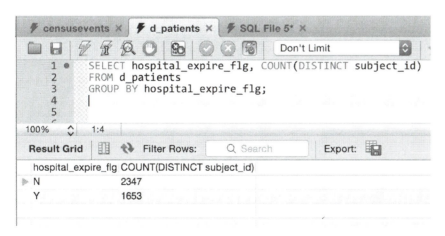

3.
SELECT expire_flg, COUNT(DISTINCT subject_id)
FROM icustay_detail
GROUP BY expire_flg;

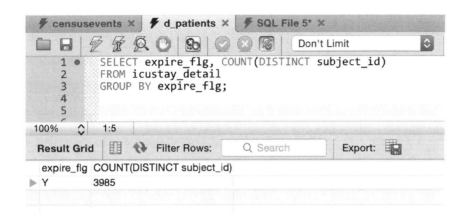

4.
SELECT hospital_expire_flg, COUNT(DISTINCT subject_id)
FROM icustay_detail
GROUP BY hospital_expire_flg;

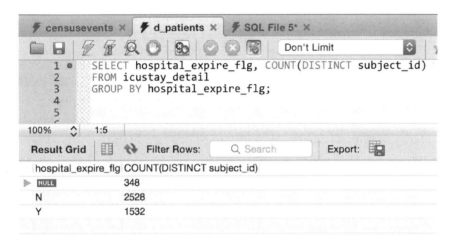

5.
SELECT icustay_expire_flg, COUNT(DISTINCT hadm_id)
FROM icustay_detail
GROUP BY icustay_expire_flg;

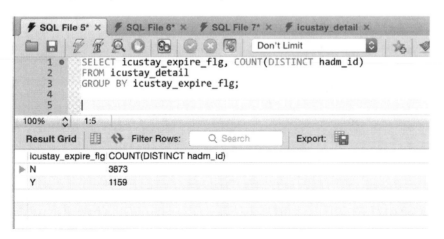

Some of the above queries return hospital mortality while counting patients and other queries reflect on ICU mortality while counting admissions. Here's a summary of the above queries on mortality in MIMIC2:

Table	Column	Deceased	Lived	Nulls	Total with Nulls	Total without Nulls	Mortality with Nulls	Mortality without Nulls
d_patients	hospital_expire_flag	1653	2347	0	4000	4000	41.3%	**41.3%**
icustay_detail	expire_flag	3985	0	0	3985	3985	100.0%	100.0%
icustay_detail	hospital_expire_flag	1532	2528	348	4408	4060	34.8%	37.7%
icustay_detail	icustay_expire_flag	1159	3873	0	5032	5032	23.0%	**23.0%**

- According to the **d_patients** table the hospital mortality is 41.3%
- All the patients in MIMIC2 are deceased per the Social Security records, so the (general) **expire_flag** in the **icustay_detail** table shows 100% mortality
- The **icustay_detail** table mortality rate is 37.7%, but we have no information on the outcomes of the 348 patients with null information, whether they lived or died. If for example, all 348 patients have died in the hospital, then the mortality would be 42.6% - not far from the 41.3% mortality calculated from the **d_patients** table.
- Finally, the ICU mortality (not hospital mortality) derived from the **icustay_detail** is 23%

Compare and corroborate results from different sources / tables and try to understand the reasons for any difference or inconsistency you may find.
Always check the number of null values, as too many nulls translates into an incomplete data set.
You do not want to reach a conclusion based on incomplete, inconsistent, biased or skewed data.

How are the above mortality results when compared to others in peer reviewed literature ?
The article *"Changes in hospital mortality for United States intensive care unit admissions from 1988 to 2012"* may provide some background information on this issue:
https://ccforum.biomedcentral.com/articles/10.1186/cc12695

Mortality by gender

As both the **sex** and the **hospital_expire_flg** are in the same table, calculating hospital mortality by sex is straightforward:

SELECT sex, COUNT(subject_id), hospital_expire_flg
FROM d_patients
GROUP BY sex, hospital_expire_flg;

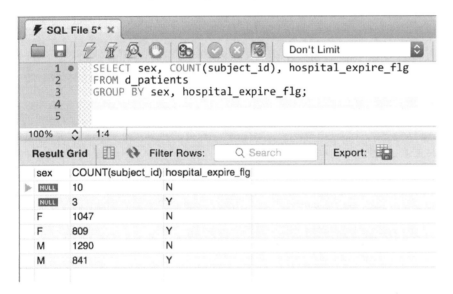

- Female hospital mortality: 809 / (1047+809) = **43.6%**
- Male hospital mortality: 841 / (1290+841) = **39.5%**

 # Question 37

Calculate the ICU mortality for each gender. Note that as one patient may have more than one admission, for this question to make sense - you'll need to count admissions and not patients.

Mortality by age

In order to calculate the age of a patient at admission, we need the patient date of birth (**dob**) and the admission date. As both parameters exist in the same table – **icustay_detail** – together with the **hospital_expire_flg**, the first exploratory query would bring all these columns in one table:

SELECT subject_id, dob, hospital_admit_dt,
TIMESTAMPDIFF(YEAR, dob, hospital_admit_dt) AS AgeAtAdmit, hospital_expire_flg
FROM icustay_detail
WHERE hospital_expire_flg IS NOT NULL
ORDER BY subject_id;

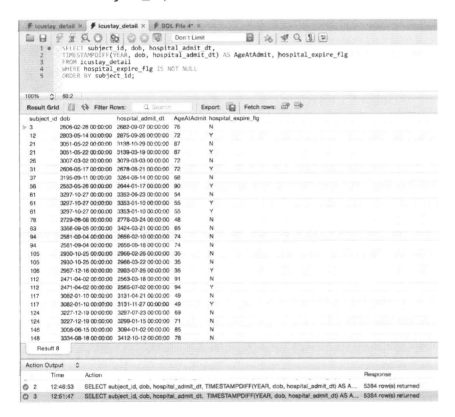

Suppose we'd like to view the mortality, grouped by decades of age. The following query will first divide the patients into those that lived or died, using the **hospital_expire_flg**, then it will count the patients in each decade age group:

SELECT hospital_expire_flg,
FLOOR(TIMESTAMPDIFF(YEAR, dob, hospital_admit_dt)/10)+1 AS DecadeAge,
COUNT(hadm_id) AS NumPts
FROM icustay_detail
WHERE TIMESTAMPDIFF(YEAR, dob, hospital_admit_dt) IS NOT NULL
GROUP BY hospital_expire_flg, DecadeAge;

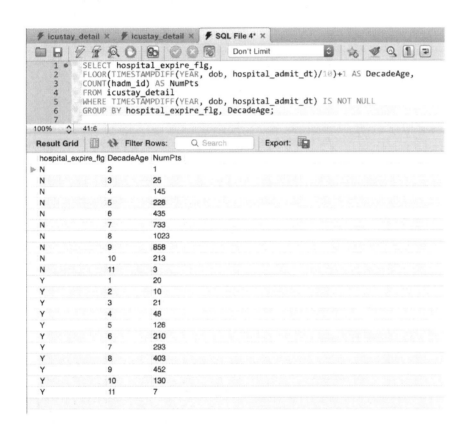

If you click on the Export icon, MySQL will create a file that you can open with a spreadsheet. While in a spreadsheet, you can calculate the total number of patients per decade and chart the mortality by decade:

hospital_expire_flg	DecadeAge	NumPts		DecadeAge	Mortality
N	1	0		1	100.0%
N	2	1		2	90.9%
N	3	25		3	45.7%
N	4	145		4	24.9%
N	5	228		5	35.6%
N	6	435		6	32.6%
N	7	733		7	28.6%
N	8	1023		8	28.3%
N	9	858		9	34.5%
N	10	213		10	37.9%
N	11	3		11	70.0%
Y	1	20			
Y	2	10			
Y	3	21			
Y	4	48			
Y	5	126			
Y	6	210			
Y	7	293			
Y	8	403			
Y	9	452			
Y	10	130			
Y	11	7			
Total	1	20			
Total	2	11			
Total	3	46			
Total	4	193			
Total	5	354			
Total	6	645			
Total	7	1026			
Total	8	1426			
Total	9	1310			
Total	10	343			
Total	11	10			

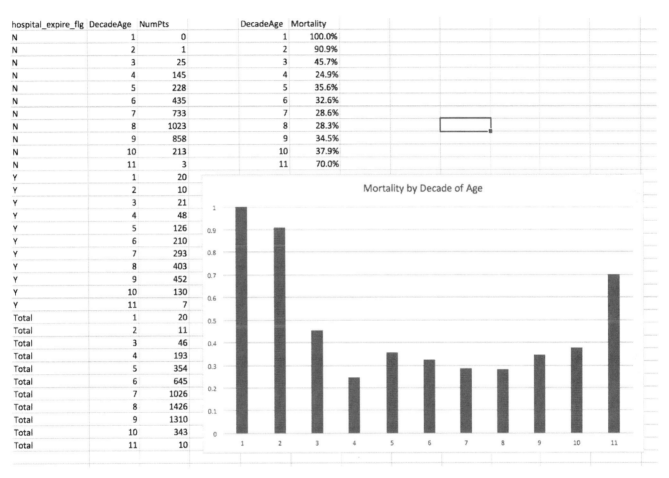

Mortality by BMI

The formula to calculate the Body Mass Index (BMI):

BMI = Weight (kg) / Height (meters) ^{2}

The following are considered accepted limits to BMI values:
- Underweight <= 18.5
- Normal 18.6 to 24.9
- Overweight 25 to 29.9
- Obese >= 30

Let's select the patients according to the above limits and for each group – we'll retrieve the number of patients that lived vs. died. Then we can compare mortality across the BMI groups.

```
SELECT hospital_expire_flg, COUNT(hadm_id) AS NumPts
FROM icustay_detail
WHERE weight_first/POWER((height/100),2) BETWEEN 10 AND 18.5
AND hospital_expire_flg IS NOT NULL
GROUP BY hospital_expire_flg;
```

Underweight: 63 Lived and 41 Died

```
SELECT hospital_expire_flg, COUNT(hadm_id) AS NumPts
FROM icustay_detail
WHERE weight_first/POWER((height/100),2) BETWEEN 18.6 AND 24.9
AND hospital_expire_flg IS NOT NULL
GROUP BY hospital_expire_flg;
```

Normal weight: 493 Lived and 240 Died

```
SELECT hospital_expire_flg, COUNT(hadm_id) AS NumPts
FROM icustay_detail
WHERE weight_first/POWER((height/100),2) BETWEEN 25 AND 29.9
AND hospital_expire_flg IS NOT NULL
GROUP BY hospital_expire_flg;
```

Overweight: 411 Lived and 199 Died

```
SELECT hospital_expire_flg, COUNT(hadm_id) AS NumPts
FROM icustay_detail
WHERE weight_first/POWER((height/100),2) BETWEEN 30 AND 100
AND hospital_expire_flg IS NOT NULL
GROUP BY hospital_expire_flg;
```

Obese: 402 Lived and 206 Died

Summarizing it all in a spreadsheet:

	Lived	Died	Total	Mortality
Underweight	63	41	104	39.4%
Normal	493	240	733	32.7%
Overweight	411	199	610	32.6%
Obese	402	206	608	33.9%
TOTAL	*1369*	*686*	*2055*	*33.4%*

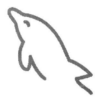

Mortality by admission type

As you may remember from previous chapters, the admission type resides in the **demographic_detail** table.

 ## Question 38

Calculate the hospital mortality for each admission type. Note that as one patient may have more than one admission, for this question to make sense - you'll need to count admissions and not patients. Summarize your results in a spreadsheet.

Mortality over time

Please refresh your knowledge about Left Join (chapter 6), as the following section makes use of this querying technique.

Using the **calendar** table that contains all the dates and a Left Join with **icustay_detail** - let's check first the number of admissions per month, grouped by **hospital_expire_flg**:

SELECT hospital_expire_flg, YEAR(datefield) AS YearAdmit, MONTH(datefield) AS MonthAdmit,
COUNT(hospital_admit_dt) AS NumAdmissions
FROM calendar LEFT JOIN icustay_detail
ON datefield = hospital_admit_dt
WHERE datefield BETWEEN '2501-01-01' AND '2511-01-01'
GROUP BY hospital_expire_flg, YEAR(datefield), MONTH(datefield)
ORDER BY YEAR(datefield), MONTH(datefield);

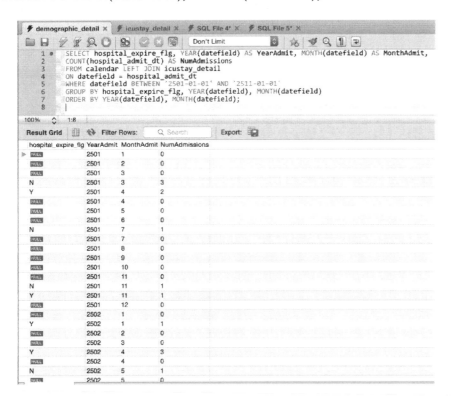

In order for the above query to run under 60 seconds, there's a limit on the time frame between the years 2501 and 2511. As a couple of months of data (4,000 patients) have been spread over 1,000 years for de-identification purposes, the results are sparsely distributed.

Question 39

Display the number of admissions per year, the number of patients that have lived thru their episode of care each year vs. those that have died. Don't limit the time frame of the query.

The results from the previous question are still sparse, and realizing that the following query is not going to be used much in real-life – let's summarize mortality over the centuries of the alleged 1,000 years in MIMIC2. As there are no centuries with zero patients or zero admissions, we can run a simple query on **icustay_detail** table, without the need of a Left Join with the **calendar** table (which was previously used to display years without any admissions).

SELECT hospital_expire_flg,
FLOOR(YEAR(hospital_admit_dt)/100) AS CenturyAdmit,
COUNT(DISTINCT subject_id) AS NumPatients
FROM icustay_detail
WHERE hospital_expire_flg IS NOT NULL
GROUP BY hospital_expire_flg, CenturyAdmit
ORDER BY CenturyAdmit;

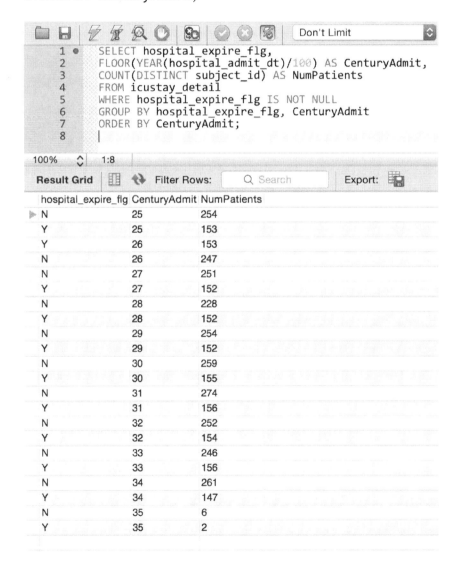

hospital_expire_flg	CenturyAdmit	NumPatients
N	25	254
Y	25	153
Y	26	153
N	26	247
N	27	251
Y	27	152
N	28	228
Y	28	152
N	29	254
Y	29	152
N	30	259
Y	30	155
N	31	274
Y	31	156
N	32	252
Y	32	154
N	33	246
Y	33	156
N	34	261
Y	34	147
N	35	6
Y	35	2

The above table could be easily summarized in a spreadsheet as:

hospital_expire_flg	CenturyAdmit	NumPatients	PtsDied	PtsTotal	PtsMortality
N	25	254		407	37.6%
Y	25	153	153		
N	26	247		400	38.3%
Y	26	153	153		
N	27	251		403	37.7%
Y	27	152	152		
N	28	228		380	40.0%
Y	28	152	152		
N	29	254		406	37.4%
Y	29	152	152		
N	30	259		414	37.4%
Y	30	155	155		
N	31	274		430	36.3%
Y	31	156	156		
N	32	252		406	37.9%
Y	32	154	154		
N	33	246		402	38.8%
Y	33	156	156		
N	34	261		408	36.0%
Y	34	147	147		
N	35	6		8	25.0%
Y	35	2	2		
TOTAL		4064	1532	4064	37.7%

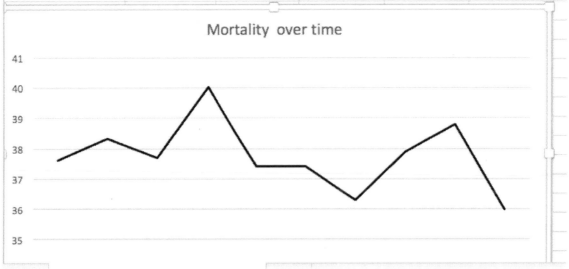

11. Length of stay (LOS)

- LOS – stored vs. calculated
- LOS by gender, age, BMI, admission type
- LOS over time

LOS – stored vs. calculated

	Average	Oct 2018
Mortality	37.7%	36.0%
LOS	13.9 days	13.7 days
Readmissions	8.0%	9.2%

Using the Information Schema, we find the LOS in **icustay_detail** table:

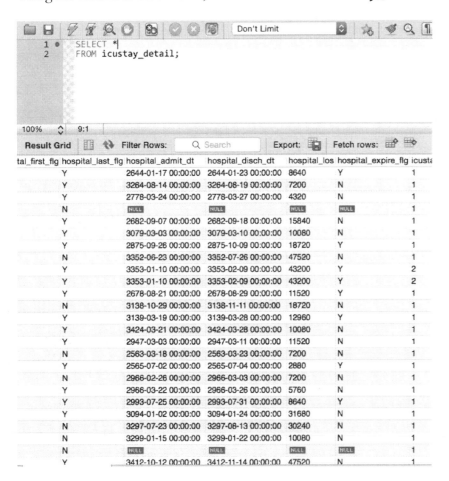

As mentioned previously, a parameter that can be calculated is usually not stored in a table. Nevertheless, the LOS is stored in **icustay_detail** table together with the **hospital_admit_dt** and **hospital_disch_dt** – even though both could be used to calculate the LOS.

Let's check the unit of the **hospital_los** and at the same time, verify whether the stored values are correct:

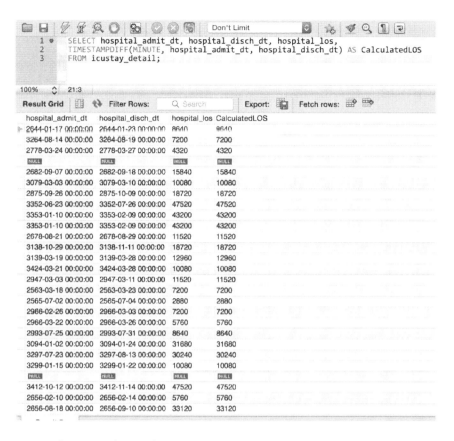

From these results we learn:
- The unit for **hospital_los** is minutes. This column is the difference in minutes between discharge and admission.
- The stored values are correct when compared to the calculated ones.

Sometimes you won't have the luxury of calculated values, like the LOS in MIMIC2. Thus, you should be able to calculate things on your own.

 Question 40

Calculate the average LOS in days.

LOS by gender, age, BMI, admission type

Gender

Having the **gender** and **hospital_los** columns in the same table should make the following question easy for you by now:

 Question 41

Calculate the average LOS in days grouped by gender.

Age

Using the same technique we've already used grouping patients by their decade age:

```
SELECT FLOOR(TIMESTAMPDIFF(YEAR, dob, hospital_admit_dt)/10)+1 AS DecadeAge,
ROUND(AVG(hospital_los/60/24),1) AvgLOSdays,
COUNT(hadm_id) AS NumAdmissions
FROM icustay_detail
WHERE TIMESTAMPDIFF(YEAR, dob, hospital_admit_dt) IS NOT NULL
GROUP BY DecadeAge;
```

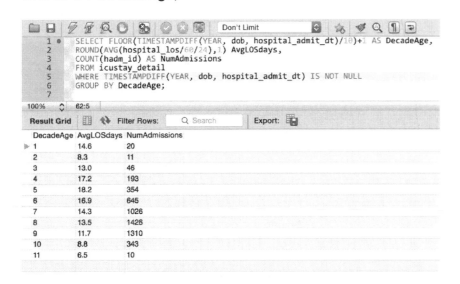

And in a spreadsheet:

DecadeAge	AvgLOSdays	NumAdmissions
1	14.6	20
2	8.3	11
3	13	46
4	17.2	193
5	18.2	354
6	16.9	645
7	14.3	1026
8	13.5	1426
9	11.7	1310
10	8.8	343
11	6.5	10
Total		5384

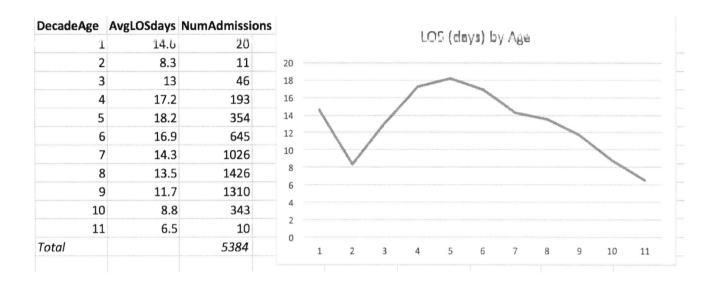

 Question 42

Calculate the average LOS and number of admissions for each of the BMI groups.
Summarize it all in a spreadsheet. 5 points bonus towards the Hero awards - if you chart the results.

Admission type

 Question 43

Calculate the average LOS and number of admissions for each type of admission.

LOS over time

 Question 44

As MIMIC2 is sparsely populated over 1,000 years – instead of the familiar monthly LOS report, calculate the LOS by century. Use the mortality over time query as a template.

12. Readmissions

- Readmissions calculation
- Readmissions by gender, age
- Readmissions over time

Readmissions calculation

	Average	Oct 2018
Mortality	37.7%	36.0%
LOS	13.9 days	13.7 days
Readmissions	8.0%	9.2%

Readmission within 30 days is one of the quality metrics any hospital needs to monitor.

There is no column in MIMIC2 related to readmission, so we have to calculate it on our own. Please refresh your knowledge about Self Join introduced earlier, as the following section makes use of this querying technique:
- As both the admission date and the discharge date reside in the same table, we need to compare the **admissions** table to itself, using the **subject_id** as the linchpin connecting the two instances of the **admissions** table – once as table X and once as table Y.
- While we use the first table instance (X) for the discharge date, we use the second table instance (Y) for the (re)admission date.
- We don't want to compare the same admission to itself, so we employ the inequality on the admission unique identifier **hadm_id**.
- Finally, we enforce the condition of the time frame between discharge (table X) and admission (table Y) to be between 0 and 30 days. If we don't use the minimum of 0, the query will return also the negative differences between dates (such as minus -122 days)

```
SELECT X.subject_id, X.hadm_id, X.admit_dt, X.disch_dt AS DISCHdate,
Y.hadm_id, Y.admit_dt AS ADMITdate, Y.disch_dt,
TIMESTAMPDIFF(DAY, X.disch_dt, Y.admit_dt)
FROM admissions X, admissions Y
WHERE X.subject_id = Y.subject_id
AND X.hadm_id <> Y.hadm_id
AND TIMESTAMPDIFF(DAY, X.disch_dt, Y.admit_dt) BETWEEN 0 AND 30;
```

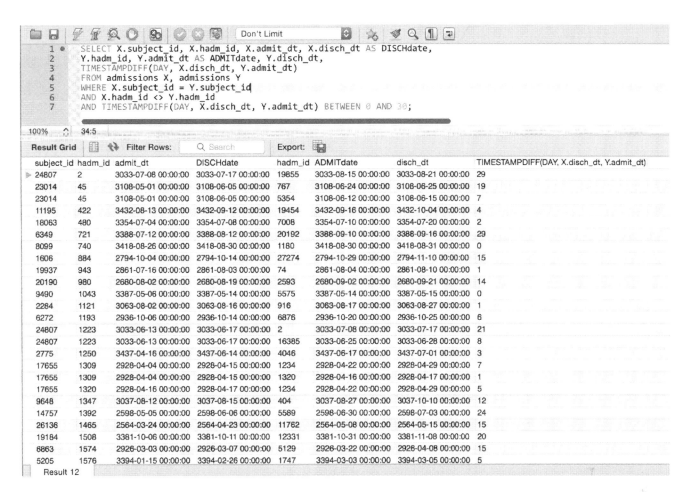

Readmissions by gender, age

As the admission and discharge dates exist in the **icustay_detail** table as well, we can calculate readmissions related to gender or age using this table only, instead of using both the **admissions** and the **icustay_detail** tables.

Gender
We'll need to calculate the number of admissions by gender (denominator) and the number of readmissions by gender (numerator). The technique used to identify readmissions was discussed in the previous paragraph.

Numerator – the number of readmissions by gender:

SELECT X.gender, COUNT(X.hadm_id) as NumPtsReadmit
FROM icustay_detail X, icustay_detail Y
WHERE X.subject_id = Y.subject_id
AND X.hadm_id <> Y.hadm_id
AND TIMESTAMPDIFF(DAY, X.hospital_disch_dt, Y.hospital_admit_dt) BETWEEN 0 AND 30
GROUP by X.gender;

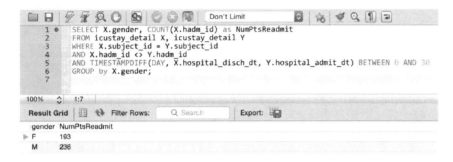

The denominator – the number of admissions per gender:

SELECT gender, COUNT(hadm_id) as NumAdmit
FROM icustay_detail
GROUP by gender;

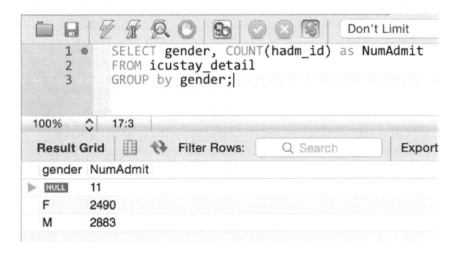

And summarized in a spreadsheet:

	Readmit	Admissions	Readmit rate
Female	193	2490	7.8%
Male	236	2883	8.2%
Total	429	5373	8.0%

Age

For the sake of brevity and clarity, we'll use the stored value of the patient's age, instead of calculating it from the date of birth and the admission date.

Using the same query technique as above, we'll first identify the patients that have been readmitted within 30 days and their age.

SELECT X.subject_id, X.hadm_id,
X.hospital_admit_dt, X.hospital_disch_dt AS DISCHdate,
Y.hadm_id, Y.hospital_admit_dt AS ADMITdate, Y.hospital_disch_dt,
TIMESTAMPDIFF(DAY, X.hospital_disch_dt, Y.hospital_admit_dt) AS DaysBetweenAdmissions,
ROUND(X.icustay_admit_age,0) AS AgeAdmit
FROM icustay_detail X, icustay_detail Y
WHERE X.subject_id = Y.subject_id
AND X.hadm_id <> Y.hadm_id
AND TIMESTAMPDIFF(DAY, X.hospital_disch_dt, Y.hospital_admit_dt) BETWEEN 0 AND 30;

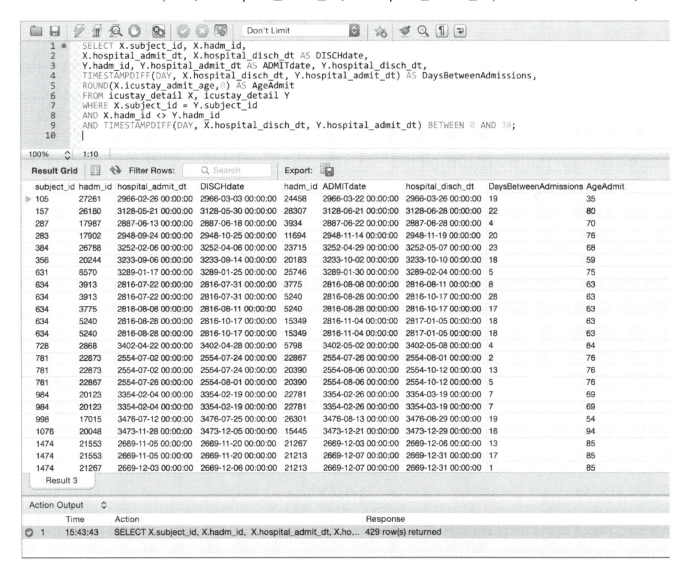

Now, we can group these results on the patients' age by decades:

```
SELECT FLOOR(X.icustay_admit_age/10)+1 AS DecadeAge, COUNT(X.hadm_id) as
NumPtsReadmit
FROM icustay_detail X, icustay_detail Y
WHERE X.subject_id = Y.subject_id
AND X.hadm_id <> Y.hadm_id
AND TIMESTAMPDIFF(DAY, X.hospital_disch_dt, Y.hospital_admit_dt) BETWEEN 0 AND 30
GROUP BY DecadeAge;
```

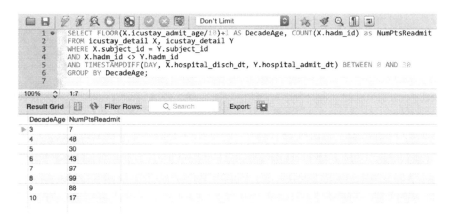

DecadeAge	NumPtsReadmit
3	7
4	48
5	30
6	43
7	97
8	99
9	88
10	17

Now that we have the number of patients readmitted within 30 days, grouped by their decades, we need the denominator – how many patients have been admitted overall in each group - so we can calculate the readmissions rate:

```
SELECT FLOOR(icustay_admit_age/10)+1 AS Decade, COUNT(hadm_id)
FROM icustay_detail
GROUP BY Decade;
```

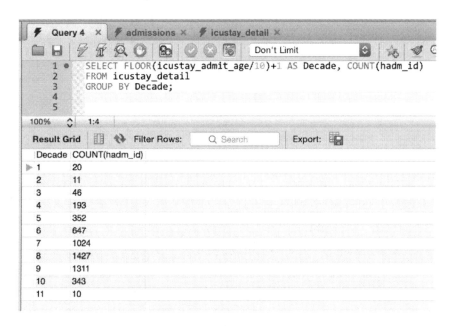

Decade	COUNT(hadm_id)
1	20
2	11
3	46
4	193
5	352
6	647
7	1024
8	1427
9	1311
10	343
11	10

And summarizing it all in a spreadsheet:

Decade Age	Readmit	Admissions	Readmit Rate
1	0	20	0.0%
2	0	11	0.0%
3	7	46	15.2%
4	48	193	24.9%
5	30	352	8.5%
6	43	647	6.6%
7	97	1024	9.5%
8	99	1427	6.9%
9	88	1311	6.7%
10	17	343	5.0%
11	0	10	0.0%
TOTAL	**429**	**5384**	**8.0%**

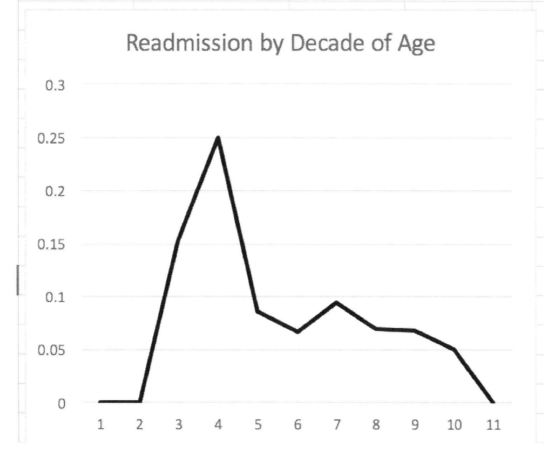

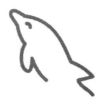

Readmissions over time

As the admissions in MIMIC2 are dispersed over 1,000 years, it doesn't make sense to create a monthly report, as most of the 12,000 months are going to be without any admissions. Instead - let's calculate the readmissions rate over the centuries and then pretend that each century is a month for reporting purposes.

Numerator - number of readmissions within 30 days, over time:

SELECT FLOOR(YEAR(X.hospital_admit_dt)/100) AS CenturyAdmit,
COUNT(X.hadm_id) as NumPtsReadmit
FROM icustay_detail X, icustay_detail Y
WHERE X.subject_id = Y.subject_id
AND X.hadm_id <> Y.hadm_id
AND TIMESTAMPDIFF(DAY, X.hospital_disch_dt, Y.hospital_admit_dt) BETWEEN 0 AND 30
GROUP by CenturyAdmit;

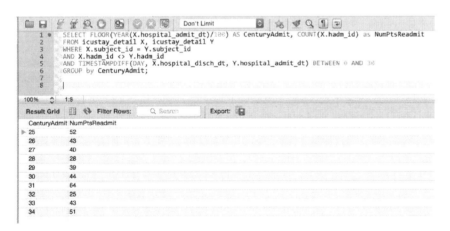

 Question 45

Calculate the number of admissions per century and then using the above query display the readmissions rate over time.

13. Diagnosis

- Patients and admissions by diagnosis
- Mortality by diagnosis
- LOS by diagnosis
- Readmission by diagnosis
- One patient - all diagnosis

Patients and admissions by diagnosis

Before you proceed with this chapter, please review the chapter on ERD, as the diagnosis, ICD, DRG and the relationships between these concepts has been thoroughly discussed in that chapter.

Diagnosis Related Grouping (DRG) summarizes one admission with one DRG code, even if multiple diagnoses / procedures have been assigned to the patient during the same episode of care.

The ERD related to diagnosis and DRG:

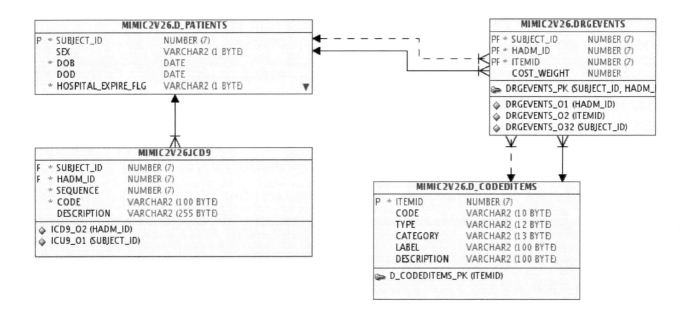

As the **ICD9** table contains the diagnosis, unique patient identifier (**subject_id**) and their unique admissions (**hadm_id**) - we can summarize around the ICD diagnosis code:

```
SELECT code, description,
COUNT(DISTINCT subject_id) AS NumPts,
COUNT(DISTINCT hadm_id) AS NumAdmis
FROM icd9
GROUP BY code
ORDER BY NumAdmis DESC;
```

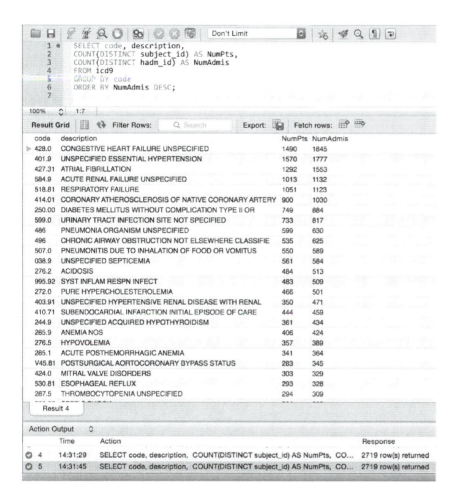

For the same type of report on DRG, we can reuse the above query, but we need to add the **d_codeditems, drgevents** tables to translate the DRG codes, using the **itemid** as the connecting link between these two tables:

SELECT code, description,
COUNT(DISTINCT subject_id) AS NumPts,
COUNT(DISTINCT hadm_id) AS NumAdmis
FROM drgevents, d_codeditems
WHERE drgevents.itemid = d_codeditems.itemid
GROUP BY code
ORDER BY NumAdmis DESC;

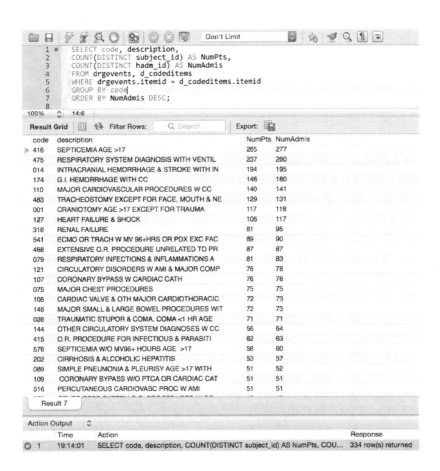

Mortality by diagnosis

We know by now that the patients' diagnoses reside in the **ICD9** table and the information on mortality can be found in the **icustay_detail** table.

Suppose we'd like to know the mortality of each and every diagnosis in MIMIC2.
The denominator would be the number of unique patients having a specific diagnosis, while the numerator would be the number of unique patients that have died having this diagnosis.

Denominator – patients with a diagnosis:

SELECT code, description, COUNT(DISTINCT icustay_detail.subject_id) AS NumPts
FROM icustay_detail, icd9
WHERE icustay_detail.subject_id = icd9.subject_id
AND hospital_expire_flg IS NOT NULL
GROUP BY code;

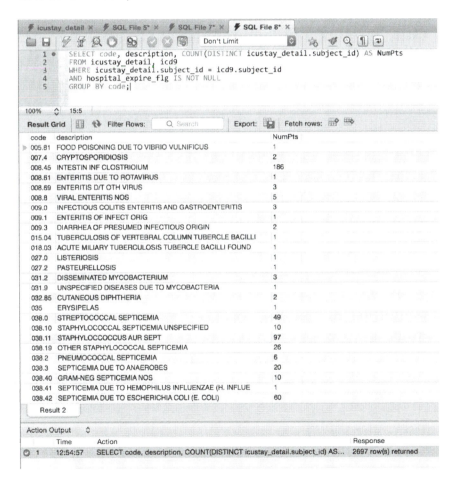

Numerator – patients that have died with a diagnosis:

SELECT code, description, COUNT(DISTINCT icustay_detail.subject_id) AS Died
FROM icustay_detail, icd9
WHERE icustay_detail.subject_id = icd9.subject_id

```
AND hospital_expire_flg ='Y'
GROUP BY code;
```

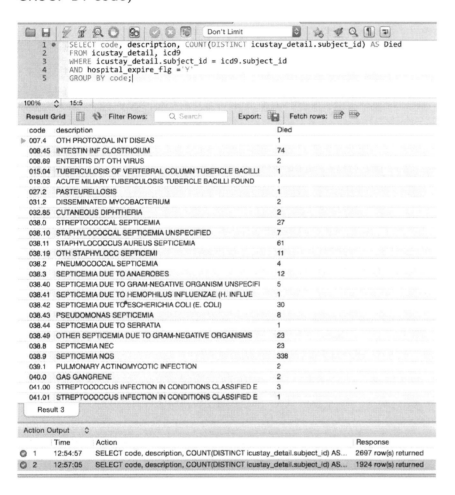

The problem at this stage is to consolidate the above results into one table.
A spreadsheet won't help, as the first list has 2,697 rows while the second has 1,924 rows.
Trying to fit the two resulting spreadsheets manually into a single one, will quickly convince you that we need to solve this problem in SQL.

We can think of the two results above as temporary tables and we can name the results accordingly using the **AS** alias mechanism – the first results set as table **TotPts** and the second results set as **DeadPts**. Once these results / tables are named, we can query them, using the diagnosis **code** as the common link between the two:

```sql
SELECT TotPts.code, TotPts.description,
NumPts, Died,
ROUND(((Died / NumPts) * 100),1) AS MortalityByDiagnosis

FROM (
SELECT code, description, COUNT(DISTINCT icustay_detail.subject_id) AS NumPts
FROM icustay_detail, icd9
WHERE icustay_detail.subject_id = icd9.subject_id
AND hospital_expire_flg IS NOT NULL
GROUP BY code) AS TotPts,

(SELECT code, description, COUNT(DISTINCT icustay_detail.subject_id) AS Died
FROM icustay_detail, icd9
WHERE icustay_detail.subject_id = icd9.subject_id
AND hospital_expire_flg ='Y'
GROUP BY code) AS DeadPts

WHERE TotPts.code = DeadPts.code
ORDER BY MortalityByDiagnosis DESC;
```

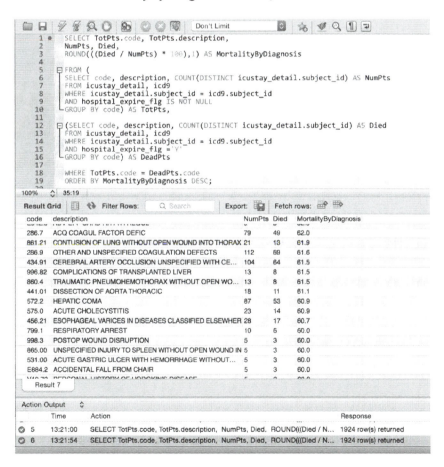

Note the above list doesn't include any diagnosis with zero mortality.

Question 46

Modify the above query to include also the diagnosis codes that have zero mortality associated.
Hint: you'd like to see all the rows from one table, even if a row doesn't correlate to any other row in the second table. Then, transform the null values into 0.

Mortality by DRG:

Similar to the mortality by diagnosis above, it would be interesting to compare mortality across all DRG codes in MIMIC2.

Using the ERD part related to DRG, let's first identify the unique admissions' DRG and their **hospital_expire_flg**. Note that the **icustay_detail** table is not part of this ERD. We connect between the **drgevents** and **d_codeditems** tables using the **itemid**. Similarly, we connect between **icustay_detail** and **drgevents** using the **hadm_id**:

SELECT icustay_detail.hadm_id, code, description, hospital_expire_flg
FROM drgevents, d_codeditems, icustay_detail
WHERE drgevents.itemid = d_codeditems.itemid
AND icustay_detail.hadm_id = drgevents.hadm_id;

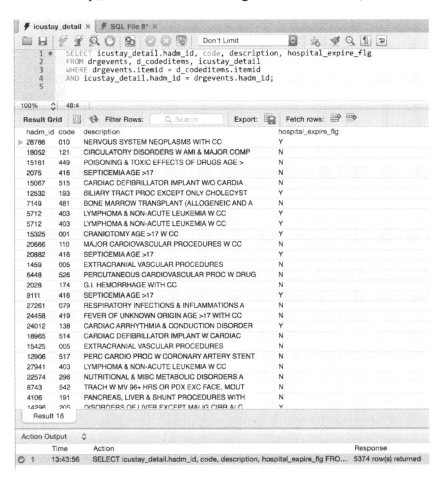

Now we can repeat the previous query for calculating mortality by diagnosis, in order to calculate mortality by DRG.

Question 47

Create two tables – one with all the DRG codes and the number of patients assigned each code (denominator).
The other table with all the DRG codes and the number of patients that have died (numerator).
Calculate mortality rate for each DRG code and arrange the results from the highest to lowest mortality.
Include DRG codes with zero mortality.

LOS by diagnosis

If we'd like to retrieve all the diagnoses in MIMIC2 and their respective average Length of Stay (LOS), the task is simple as **hospital_los** resides in the **icustay_detail** table, while the diagnosis exist in the **ICD9** table. What connects between the two is **hadm_id** – the unique identifier of an admission:

```
SELECT code, description, AVG(hospital_los/60/24) AS AvgLOS,
COUNT(icustay_detail.hadm_id) AS NumAdmit
FROM icustay_detail, icd9
WHERE icustay_detail.hadm_id = icd9.hadm_id
GROUP BY code
ORDER BY AvgLos DESC;
```

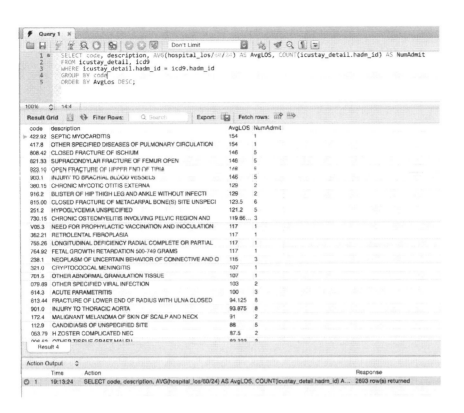

If however, we sort the above on the number of admissions, a different picture emerges:

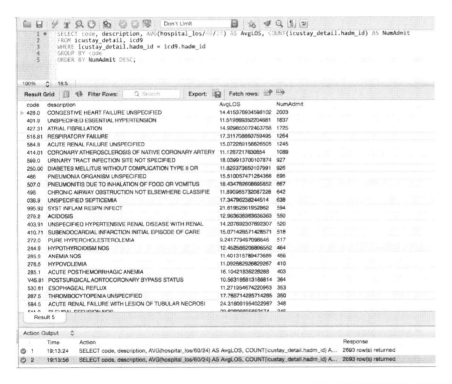

Question 48

Calculate the average LOS for each DRG code in MIMIC2.
Retrieve also the number of admissions and arrange it from the most frequent DRG code to the least used.

Readmissions by diagnosis

As we know already how to identify patients that have been readmitted within 30 days of a previous discharge, it would be interesting to know these patients' diagnoses – both at the time of discharge and at the time of readmission:

- What is the percentage of patients readmitted within 30 days for each discharge diagnosis ?
- Which diagnosis at discharge has the highest rate of readmission ?
- How many days on average it takes from discharge to readmission for each discharge diagnosis ?
- When patients are readmitted, what are their main diagnosis (at readmission) ?

Having information based on data, can help a quality-driven healthcare organization focus on those patients that are most likely to be readmitted, and pro-actively implement steps to reduce their readmission rate.

The query design steps:

- Identify all the patients admitted by diagnosis – the denominator
- Identify the patients that have been readmitted within 30 days and their diagnoses at discharge – the numerator
- Calculate the percentage of readmission per diagnosis and the average time to readmit
- For patients readmitted within 30 days – find the most common diagnosis at readmission

Patients admitted by diagnosis – the denominator

```
SELECT code, description,
COUNT(admissions.hadm_id) AS NumAdmit
FROM admissions, icd9
WHERE admissions.hadm_id = icd9.hadm_id
GROUP BY code
ORDER by NumAdmit DESC;
```

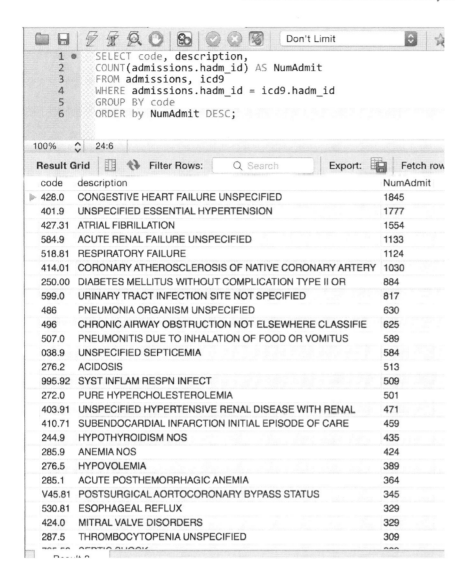

Patients readmitted within 30 days by diagnosis – the numerator

The technique to identify readmissions, relies on a self-join which basically compares a table to itself . Self-join was introduced and thoroughly discussed in previous chapters.

In the following query, we are going to compare the **admissions** table to itself – once as table **X** (discharge) and once as table **Y** (readmissions), while the **subject_id** is the link between the two instances of this table.

SELECT code, description,
AVG(TIMESTAMPDIFF(DAY, X.disch_dt, Y.admit_dt)) AS AvgDays2Readmit,
COUNT(X.hadm_id) AS NumReAdmit
FROM admissions X, admissions Y, icd9
WHERE X.subject_id = Y.subject_id
AND X.hadm_id <> Y.hadm_id
AND TIMESTAMPDIFF(DAY, X.disch_dt, Y.admit_dt) BETWEEN 0 AND 30
AND X.hadm_id = icd9.hadm_id
GROUP BY code
ORDER by NumReAdmit DESC, AvgDays2Readmit ASC;

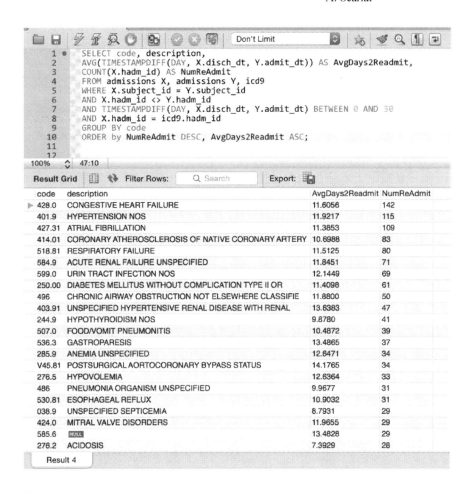

Calculate the readmission rates and time to readmission for each diagnosis

Next step is to consolidate the denominator and numerator results from the previous queries.
In order to do that, we're going to consider each result as a temporary table – **AdmitTb**, **ReadmitTb** and link the two tables with the diagnosis **code**:

SELECT AdmitTb.code, AdmitTb.description, AvgDays2Readmit, NumReAdmit, NumAdmit,
ROUND(100 * NumReAdmit/NumAdmit,1) AS PercentReadmit
FROM (
SELECT code, description,
COUNT(admissions.hadm_id) AS NumAdmit
FROM admissions, icd9
WHERE admissions.hadm_id = icd9.hadm_id
GROUP BY code
) AS AdmitTb,
(
SELECT code, description,
ROUND(AVG(TIMESTAMPDIFF(DAY, X.disch_dt, Y.admit_dt)),1) AS AvgDays2Readmit,
COUNT(X.hadm_id) AS NumReAdmit
FROM admissions X, admissions Y, icd9
WHERE X.subject_id = Y.subject_id
AND X.hadm_id <> Y.hadm_id
AND TIMESTAMPDIFF(DAY, X.disch_dt, Y.admit_dt) BETWEEN 0 AND 30

AND X.hadm_id = icd9.hadm_id
GROUP BY code
) AS ReadmitTb

WHERE AdmitTb.code = ReadmitTb.code
ORDER BY NumReAdmit DESC;

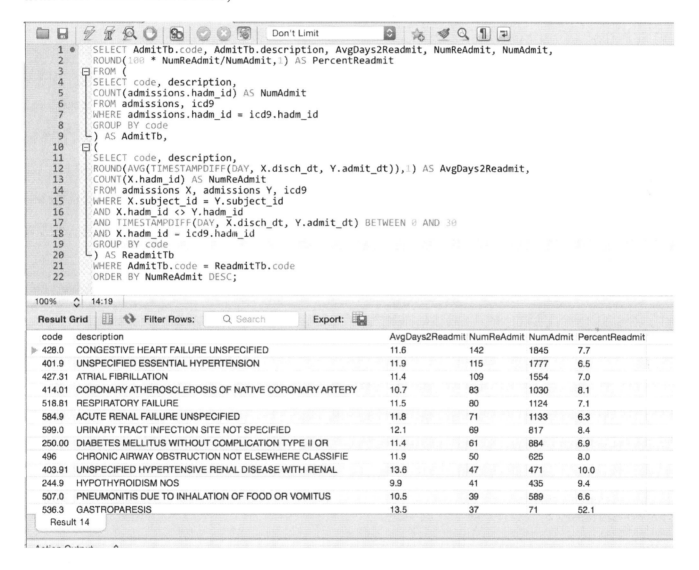

Question 49

Similar to the above, summarize all the diagnoses at **readmission** – number of readmissions (descending order) and average time to readmission (ascending order).

Readmission rate by DRG

The query design for calculating readmission rates by DRG is similar to the previous query, except that instead of the one **ICD9** table we've used for the diagnosis, we need to use two tables: **drgevents** table and **d_codeditems** table for the DRG codes and descriptions.

The technique to identify those readmitted within 30 days of discharge and the consolidation of the denominator and numerator, remains the same as in the previous query.

Denominator - all DRG:

SELECT code, description,
COUNT(admissions.hadm_id) AS NumAdmit
FROM admissions, drgevents, d_codeditems
WHERE admissions.hadm_id = drgevents.hadm_id
AND drgevents.itemid = d_codeditems.itemid
GROUP BY code
ORDER by NumAdmit DESC;

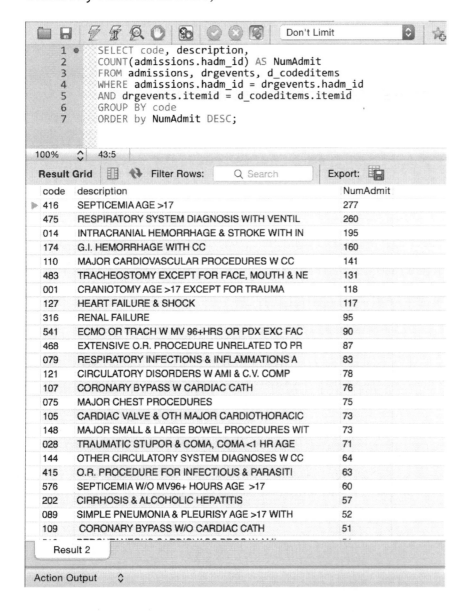

Numerator – DRG at discharge for patients readmitted within 30 days:

```
SELECT code, description,
ROUND(AVG(TIMESTAMPDIFF(DAY, X.disch_dt, Y.admit_dt)),1) AS AvgDays2Readmit,
COUNT(X.hadm_id) AS NumReAdmit
FROM admissions X, admissions Y, drgevents, d_codeditems
WHERE X.subject_id = Y.subject_id
AND X.hadm_id <> Y.hadm_id
AND X.hadm_id = drgevents.hadm_id
AND drgevents.itemid = d_codeditems.itemid
AND TIMESTAMPDIFF(DAY, X.disch_dt, Y.admit_dt) BETWEEN 0 AND 30
GROUP BY code
ORDER by NumReAdmit DESC, AvgDays2Readmit ASC;
```

code	description	AvgDays2Readmit	NumReAdmit
475	RESPIRATORY SYSTEM DIAGNOSIS WITH VENTIL	13.4	30
483	TRACHEOSTOMY EXCEPT FOR FACE, MOUTH & NE	10.9	21
316	RENAL FAILURE	11.9	20
541	ECMO OR TRACH W MV 96+HRS OR PDX EXC FAC	6.1	17
416	SEPTICEMIA AGE >17	8.8	13
001	CRANIOTOMY AGE >17 EXCEPT FOR TRAUMA	8.5	10
110	MAJOR CARDIOVASCULAR PROCEDURES W CC	13.6	9
174	G.I. HEMORRHAGE WITH CC	9.9	8
148	MAJOR SMALL & LARGE BOWEL PROCEDURES WIT	13.6	8
415	O.R. PROCEDURE FOR INFECTIOUS & PARASITI	12.3	7
079	RESPIRATORY INFECTIONS & INFLAMMATIONS A	12.6	7
294	DIABETES AGE >35	12.7	7
075	MAJOR CHEST PROCEDURES	6.8	6
107	CORONARY BYPASS W CARDIAC CATH	8.3	6
127	HEART FAILURE & SHOCK	12.2	6
121	CIRCULATORY DISORDERS W AMI & MAJOR COMP	12.5	6
202	CIRRHOSIS & ALCOHOLIC HEPATITIS	12.7	6
087	PULMONARY EDEMA & RESPIRATORY FAILURE	9.8	5
207	DISORDERS OF THE BILIARY TRACT WITH CC	11.2	5
109	CORONARY BYPASS W/O CARDIAC CATH	12.0	5
134	HYPERTENSION	12.0	5

Consolidate the previous results and calculate readmission rate and time to readmission by DRG:

SELECT AdmitTb.code, AdmitTb.description, AvgDays2Readmit, NumReAdmit, NumAdmit,
ROUND(100*NumReAdmit/NumAdmit,1) AS PercentReadmit
FROM

(SELECT code, description,
ROUND(AVG(TIMESTAMPDIFF(DAY, X.disch_dt, Y.admit_dt)),1) AS AvgDays2Readmit,
COUNT(X.hadm_id) AS NumReAdmit
FROM admissions X, admissions Y, drgevents, d_codeditems
WHERE X.subject_id = Y.subject_id
AND X.hadm_id <> Y.hadm_id
AND X.hadm_id = drgevents.hadm_id
AND drgevents.itemid = d_codeditems.itemid
AND TIMESTAMPDIFF(DAY, X.disch_dt, Y.admit_dt) BETWEEN 0 AND 30
GROUP BY code) AS ReAdmitTb,

(SELECT code, description,
COUNT(admissions.hadm_id) AS NumAdmit
FROM admissions, drgevents, d_codeditems
WHERE admissions.hadm_id = drgevents.hadm_id
AND drgevents.itemid = d_codeditems.itemid
GROUP BY code) AS AdmitTb

WHERE AdmitTb.code = ReAdmitTb.code
ORDER BY NumReAdmit DESC;

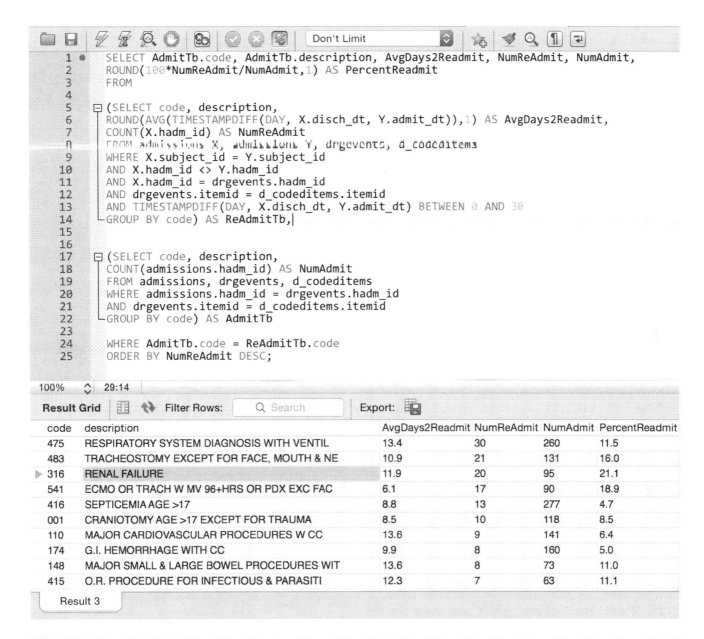

Question 50

Similar to the above, summarize all the DRG codes at **readmission** within 30 days – number of readmissions (descending order) and average time to readmission (ascending order).

One patient - all diagnoses

Using the previous ERD, retrieving all the ICD9 codes for a single patient should be no problem by now. In previous chapters we've learned how to retrieve all the admissions for a single patient.

As the timing of a diagnosis on a patient's clinical time line is important, we'd like to see one patient's diagnoses (ICD9 codes) arranged from the newest on top to the oldest at the bottom.
The goal is to retrieve for one patient, all the admission dates and the ICD9 codes that have been attributed at each admission.

It's good to know whether a date and time column for a parameter is the actual time that parameter happened - or - it represents the time of the documentation in the system.

The initial obstacle is that none of the tables in the above ERD have any date or time column on the date of the ICD9 code assignment. When was the patient diagnosed with those ICD9 codes ?

The plan is to use the **admissions** table with its date of admission and link it to the **IC9** codes table for a specific patient (**subject_id** = 4410) using the **subject_id** as the link between the tables:

```
SELECT DISTINCT admit_dt, code, description
FROM ICD9, admissions
WHERE admissions.subject_id =icd9.subject_id
AND admissions.subject_id = 4410
ORDER BY admit_dt DESC;
```

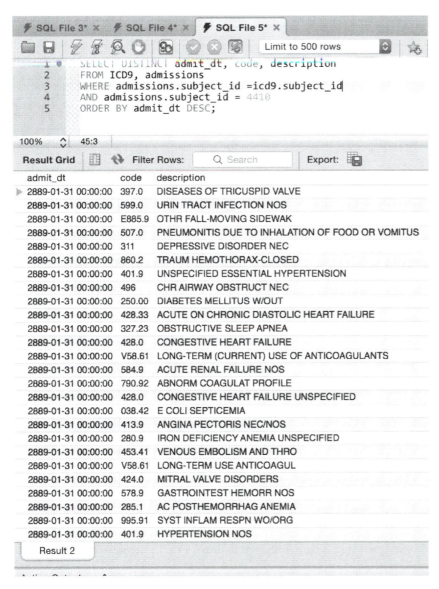

 Question 51

Similar to the above, retrieve this patient's DRG codes and the admissions dates for the assigned DRG codes. Arrange results from most recent on top to oldest at the bottom.

14. Sepsis profile

- Profile structure
- Sepsis related diagnosis
- Volumes: with and without sepsis
- Gender and age: with and without sepsis
- Mortality: with and without sepsis
- LOS: with and without sepsis
- Readmissions: with and without sepsis

Profile structure

A profile of a condition, a specific diagnosis like sepsis may include:

1. **Volumes** of patients / admissions: Sepsis related vs total, Current (last month), Over time
2. **Age** Average age and the age distribution of patients with / without sepsis
3. **Gender** distribution of patients with / without sepsis
4. **Mortality**
    a. Average mortality of patients with / without sepsis
    b. Mortality over time of patients with / without sepsis
5. **LOS**
    a. Average LOS of patients with / without sepsis
    b. LOS over time of patients with / without sepsis
6. **Readmissions**
    a. Average readmission rate of patients with / without sepsis
    b. Readmission rate over time of patients with / without sepsis

In the next chapters we'll learn how to extract information on Procedures, Drugs, Labs, Imaging, etc. which could be added to the Sepsis profile.

A sepsis profile, based on MIMIC2, may be visualized as:

Sepsis Profile. October 2018

printed Nov 15, 2018 by Alex Scarlat MD

Volumes	Total	Oct 2018
Patients w Sepsis	907 (23%)	82 (20.4%)
Admissions w Sepsis	976 (19.3%)	85 (16.4%)

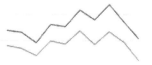

Mortality	Total	Oct 2018
With Sepsis	54.8%	53.7%
Without Sepsis	25.4%	24.4%

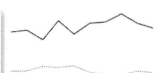

LOS	Total	Oct 2018
With Sepsis	19.5 days	21.8 days
Without Sepsis	13.6 days	13.6 days

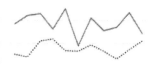

Readmissions	Total	Oct 2018
With Sepsis	5.2%	4.9%
Without Sepsis	7.2%	9.5%

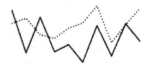

	Female : Male	Average Age
With Sepsis	1 : 1.13	69.8
Without Sepsis	1 : 1.15	70.5

ICD9 Codes - 92% of admissions

- 038.9 Unspecified septicemia
- 785.52 Septic shock
- 38.11 Staph aur septicemia
- 38.42 E Coli septicemia
- 38.49 Other Gram Neg septicemia
- 38   Streptococcal septicemia

Procedures, Lab, Drugs, etc
Following chapters

Sepsis related diagnosis

We need first to identify the ICD9 codes related to sepsis:

```
SELECT DISTINCT code, description
FROM icd9
WHERE description LIKE '%sep%';
```

This query will return 38 ICD9 codes that have the three characters **sep** in their description.
As it contains unrelated diagnoses, such as **aseptic necrosis of head and neck of femur**, we need to refine the query to return only sepsis or septicemia related diagnoses:

```
SELECT DISTINCT code, description
FROM mimic2.icd9
WHERE description LIKE '%sep%'
AND description NOT LIKE '%septal%'
AND description NOT LIKE '%aseptic%'
AND description NOT LIKE '%sept def%'
AND description NOT LIKE '%separation%';
```

It's considered good practice to identify the relevant instances before counting or calculating any aggregate functions.

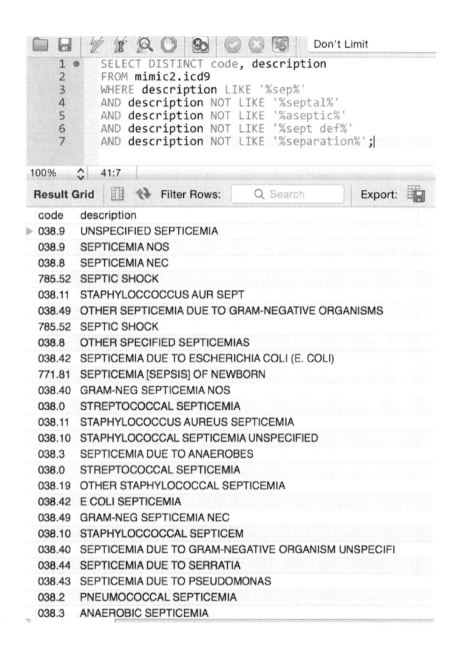

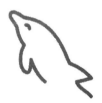

Volumes: with / without sepsis

Volumes	Total	Oct 2018
Patients w Sepsis	907 (23%)	**82** (20.4%)
Admissions w Sepsis	976 (19.3%)	**85** (16.4%)

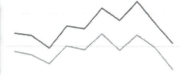

Having identified the ICD9 diagnosis codes related to sepsis, we can move to the next step, calculating the volumes of patients and admissions related to sepsis.

Basically, we need to count the number of patients and the number of admissions, where one of the 30 ICD9 diagnosis codes above have been assigned:

```
SELECT code, description,
COUNT(DISTINCT subject_id) AS NumPts,
COUNT(DISTINCT hadm_id) AS NumAdmit
FROM mimic2.icd9
WHERE description LIKE '%sep%'
AND description NOT LIKE '%septal%'
AND description NOT LIKE '%aseptic%'
AND description NOT LIKE '%sept def%'
AND description NOT LIKE '%separation%'
GROUP BY code;
```

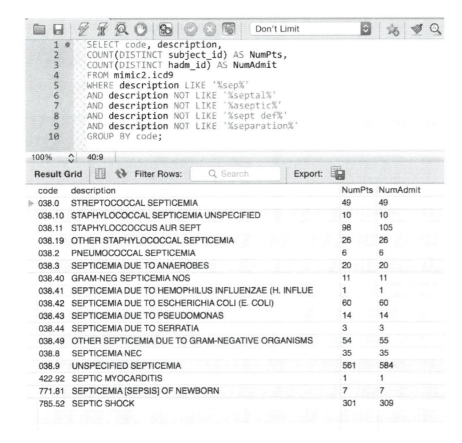

If we are interested only in the total numbers for sepsis related admissions and patients, without the subgroups – then we need only remove the grouping from the query:

SELECT COUNT(DISTINCT subject_id) AS NumPts,
COUNT(DISTINCT hadm_id) AS NumAdmit
FROM mimic2.icd9
WHERE description LIKE '%sep%'
AND description NOT LIKE '%septal%'
AND description NOT LIKE '%aseptic%'
AND description NOT LIKE '%sept def%'
AND description NOT LIKE '%separation%';

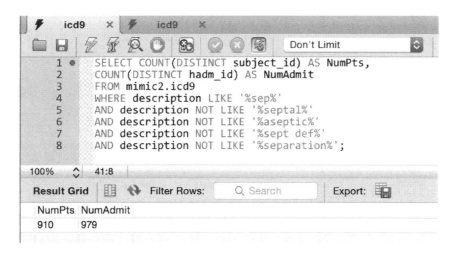

Always try to calculate numerator and denominator from the same table sources.
If you calculate the numerator and denominator from different sources, the results may prove inconsistent.

How are the numbers related to sepsis when compared to the whole population of MIMIC2 ?
In order to have the totals – the whole MIMIC2 patients and admissions - we need only to remove the condition in the previous query:

SELECT COUNT(DISTINCT subject_id) AS NumPts,
COUNT(DISTINCT hadm_id) AS NumAdmit
FROM mimic2.icd9;

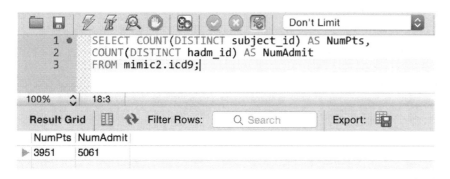

Thus, the percentage of sepsis related:
- **Patients**: 910 / 3951 = **23.0**%
- **Admissions**: 979 / 5061 = **19.3**%

Is there a recent increase or decrease in the number of patients or admissions related to sepsis ?
A chart, plot, a trend of the percentage of patients with sepsis may come in handy when answering this kind of questions. For such a time series calculation, we'll need the number of admissions with a sepsis diagnosis vs. the total number of admissions – for each century (month).

Denominator – total number of patients / admissions - by century:

SELECT FLOOR(YEAR(admit_dt)/100) AS CenturyAdmit,
COUNT(DISTINCT admissions.subject_id) AS NumPts,
COUNT(DISTINCT admissions.hadm_id) AS NumAdmit
FROM admissions, icd9
WHERE admissions.hadm_id = icd9.hadm_id
GROUP BY CenturyAdmit;

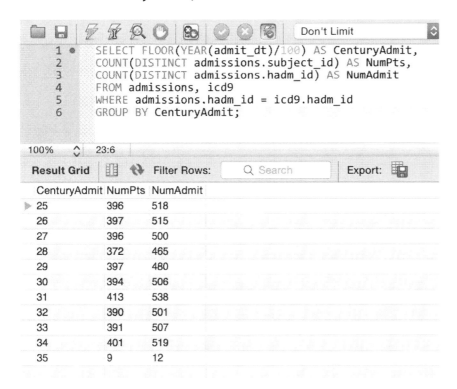

CenturyAdmit	NumPts	NumAdmit
25	396	518
26	397	515
27	396	500
28	372	465
29	397	480
30	394	506
31	413	538
32	390	501
33	391	507
34	401	519
35	9	12

Numerator – sepsis related patients / admissions by century:

SELECT FLOOR(YEAR(admit_dt)/100) AS CenturyAdmit,
COUNT(DISTINCT admissions.subject_id) AS NumPts,
COUNT(DISTINCT admissions.hadm_id) AS NumAdmit
FROM admissions, icd9
WHERE admissions.hadm_id = icd9.hadm_id
AND description LIKE '%sep%'
AND description NOT LIKE '%septal%'
AND description NOT LIKE '%aseptic%'

AND description NOT LIKE '%sept def%'
AND description NOT LIKE '%separation%'
GROUP BY CenturyAdmit;

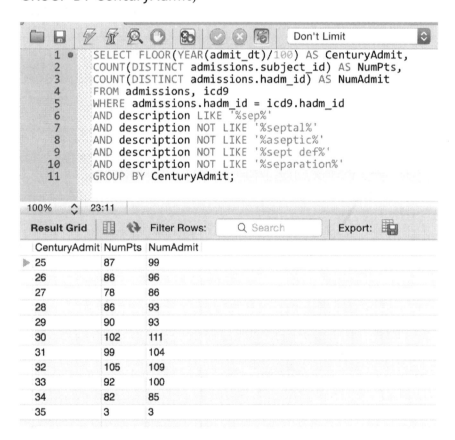

Summarizing it all in a spreadsheet, while substituting the 25th to 35th centuries with the months of 2018 for beautification purposes:

MonthYearAdmit	NumPts	NumAdmit	SepsisPts	SepsisAdmit	PercentPts	PercentAdmit
Jan-18	396	518	87	99	22.0%	19.1%
Feb-18	397	515	86	96	21.7%	18.6%
Mar-18	396	500	78	86	19.7%	17.2%
Apr-18	372	465	86	93	23.1%	20.0%
May-18	397	480	90	93	22.7%	19.4%
Jun-18	394	506	102	111	25.9%	21.9%
Jul-18	413	538	99	104	24.0%	19.3%
Aug-18	390	501	105	109	26.9%	21.8%
Sep-18	391	507	92	100	23.5%	19.7%
Oct-18	401	519	82	85	20.4%	16.4%
Nov-18	9	12	3	3	33.3%	25.0%
Total	**3956**	**5061**	**910**	**979**	**23.0%**	**19.3%**

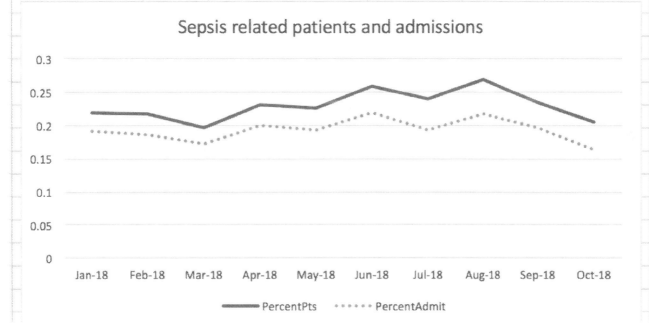

Question 52

The patients in MIMIC2 are dispersed over 1,000 years – thus, we have grouped them by centuries for a meaningful trend. As most probably you won't have to group your own data into centuries in order to see a trend for a condition – modify the above query to return data on the total number of patients and admissions, over time, by year and month instead of century. No need to display the months without data as 0.

In the following queries, we are going to count admissions and not patients.

As one patient may have many admissions, some may be related to and some may be unrelated to sepsis. We cannot logically label such a patient as sepsis, as the patient had sepsis unrelated admissions.
For the same reason, we can't label such a patient as sepsis unrelated, as the patient had admissions that were actually sepsis related.

When we count or calculate averages – we'd like to have the information about all the admissions unrelated to sepsis to be grouped in one haystack. We'd like all the information about sepsis related admissions in the other haystack.
If a patient appears in both groups – that's ok. The patient's admissions related to sepsis will be accounted for in one group, while the same patient's other admissions - unrelated to sepsis - will be counted for in a separate group.

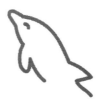

Gender and age: with / without sepsis

	Female : Male	Average Age
With Sepsis	1 : 1.13	69.8
Without Sepsis	1 : 1.15	70.5

Let's compare the average age of the patients with sepsis vs. the patients without sepsis.

First let's calculate the average age at admission of the patients with a diagnosis of sepsis:

```
SELECT ROUND(AVG(icustay_admit_age),1) AS AvgAge
FROM icustay_detail, icd9
WHERE icustay_detail.hadm_id = icd9.hadm_id
AND description LIKE '%sep%'
AND description NOT LIKE '%septal%'
AND description NOT LIKE '%aseptic%'
AND description NOT LIKE '%sept def%'
AND description NOT LIKE '%separation%';
```

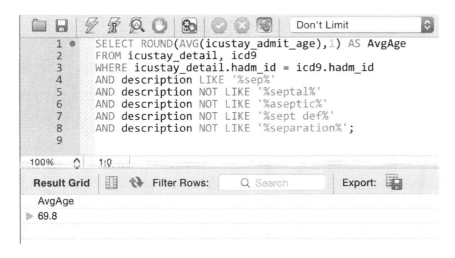

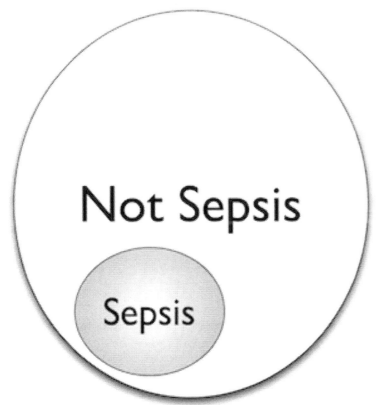

From the Venn diagram: **Not Sepsis = Total - Sepsis**

The Venn diagram also explains why you should always check your results when two mutually exclusive groups exist - either by SQL or by summarizing it in a spreadsheet: **Total = Sepsis + Not Sepsis**

In order to calculate the average age of the patients without sepsis, we need to reuse the above query and eliminate the admissions that had a sepsis related diagnosis.
Who are the patients with a diagnosis of sepsis ? What are their admission unique identifiers ?

SELECT DISTINCT icustay_detail.hadm_id
FROM icustay_detail, icd9
WHERE icustay_detail.hadm_id = icd9.hadm_id

AND description LIKE '%sep%'
AND description NOT LIKE '%septal%'
AND description NOT LIKE '%aseptic%'
AND description NOT LIKE '%sept def%'
AND description NOT LIKE '%separation%';

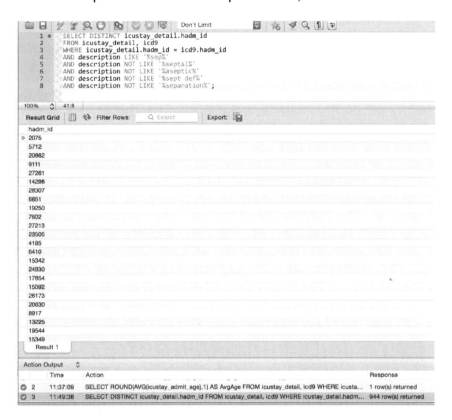

Knowing the admissions unique identifiers related to sepsis, we can now use the **NOT IN** SQL operator, on a subquery (the sepsis related admissions) - in order to implement the **Not Sepsis = Total - Sepsis** from the Venn diagram above:

SELECT ROUND(AVG(icustay_admit_age),1) AS AvgAge
FROM icustay_detail
WHERE icustay_detail.hadm_id NOT IN
(SELECT DISTINCT icustay_detail.hadm_id
FROM icustay_detail, icd9
WHERE icustay_detail.hadm_id = icd9.hadm_id
AND description LIKE '%sep%'
AND description NOT LIKE '%septal%'
AND description NOT LIKE '%aseptic%'
AND description NOT LIKE '%sept def%'
AND description NOT LIKE '%separation%');

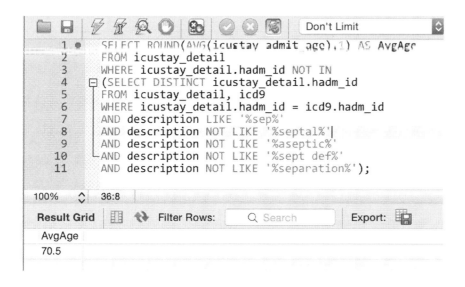

Average age:
- With sepsis: **69.8** years
- Without sepsis: **70.5** years

We can also compare the age distributions between these two groups, while reusing the group by decade of age technique, introduced in previous chapters.

Age distribution of patients with sepsis related diagnosis:

```
SELECT FLOOR(icustay_admit_age/10)+1 AS Decade,
COUNT(DISTINCT icustay_detail.hadm_id)
FROM icustay_detail, icd9
WHERE icustay_detail.hadm_id = icd9.hadm_id
AND description LIKE '%sep%'
AND description NOT LIKE '%septal%'
AND description NOT LIKE '%aseptic%'
AND description NOT LIKE '%sept def%'
AND description NOT LIKE '%separation%'
GROUP BY Decade;
```

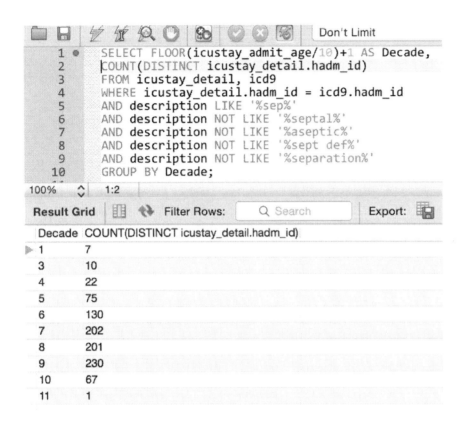

For the age distribution of the **Not Sepsis** patients, we'll use the same **NOT IN** technique as described above on the Venn diagram:

SELECT FLOOR(icustay_admit_age/10)+1 AS Decade,
COUNT(DISTINCT icustay_detail.hadm_id)
FROM icustay_detail
WHERE icustay_detail.hadm_id NOT IN
(SELECT DISTINCT icustay_detail.hadm_id
FROM icustay_detail, icd9
WHERE icustay_detail.hadm_id = icd9.hadm_id
AND description LIKE '%sep%'
AND description NOT LIKE '%septal%'
AND description NOT LIKE '%aseptic%'
AND description NOT LIKE '%sept def%'
AND description NOT LIKE '%separation%')
GROUP BY Decade;

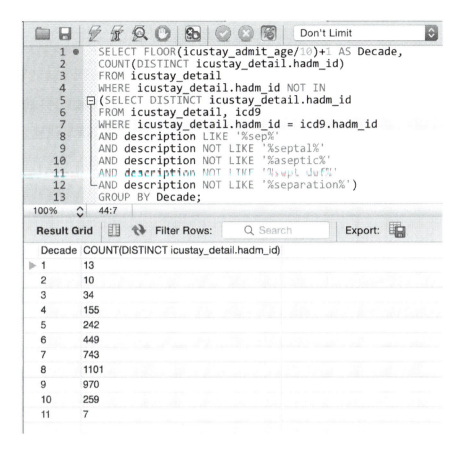

And summarizing the age distributions of the two populations in a spreadsheet:

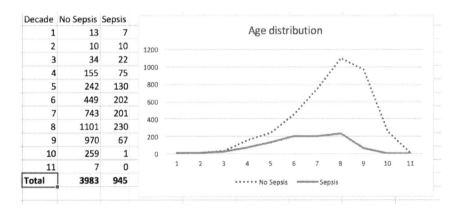

Question 53

Calculate and compare the gender distributions of the admissions with sepsis related diagnosis vs. the admissions without sepsis diagnosis.

Mortality: with / without sepsis

Mortality	Total	Oct 2018
With Sepsis	54.8%	53.7%
Without Sepsis	25.4%	24.4%

For the sepsis related admissions, the mortality is derived by grouping the admissions related to sepsis on - **hospital_expire_flg** (the column with the information on the patients' deaths):

```
SELECT hospital_expire_flg,
COUNT(DISTINCT icustay_detail.hadm_id) AS NumAdmit
FROM icustay_detail, icd9
WHERE icustay_detail.hadm_id = icd9.hadm_id
AND description LIKE '%sep%'
AND description NOT LIKE '%septal%'
AND description NOT LIKE '%aseptic%'
AND description NOT LIKE '%sept def%'
AND description NOT LIKE '%separation%'
GROUP BY hospital_expire_flg;
```

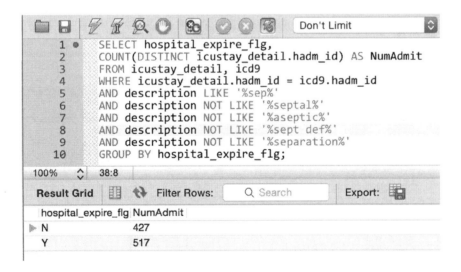

Reusing the above query with the **NOT IN** operator, we can retrieve the mortality for the sepsis unrelated admissions:

```
SELECT hospital_expire_flg,
COUNT(DISTINCT icustay_detail.hadm_id) AS NumAdmit
FROM icustay_detail
WHERE icustay_detail.hadm_id NOT IN
(SELECT DISTINCT icustay_detail.hadm_id
FROM icustay_detail, icd9
```

```
WHERE icustay_detail.hadm_id = icd9.hadm_id
AND description LIKE '%sep%'
AND description NOT LIKE '%septal%'
AND description NOT LIKE '%aseptic%'
AND description NOT LIKE '%sept def%'
AND description NOT LIKE '%separation%')
GROUP BY hospital_expire_flg;
```

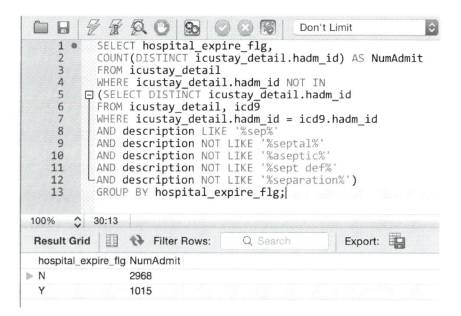

Mortality:
- With sepsis: 517 / (517 +427) = **54.8%**
- Without sepsis: 1,015 / (1,015 +2,968) = **25.4%**

For the mortality over time charts, we are going to reuse the grouping by the century technique twice: once for the sepsis related admissions and once for the sepsis unrelated admissions.

Sepsis related admissions mortality over time:

```
SELECT hospital_expire_flg,
FLOOR(YEAR(hospital_admit_dt)/100) AS CenturyAdmit,
COUNT(DISTINCT icustay_detail.hadm_id) AS NumAdmit
FROM icustay_detail, icd9
WHERE icustay_detail.hadm_id = icd9.hadm_id
AND description LIKE '%sep%'
AND description NOT LIKE '%septal%'
AND description NOT LIKE '%aseptic%'
AND description NOT LIKE '%sept def%'
AND description NOT LIKE '%separation%'
GROUP BY hospital_expire_flg, CenturyAdmit;
```

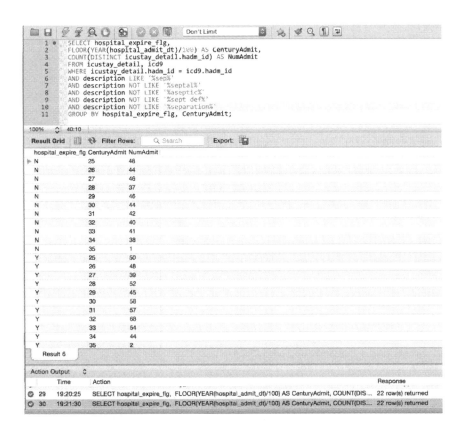

Sepsis unrelated admissions mortality over time:

SELECT hospital_expire_flg,
FLOOR(YEAR(hospital_admit_dt)/100) AS CenturyAdmit,
COUNT(DISTINCT icustay_detail.hadm_id) AS NumAdmit
FROM icustay_detail, icd9
WHERE icustay_detail.hadm_id = icd9.hadm_id
AND icustay_detail.hadm_id NOT IN
(SELECT DISTINCT icustay_detail.hadm_id
FROM icustay_detail, icd9
WHERE icustay_detail.hadm_id = icd9.hadm_id
AND description LIKE '%sep%'
AND description NOT LIKE '%septal%'
AND description NOT LIKE '%aseptic%'
AND description NOT LIKE '%sept def%'
AND description NOT LIKE '%separation%')
GROUP BY hospital_expire_flg, CenturyAdmit;

Medical Information Extraction and Analysis

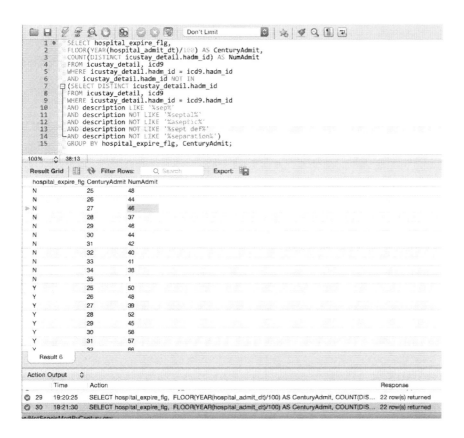

Summarizing the above two queries and substituting the 25th – 35th centuries with the months of 2018:

Month Admit	Sepsis Live	Sepsis Expired	Sepsis Total	Sepsis Mortality	No Sepsis Live	No Sepsis Expired	No Sepsis Total	No Sepsis Mortality
Jan-18	48	50	98	51.0%	305	103	408	25.2%
Feb-18	44	48	92	52.2%	304	104	408	25.5%
Mar-18	46	39	85	45.9%	287	113	400	28.3%
Apr-18	37	52	89	58.4%	260	100	360	27.8%
May-18	46	45	91	49.5%	266	107	373	28.7%
Jun-18	44	58	102	56.9%	294	96	390	24.6%
Jul-18	42	57	99	57.6%	329	97	426	22.8%
Aug-18	40	68	108	63.0%	295	86	381	22.6%
Sep-18	41	54	95	56.8%	298	102	400	25.5%
Oct-18	38	44	82	53.7%	319	103	422	24.4%
Nov-18	1	2	3	66.7%	8	0	8	0.0%
TOTAL	427	517	944	54.8%	2965	1011	3976	25.4%

Mortality - with & without sepsis

LOS: with / without sepsis

LOS	Total	Oct 2018
With Sepsis	19.5 days	21.8 days
Without Sepsis	13.6 days	13.6 days

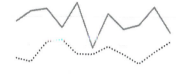

The average length of stay for admissions related to sepsis:

```
SELECT ROUND(AVG(hospital_los/60/24),1) AS AvgLOS
FROM icustay_detail, icd9
WHERE icustay_detail.hadm_id = icd9.hadm_id
AND description LIKE '%sep%'
AND description NOT LIKE '%septal%'
AND description NOT LIKE '%aseptic%'
AND description NOT LIKE '%sept def%'
AND description NOT LIKE '%separation%';
```

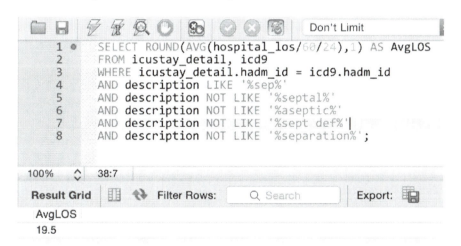

 ## Question 54

Calculate the average LOS for admissions unrelated to sepsis.

 ## Question 55

Calculate the average LOS for admissions related to sepsis, over time, grouped by century. Repeat the same query for the admissions unrelated to sepsis.

Readmissions: with / without sepsis

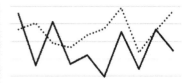

Readmissions	Total	Oct 2018
With Sepsis	5.2%	4.9%
Without Sepsis	7.2%	9.5 %

In order to compare the readmission rates between sepsis related and sepsis unrelated admissions, we need to calculate both:

- Readmission rate for sepsis = Number of readmissions / all the admissions related to sepsis
- Readmission rate for sepsis unrelated = Number of readmissions / all the admissions unrelated to sepsis

Note that the reason for admission is sepsis related, while the reason for readmission is not important in this quality metric calculation. Thus, a readmission due to sepsis will not be counted in this query, if the discharge diagnosis was not sepsis related.

Denominator – admissions related to sepsis:

```
SELECT FLOOR(YEAR(X.hospital_admit_dt)/100) AS CenturyAdmit,
COUNT(DISTINCT X.hadm_id) as NumPtsAdmit
FROM icustay_detail X, icd9
WHERE X.hadm_id = icd9.hadm_id
AND description LIKE '%sep%'
AND description NOT LIKE '%septal%'
AND description NOT LIKE '%aseptic%'
AND description NOT LIKE '%sept def%'
AND description NOT LIKE '%separation%'
GROUP BY CenturyAdmit;
```

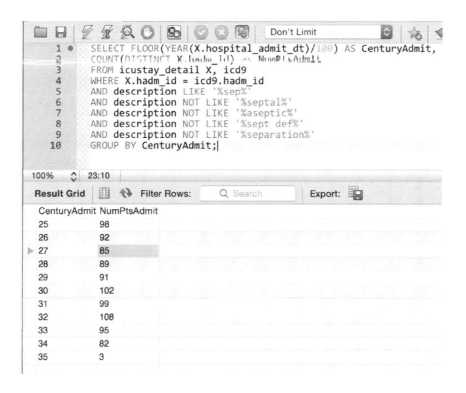

Numerator – readmissions of patients discharged with sepsis related diagnosis:

SELECT FLOOR(YEAR(X.hospital_admit_dt)/100) AS CenturyAdmit,
COUNT(DISTINCT X.hadm_id) as NumPtsReadmit
FROM icustay_detail X, icustay_detail Y, icd9
WHERE X.subject_id = Y.subject_id
AND X.hadm_id <> Y.hadm_id
AND TIMESTAMPDIFF(DAY, X.hospital_disch_dt, Y.hospital_admit_dt) BETWEEN 0 AND 30
AND X.hadm_id = icd9.hadm_id
AND description LIKE '%sep%'
AND description NOT LIKE '%septal%'
AND description NOT LIKE '%aseptic%'
AND description NOT LIKE '%sept def%'
AND description NOT LIKE '%separation%'
GROUP BY CenturyAdmit;

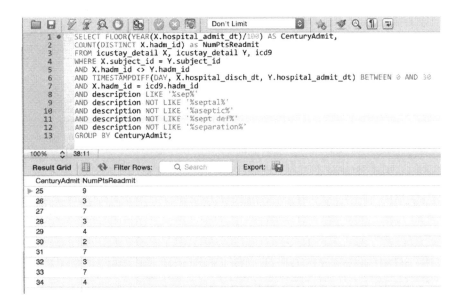

 Question 56

Calculate and compare the average readmission rate related to sepsis vs the average readmission rate unrelated to sepsis.

 Question 57

Calculate the readmission rate, unrelated to sepsis, over time, grouped by century and display them as months.

Exporting to a spreadsheet and summarizing the above with the results from question 57:

CenturyAdmit	SepsisReadmit	SepsisAdmit	NoSepsisReadmit	NoSepsisAdmit	Sepsis Readmit	No Sepsis Readmit
Jan-18	9	98	30	408	9.2%	7.4%
Feb-18	3	92	33	408	3.3%	8.1%
Mar-18	7	85	23	400	8.2%	5.8%
Apr-18	3	89	19	360	3.4%	5.3%
May-18	4	91	25	373	4.4%	6.7%
Jun-18	2	102	29	390	2.0%	7.4%
Jul-18	7	99	42	426	7.1%	9.9%
Aug-18	3	108	18	381	2.8%	4.7%
Sep-18	7	95	29	400	7.4%	7.3%
Oct-18	4	82	40	422	4.9%	9.5%
Nov-18	0	3	0	8	0.0%	0.0%
TOTAL	49	944	288	3976	5.2%	7.2%

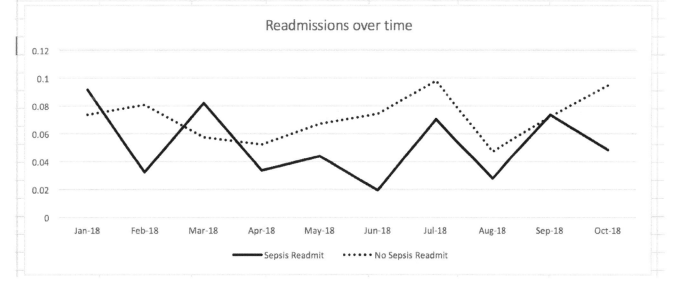

Question 58

Retrieve the DRG codes used to summarize the sepsis related admissions. Arrange the results from the most common to the least used DRG code.

15. Lab

- Non-microbiology vs. microbiology
- One patient – all labs
- MRSA patients
- Lab utilization
- Hypoglycemia in diabetics
- Hypoglycemia – time to next lab

Non-microbiology vs. microbiology

Figure 2.15 in the MIMIC2 guide offers the following ERD related to laboratory results:

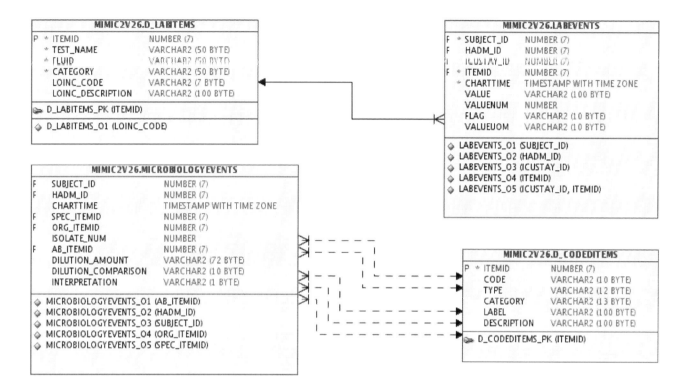

Figure 2.15: Laboratory and microbiology tests. These data are stored in the labevents and microbiologyevents tables. d_labitems and d_coded items contain full descriptions of the lab tests (with LOINC codes) and microbiology tests (specimin, organism and antibiotic).

We can identify two main areas in this ERD:
- Chemistry, hematology, serology, etc. - non-microbiology - labs (upper part of ERD): **labevents** table contains the actual lab results, while the **d_labitems** is the dictionary used to translate the lab name and description. The link between the two tables is a simple 1:M relationship.
- Microbiology labs (lower part): **microbiologyevents** table contains the actual microbiology lab results, while the **d_codeditems** is the dictionary used to translate the microbiology parameters. The link between the two tables is a complex, multiple 1:M relationships for specimen, organism and its antibiotic sensitivity.

One patient – all labs

Retrieving the chemistry, hematology and other non-microbiology lab results for one patient is straight forward: we'll use the **itemid** as the PK/FK link between the results in the **labevents** table and their descriptions in the **d_labitems** table:

SELECT * FROM labevents, d_labitems
WHERE subject_id = 61
AND labevents.itemid = d_labitems.itemid
ORDER BY charttime DESC;

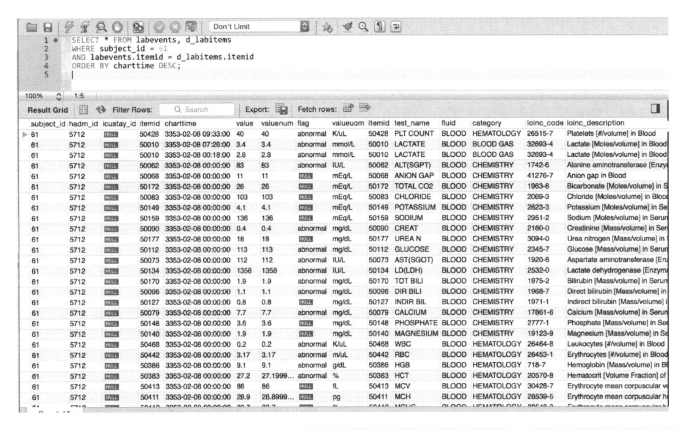

 ## Question 59

Retrieve all the abnormal lab results of the patient in the previous query.

Retrieving the microbiology results without their descriptions, for one patient:

SELECT * FROM mimic2.microbiologyevents
WHERE subject_id = 61
ORDER BY charttime DESC;

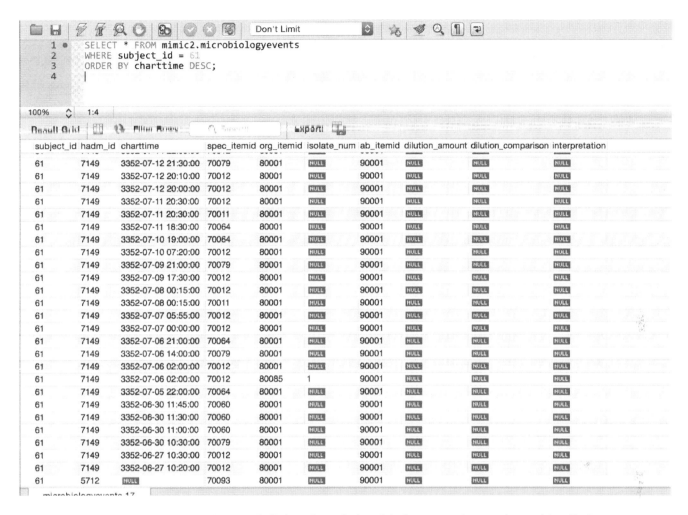

Note that each row has three columns defining the relationship between the results and its dictionary:
- Specimen - **spec_itemid**
- Organism - **org_itemid**
- Antibiotic sensitivity - **ab_itemid**

As mentioned, the relationship between the **microbiologyevents** table and the **d_codeditems** is complex, as it has multiple 1:M relationships between the results table and its dictionary table. In order to retrieve three descriptions for each row - Specimen, Organism, Antibiotic - we have to compare the **microbiologyevents** table to the **d_codeditems** (dictionary) table - three times. Each time we search for a different map to the same itemid in **d_codeditems:** once with **spec_itemid**, once with **org_itemid** and finally with **ab_itemid**:

- Specimen.itemid = spec_itemid
- Organism.itemid = org_itemid
- Ab.itemid = ab_itemid

```
SELECT * FROM
(SELECT subject_id, hadm_id, spec_itemid, org_itemid, ab_itemid FROM microbiologyevents)
AS Patient,
(SELECT itemid, label AS Specimen FROM d_codeditems) AS Specimen,
(SELECT itemid, label AS Organism FROM d_codeditems) AS Organism,
(SELECT itemid, label AS Antibiotic FROM d_codeditems) AS Ab
WHERE subject_id = 19213
AND Specimen.itemid = spec_itemid
AND Organism.itemid = org_itemid
AND Ab.itemid = ab_itemid
ORDER BY hadm_id, spec_itemid;
```

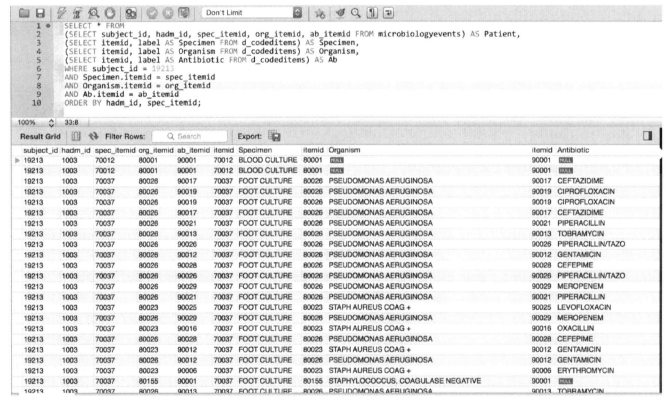

MRSA patients

Using the same mechanism of comparing the microbiology results table three times to its dictionary (Specimen, Organism, Antibiotic), while restricting the query to the very nasty organisms labeled as "Methicillin Resistant Staph Aureus" (MRSA):

SELECT * FROM
(SELECT charttime, subject_id, hadm_id, spec_itemid, org_itemid, ab_itemid FROM microbiologyevents) AS Patient,
(SELECT itemid, label AS Specimen FROM d_codeditems) AS Specimen,
(SELECT itemid, label AS Organism FROM d_codeditems WHERE label LIKE '%Meth%Resist%Staph%Aureus%') AS Organism,
(SELECT itemid, label AS Antibiotic FROM d_codeditems) AS Ab
WHERE Specimen.itemid = spec_itemid
AND Organism.itemid = org_itemid
AND Ab.itemid = ab_itemid
ORDER BY charttime DESC;

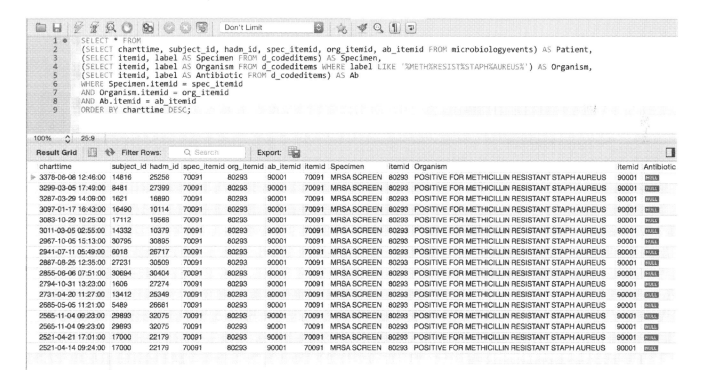

 Question 60

Retrieve all the patients with the quite unfriendly bug Clostridium Difficile in their microbiology lab result.

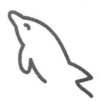

Lab utilization

Let's see how often are the various lab tests being used:

SELECT loinc_description, COUNT(labevents.itemid) AS CountLabs
FROM labevents, d_labitems
WHERE labevents.itemid = d_labitems.itemid
GROUP BY loinc_description
ORDER BY CountLabs DESC;

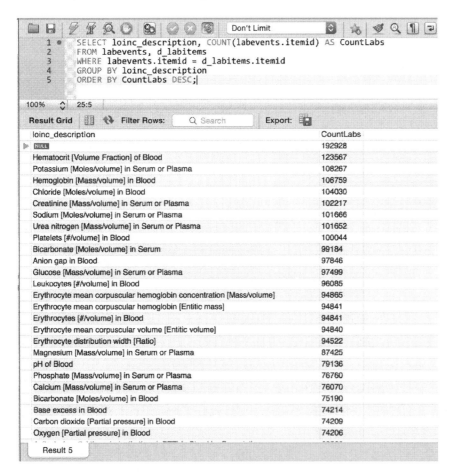

If we'd like to see the ratio of abnormal results to the total volume of lab tests, we need to consolidate two queries: one that retrieves all the lab tests and the number of times they have been used, and the other query to retrieve the same, but only for abnormal results. The link between the two temporary tables is the lab LOINC description:

```sql
SELECT AllLabs.loinc_description, CountLabs, AbnormalLabs,
ROUND(100*AbnormalLabs/CountLabs, 1) AS AbnormalRatio
FROM

(SELECT loinc_description, COUNT(labevents.itemid) AS CountLabs
FROM labevents, d_labitems
WHERE labevents.itemid = d_labitems.itemid
GROUP BY loinc_description) AS AllLabs,

(SELECT loinc_description, COUNT(labevents.itemid) AS AbnormalLabs
FROM labevents, d_labitems
WHERE labevents.itemid = d_labitems.itemid
AND flag = 'abnormal'
GROUP BY loinc_description) AS AbLabs

WHERE AbLabs.loinc_description = AllLabs.loinc_description
ORDER BY AbnormalRatio DESC;
```

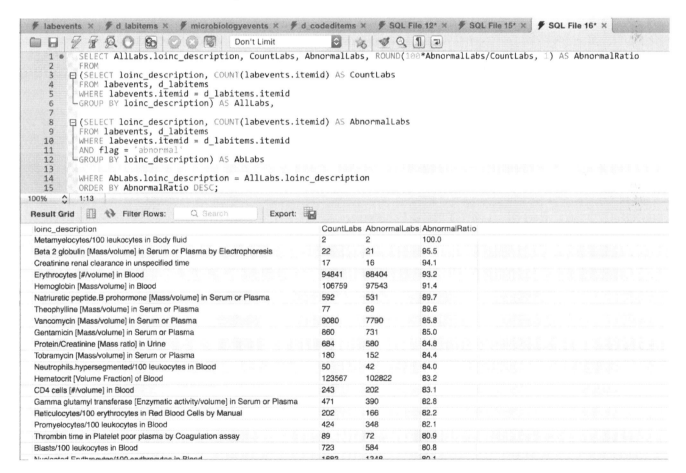

Hypoglycemia in diabetics

One of the quality metrics related to the diabetic patients' management in an intensive care unit is the frequency of hypoglycemia or low blood sugar - life threatening events these patients may experience. In order to get an overview on the prevalence of this life threatening event in the population of diabetics, we need:

- Identify all the diagnosis related to diabetes
- Identify the admissions of the patients diagnosed as diabetics
- Identify the lab tests that may indicate hypoglycemia
- Count the number of admissions of diabetic patients that had at least one hypoglycemic event
- Calculate the ratio between the number of diabetic admissions with a hypoglycemic event over all diabetic admissions

Diagnosis related to diabetes:

First we need identify all the diagnosis in the ICD9 table that are related to diabetes.
As diabetes insipidus is unrelated to diabetes mellitus, we remove these diagnosis from our list. We also remove from our query the "Family history of diabetes":

```
SELECT DISTINCT(description) FROM mimic2.icd9
WHERE description LIKE '%DIABETES%'
AND description NOT LIKE '%INSIPIDUS%'
AND description NOT LIKE '%FAM%'
ORDER BY description;
```

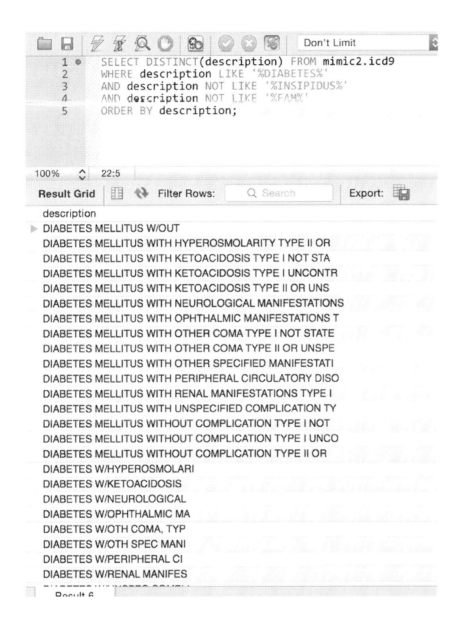

Admissions of patients diagnosed as diabetics:

SELECT hadm_id, description FROM icd9
WHERE description LIKE '%DIABETES%'
AND description NOT LIKE '%INSIPIDUS%'
AND description NOT LIKE '%FAM%'
ORDER BY hadm_id;

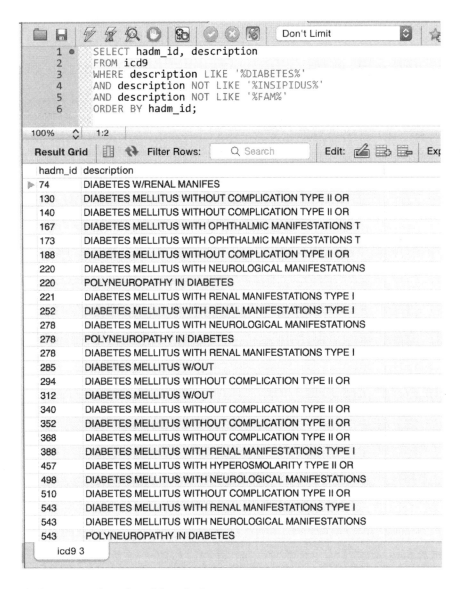

Lab tests related to blood glucose:

SELECT DISTINCT(loinc_description)
FROM d_labitems
WHERE loinc_description LIKE '%glucose %'
AND fluid = 'BLOOD';

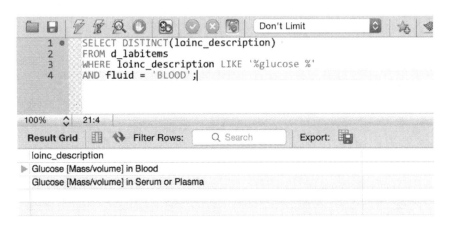

Number of diabetic admissions with at least one hypoglycemic event

SELECT COUNT(DISTINCT(icd9.hadm_id)) AS HypoDiabAdmis
FROM icd9, d_labitems, labevents
WHERE icd9.hadm_id = labevents.hadm_id
AND d_labitems.itemid = labevents.itemid
AND description LIKE '%DIABETES%'
AND description NOT LIKE '%INSIPIDUS%'
AND description NOT LIKE '%FAM%'
AND loinc_description LIKE '%glucose %'
AND fluid = 'BLOOD'
AND value < 60;

```
 1  SELECT COUNT(DISTINCT(icd9.hadm_id)) AS HypoDiabAdmis
 2  FROM icd9, d_labitems, labevents
 3  WHERE icd9.hadm_id = labevents.hadm_id
 4  AND d_labitems.itemid = labevents.itemid
 5  AND description LIKE '%DIABETES%'
 6  AND description NOT LIKE '%INSIPIDUS%'
 7  AND description NOT LIKE '%FAM%'
 8  AND loinc_description LIKE '%glucose %'
 9  AND fluid = 'BLOOD'
10  AND value < 60;
```

HypoDiabAdmis
▶ 345

Number of all diabetic admissions:

SELECT COUNT(DISTINCT(icd9.hadm_id)) AS AllDiabAdmis
FROM icd9, d_labitems, labevents
WHERE icd9.hadm_id = labevents.hadm_id
AND d_labitems.itemid = labevents.itemid
AND description LIKE '%DIABETES%'
AND description NOT LIKE '%INSIPIDUS%'
AND description NOT LIKE '%FAM%'
AND loinc_description LIKE '%glucose %'
AND fluid = 'BLOOD';

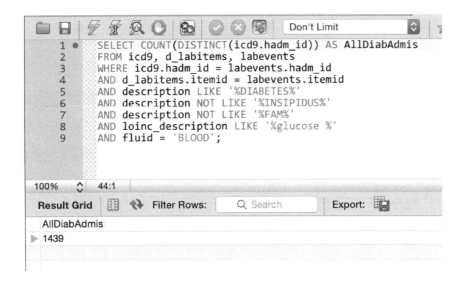

345 admissions of diabetics with a hypo event / **1439** admissions of diabetics = **24%** of diabetic admissions experience at least one hypoglycemic event.

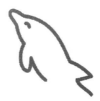

Hypoglycemia – time to next lab

Another quality metric related to diabetic patients' management is the time interval between a hypoglycemic lab result and the second lab documentation. This type of query, requires the following strategy:

- Identify the hypoglycemic lab results of diabetics
- Identify all the blood glucose results of diabetics
- Link the two temporary tables using the **hadm_id**
- Filter the above so the initial hypoglycemic results are compared only to their next glucose measurement

Hypoglycemic results of diabetics:

```
SELECT DISTINCT icd9.hadm_id, value AS HypoValue, charttime AS HypoDT
FROM icd9, d_labitems, labevents
WHERE icd9.hadm_id = labevents.hadm_id
AND d_labitems.itemid = labevents.itemid
AND description LIKE '%DIABETES%'
AND description NOT LIKE '%INSIPIDUS%'
AND description NOT LIKE '%FAM%'
AND loinc_description LIKE '%glucose %'
AND fluid = 'BLOOD'
AND value < 60;
```

Medical Information Extraction and Analysis

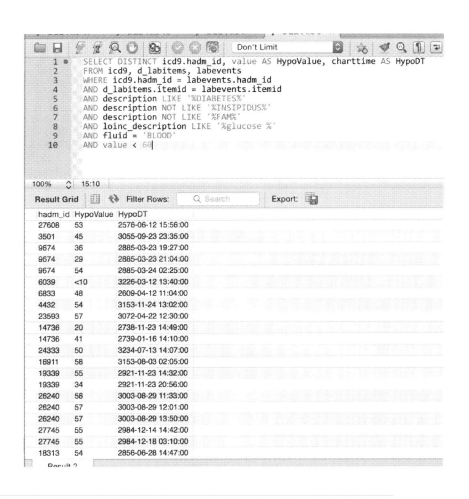

Blood glucose results of diabetics:

SELECT DISTINCT icd9.hadm_id, value AS NextValue, charttime AS NextDT
FROM icd9, d_labitems, labevents
WHERE icd9.hadm_id = labevents.hadm_id
AND d_labitems.itemid = labevents.itemid
AND description LIKE '%DIABETES%'
AND description NOT LIKE '%INSIPIDUS%'
AND description NOT LIKE '%FAM%'
AND loinc_description LIKE '%glucose %'
AND fluid = 'BLOOD';

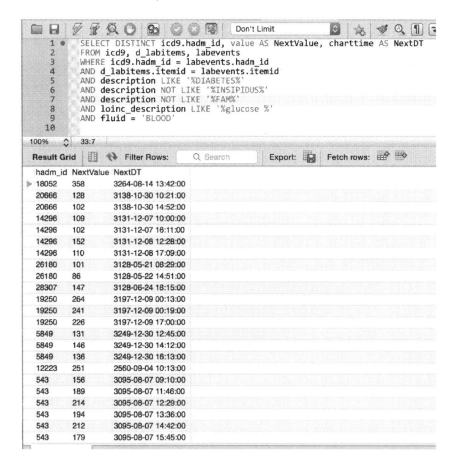

Consolidate the above results, while comparing the hypo with the next glucose lab:

We are going to use the previous results as temporary tables:
- HypoEvents - hypoglycemic labs of diabetics
- GlucEvents - all glucose labs of diabetics

The link between these two temporary tables is the **hadm_id,** while the next glucose measurement is assured by the grouping around the hypoglycemic value:

SELECT DISTINCT *, TIMESTAMPDIFF(MINUTE, HypoDT, NextDT) AS MinutesBetweenLabs
FROM

(SELECT DISTINCT icd9.hadm_id, value AS HypoValue, charttime AS HypoDT
FROM icd9, d_labitems, labevents
WHERE icd9.hadm_id = labevents.hadm_id
AND d_labitems.itemid = labevents.itemid
AND description LIKE '%DIABETES%'
AND description NOT LIKE '%INSIPIDUS%'
AND description NOT LIKE '%FAM%'
AND loinc_description LIKE '%glucose %'
AND fluid = 'BLOOD'
AND value < 60) AS HypoEvents,

(SELECT DISTINCT icd9.hadm_id, value AS NextValue, charttime AS NextDT
FROM icd9, d_labitems, labevents
WHERE icd9.hadm_id = labevents.hadm_id
AND d_labitems.itemid = labevents.itemid
AND description LIKE '%DIABETES%'
AND description NOT LIKE '%INSIPIDUS%'
AND description NOT LIKE '%FAM%'
AND loinc_description LIKE '%glucose %'
AND fluid = 'BLOOD') AS GlucEvents

WHERE HypoEvents.hadm_id = GlucEvents.hadm_id
AND GlucEvents.NextDT > HypoEvents.HypoDT
GROUP BY HypoEvents.hadm_id, HypoValue;

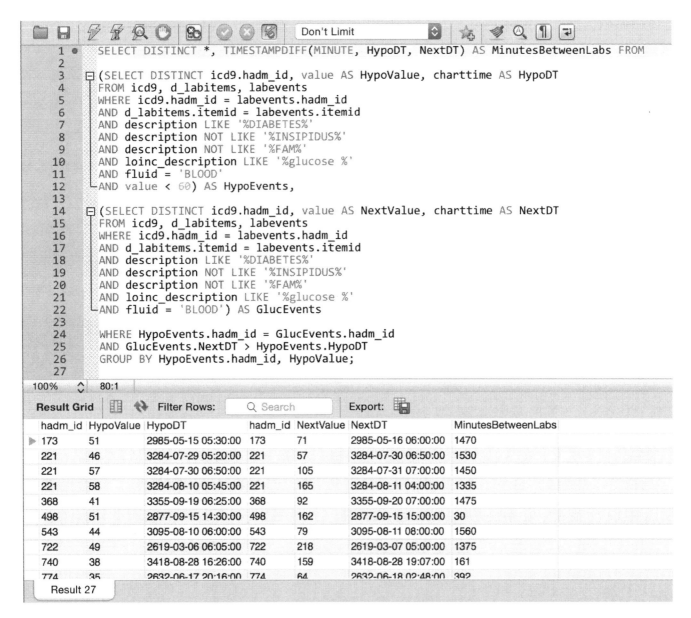

Question 61

Calculate for diabetic patients that have experienced a hypoglycemic event - the average value of the hypoglycemic blood glucose results, the average time to the next blood glucose lab charting and the average blood glucose of the second lab after the hypo event.

16. Drug

- IV vs. Non-IV
- One patient – all drugs and medications
- Drugs utilization: ordered vs. administered
- Average time to execute an order
- Nitroprusside toxicity

IV vs. Non-IV

There are two main categories of drugs and medications in MIMIC2: IV (intra-venous) and non-IV. Each category has its own set of tables and parameters.

IV drugs and meds:

The MIMIC2 guide offers the following ERD for the intra-venous drugs that have been administered. Note that these tables have no information on the actual orders that have preceded these meds administration.

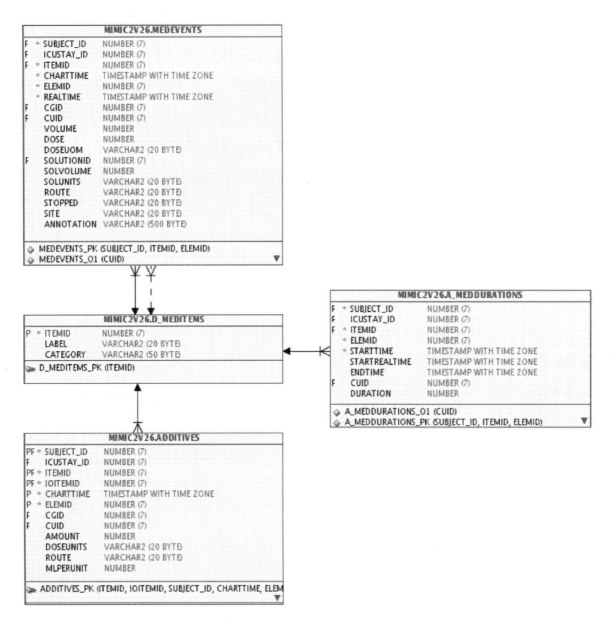

Figure 2.9: Patient medication is stored in 4 tables. The medevents, d_meditems, a_meddurations and additives tables record all data related to patient medication.

Non-IV drugs and meds:

The MIMIC2 guide offers no ERD for Non-IV drugs. Thus, we query the database
INFORMATION_SCHEMA for columns that may have the term **drug** or **med** in their names:

SELECT * FROM INFORMATION_SCHEMA.COLUMNS
WHERE COLUMN_NAME LIKE '%med%'
OR COLUMN_NAME LIKE '%drug%';

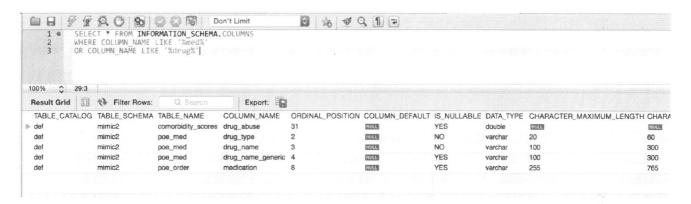

 # Question 62

Browse the **poe_order** and **poe_med** tables and identify the relationship between these tables and the relevant PK/FK that connects the tables.

One patient – all drugs and medications

All IV drugs for one patient:

The main parameters of interest for an IV administered drug are:
- Drug name
- Dose or rate of infusion
- Route
- Additives or other fluids used for dilution purposes
- Start and end date time stamps
- Duration of infusion

If we need only the names of the drugs a patient has been administered, we can query the **medevents** and the **d_meditems** dictionary tables:

```
SELECT DISTINCT d_meditems.label AS DrugName
FROM medevents, d_meditems
WHERE medevents.itemid = d_meditems.itemid
AND medevents.subject_id = 11710
and stopped IS NULL
ORDER BY DrugName;
```

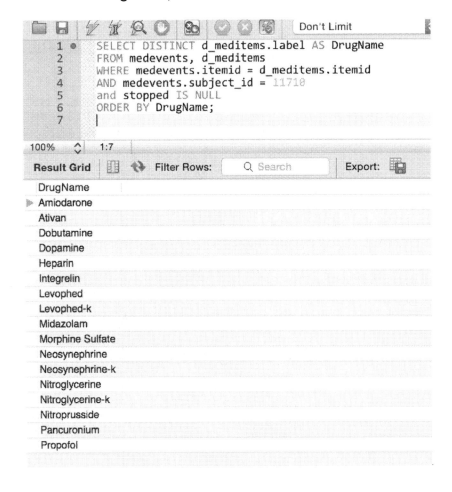

DrugName
Amiodarone
Ativan
Dobutamine
Dopamine
Heparin
Integrelin
Levophed
Levophed-k
Midazolam
Morphine Sulfate
Neosynephrine
Neosynephrine-k
Nitroglycerine
Nitroglycerine-k
Nitroprusside
Pancuronium
Propofol

If we'd like more information about these IV medications, such as the route, dose, dose unit, start time, solution volume and additives:

```
SELECT DISTINCT medevents.icustay_id, medevents.itemid, d_meditems.label AS DrugName,
realtime, dose, doseuom, ioitemid, solvolume, solunits, medevents.route
FROM medevents, d_meditems, additives
WHERE medevents.itemid = d_meditems.itemid
AND additives.itemid = medevents.itemid
AND additives.icustay_id = medevents.icustay_id
AND medevents.subject_id = 11710
and stopped IS NULL
ORDER BY realtime;
```

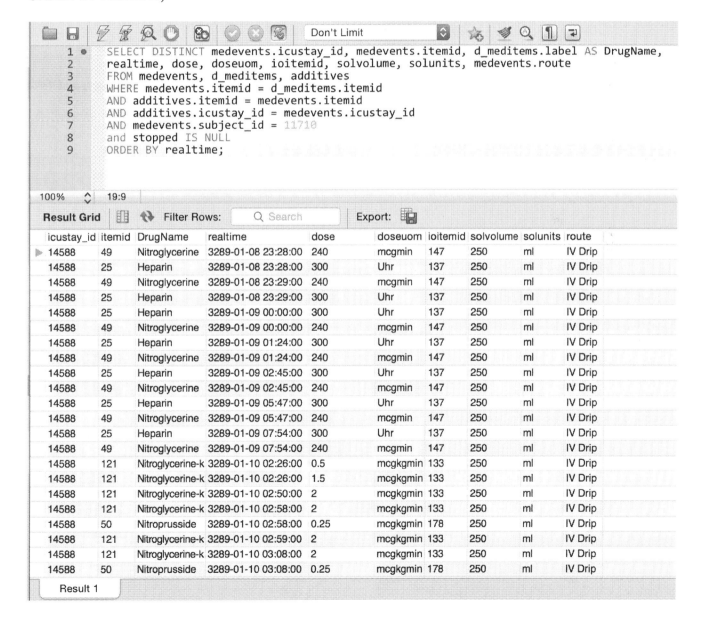

Question 63

One column in the above results is still showing a code instead of its description – **ioitemid**.
Find the dictionary table to translate this column into its description. Hint: this dictionary table is not in the above ERD.

Let's add the start and end times of these IV drugs as well as their durations:

SELECT DISTINCT medevents.icustay_id, d_meditems.label AS DrugName,
dose, doseuom, d_ioitems.label AS SolnName, solvolume, solunits, medevents.route,
startrealtime, endtime, TIMESTAMPDIFF(MINUTE, startrealtime, endtime) AS DurationMins
FROM medevents, d_meditems, additives, d_ioitems, a_meddurations
WHERE medevents.itemid = d_meditems.itemid
AND additives.itemid = medevents.itemid
AND additives.icustay_id = medevents.icustay_id
AND d_ioitems.itemid = ioitemid
AND a_meddurations.icustay_id = medevents.icustay_id
AND a_meddurations.itemid = medevents.itemid
AND medevents.subject_id = 11710
and stopped IS NULL
ORDER BY startrealtime;

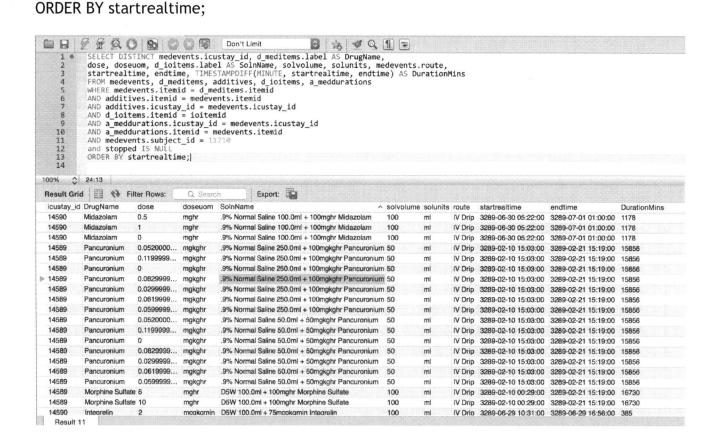

All the orders and non-IV drugs for one patient:

Using the link between the orders table **poe_order** and the non-iv meds **poe_med**, we can retrieve all the orders and non-iv drugs related to one patient:

```
SELECT * FROM poe_med, poe_order
WHERE poe_med.poe_id = poe_order.poe_id
AND subject_id = 20324
ORDER BY start_dt;
```

poe_id	drug_type	drug_name	drug_name_generic	prod_strength	form_rx	dose_val_rx	dose_unit_rx	form_val_disp	form_unit_disp	dose_val_disp	dose_unit_disp
90	MAIN	Artificial Tears	Artificial Tears	1.4%;15ML BTL	OPSOL	1-2	DROP	0.05-0.1	DBTL	20	DROP
91	MAIN	Acetaminophen	Acetaminophen	325MG TAB	TAB	325-650	mg	1-2	TAB	325	mg
92	BASE	D5W	NULL	1 BAG	INJ	250	ml	250	ml	1	ml
92	MAIN	DopAmine	NULL	400MG PREMIX	BAG	400	mg	1	BAG	400	mg
94	MAIN	Nystatin Ointment	Nystatin Ointment	100KU/GM OINT	OINT	1	Appl	1	Appl	1	Appl
95	MAIN	Lorazepam	Lorazepam	2MG/ML SYR	SYR	0.5-2	mg	0.25-1	ml	2	mg
96	MAIN	Lorazepam	Lorazepam	0.5MG TAB	TAB	0.5-2	mg	1-4	TAB	0.5	mg
4137	MAIN	Albuterol-Ipratropium	Albuterol Sulfate/Ipratropium	14.7gm Inhaler	AERO	1-2	PUFF	0.01-0.02	CAN	100	PUFF
97	MAIN	Miconazole Powder 2%	Miconazole Powder 2%	30GM BOTTLE	PWDR	1	Appl	1	BTL	1	Appl
98	MAIN	Furosemide	Furosemide	40MG/4ML VIAL	INJ	40	mg	4	VIAL	10	mg
99	MAIN	Oxymetazoline HCl	Oxymetazoline Hcl	0.05%;3ML SPRAY BOTTLE	SOLN	1	SPRY	0.01	BTL	100	SPRY
100	MAIN	Sodium Chloride Nasal	Sodium Chloride Nasal	45ML BOTTLE	SPR	1-2	SPRY	1-2	SPRY	1	SPRY
101	MAIN	Albuterol-Ipratropium	Albuterol Sulfate/Ipratropium	14.7gm Inhaler	AERO	1-2	PUFF	0.01-0.02	CAN	100	PUFF
102	BASE	SW	NULL	50ml Bag	INJ	50	ml	50	ml	1	ml
102	MAIN	Potassium Chloride	NULL	20mEq/50ml Premix	BAG	20	mEq	1	BAG	20	mEq
103	BASE	D5W	NULL	HEPARIN BASE	INJ	250	ml	250	ml	1	ml
103	MAIN	Heparin Sodium	NULL	25,000 unit Premix Bag	INJ	25000	UNIT	1	BAG	25000	UNIT
13481	MAIN	Furosemide	Furosemide	40MG/4ML VIAL	INJ	40	mg	1	VIAL	40	mg
4066	MAIN	Sodium Chloride Nasal	Sodium Chloride Nasal	45ML BOTTLE	SPR	1-2	SPRY	1-2	SPRY	1	SPRY
93	MAIN	Lansoprazole Oral Solution	Lansoprazole Oral Solution	30mg/10ml Udcup	CAP	30	mg	1	UDCUP	30	mg
4250	BASE	SW	NULL	50ml Bag	INJ	50	ml	50	ml	1	ml
4250	MAIN	Potassium Chloride	NULL	20mEq/50ml Premix	BAG	20	mEq	1	BAG	20	mEq
4402	BASE	NS	NULL	100ML BAG	INJ	100	ml	100	ml	1	ml
4402	MAIN	Pantoprazole Sodium	NULL	40mg Vial	INJ	40	mg	1	VIAL	40	mg
8142	BASE	NS	NULL	100ML BAG	INJ	100	ml	100	ml	1	ml
8142	MAIN	Pantoprazole Sodium	NULL	40mg Vial	INJ	40	mg	1	VIAL	40	mg
5398	BASE	SW	NULL	50ml Bag	INJ	50	ml	50	ml	1	ml

Drugs utilization: ordered vs. administered

We can count the number of patients and admissions where an order for a medication exists, using only the **poe_order** table:

SELECT medication, COUNT(DISTINCT subject_id) AS Patients, COUNT(DISTINCT hadm_id) AS Admissions
FROM poe_order
GROUP BY medication
ORDER BY Admissions DESC;

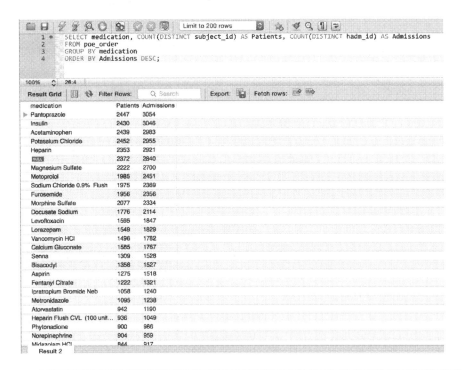

It's important to distinguish between drugs that have been ordered vs. drugs that have been administered.

 Question 64

The above query summarizes the orders of drugs by patient and admission.
Summarize the same for the medications which have actually been administered.

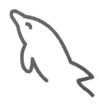

Average time to execute an order

The time stamp of an order and the start of a drug administration are in the same table: **poe_order**, making the calculation of the average time to execute an order, a breeze:

```
SELECT ROUND(AVG(TIMESTAMPDIFF(MINUTE, enter_dt, start_dt)),0) AS AVGTime2Exec,
COUNT(DISTINCT hadm_id) AS Admissions
FROM poe_order
ORDER BY AVGTime2Exec;
```

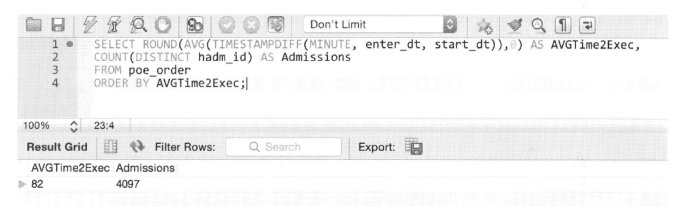

AVGTime2Exec	Admissions
82	4097

 ## Question 65

Calculate the average time to execute a med order by route of administration.
Count also the number of admissions where a route of administration was employed.

Nitroprusside toxicity

Nitroprusside is used extensively in the ICU to control blood pressure and induce vasodilation. This drug has a limit of 0.5 mg/kg/hour which should not be exceeded as it may cause cyanide toxicity.
Let's identify the instances and percentage of the higher than recommended doses of nitroprusside in MIMIC2.

First step – let's identify all the instances that nitroprusside was administered. As nitroprusside is administered IV, we are going to reuse a slightly modified previous query that retrieves information on IV drips:

```
SELECT DISTINCT medevents.icustay_id, d_meditems.label AS DrugName,
startrealtime, endtime, TIMESTAMPDIFF(MINUTE, startrealtime, endtime) AS DurationMins,
dose, doseuom
FROM medevents, d_meditems, additives, a_meddurations
WHERE medevents.itemid = d_meditems.itemid
AND additives.itemid = medevents.itemid
AND additives.icustay_id = medevents.icustay_id
AND a_meddurations.icustay_id = medevents.icustay_id
AND a_meddurations.itemid = medevents.itemid
AND d_meditems.label LIKE '%nitroprusside%'
AND dose IS NOT NULL
ORDER BY icustay_id, startrealtime;
```

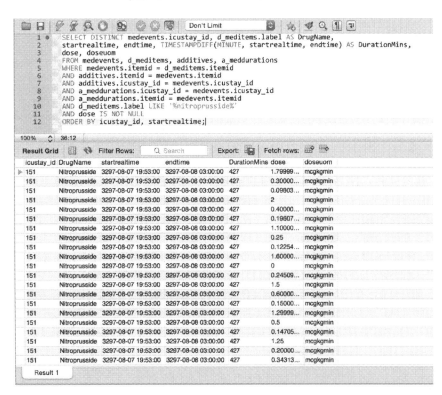

In these results there are instances with the same **icustay_id, starttime** and **endtime** – but with different doses. That's expected as nitroprusside is a drug titrated to effect - clinicians change the dose frequently as the blood pressure and other cardio vascular parameters are monitored continuously. We need to average the dose for the time frame nitroprusside was used:

SELECT DISTINCT medevents.icustay_id, d_meditems.label AS DrugName,
startrealtime, endtime, TIMESTAMPDIFF(MINUTE, startrealtime, endtime) AS DurationMins,
ROUND(AVG(dose),3) AS AVGdose, doseuom
FROM medevents, d_meditems, additives, a_meddurations
WHERE medevents.itemid = d_meditems.itemid
AND additives.itemid = medevents.itemid
AND additives.icustay_id = medevents.icustay_id
AND a_meddurations.icustay_id = medevents.icustay_id
AND a_meddurations.itemid = medevents.itemid
AND d_meditems.label LIKE '%nitroprusside%'
AND dose IS NOT NULL
GROUP BY icustay_id, startrealtime;

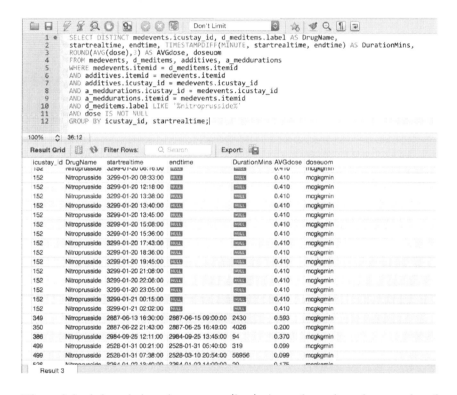

The original dose is in micrograms/kg/min and needs to be translated to mg/kg/hour:

Dose in mcg/kg/min X 60 / 1000 = Dose in mg/kg/hour

SELECT DISTINCT medevents.icustay_id, d_meditems.label AS DrugName,
ROUND(AVG(dose),3) AS AVGdose, doseuom,
startrealtime, endtime, TIMESTAMPDIFF(MINUTE, startrealtime, endtime) AS DurationMins,
ROUND(AVG(dose) * 60 /1000,2) AS DoseMgPerKgPerHour
FROM medevents, d_meditems, additives, a_meddurations
WHERE medevents.itemid = d_meditems.itemid
AND additives.itemid = medevents.itemid
AND additives.icustay_id = medevents.icustay_id
AND a_meddurations.icustay_id = medevents.icustay_id

AND a_meddurations.itemid = medevents.itemid
AND d_meditems.label LIKE '%nitroprusside%'
AND dose IS NOT NULL
GROUP BY icustay_id, startrealtime;

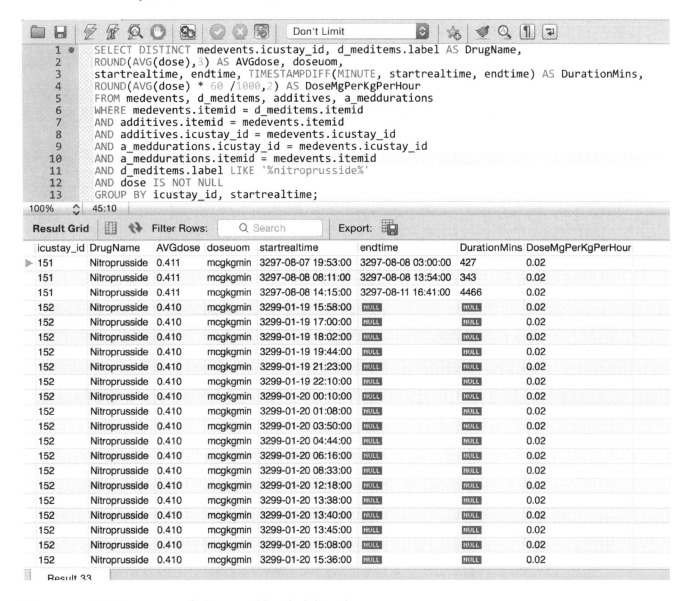

There were 736 instances of nitroprusside administrations.

Lastly, we filter the results for those above the maximum recommended dose of 0.5 mg/kg/hour:

SELECT DISTINCT medevents.icustay_id, d_meditems.label AS DrugName,
ROUND(AVG(dose),3) AS AVGdose, doseuom,
startrealtime, endtime, TIMESTAMPDIFF(MINUTE, startrealtime, endtime) AS DurationMins,
ROUND(AVG(dose) * 60 /1000,2) AS DoseMgPerKgPerHour
FROM medevents, d_meditems, additives, a_meddurations
WHERE medevents.itemid = d_meditems.itemid
AND additives.itemid = medevents.itemid
AND additives.icustay_id = medevents.icustay_id
AND a_meddurations.icustay_id = medevents.icustay_id

```
AND a_meddurations.itemid = medevents.itemid
AND d_meditems.label LIKE '%nitroprusside%'
AND dose IS NOT NULL
GROUP BY icustay_id, startrealtime
HAVING DoseMgPerKgPerHour > 0.5;
```

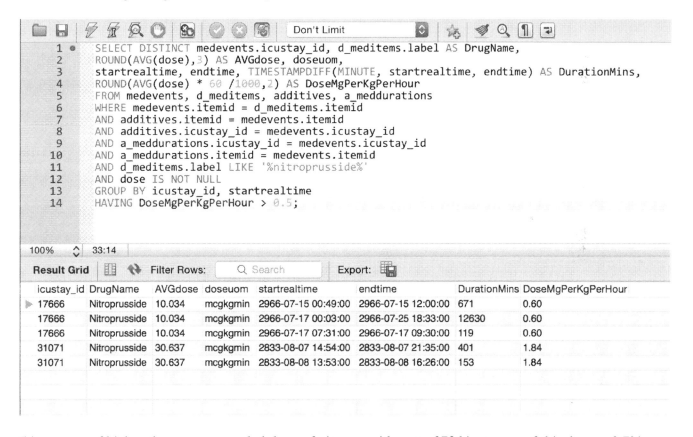

5 instances of higher than recommended dose of nitroprusside out of **736** instances of this drug = **0.7%**

17. Procedure

- One patient: all procedures
- Volumes by procedure
- Mortality by procedure
- LOS by procedure
- Readmissions by procedure

One patient: all procedures

The MIMIC2 ERD on procedures:

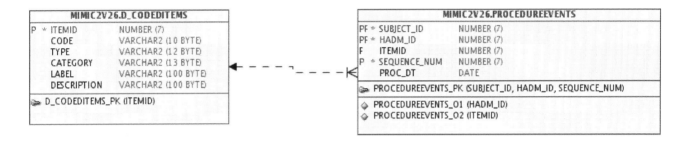

Figure 2.14: Procedures performed on a patient. The d_codeditems and procedureevents tables record all data related to patient procedures.

Question 66

Retrieve all the procedures performed on patient subject_id = 11710, the relevant hadm_id, procedure description and order results by their procedure date.

One procedure: all patients

Using the ERD, finding all the patients that underwent extra-corporeal circulation should be easy:

SELECT subject_id, hadm_id, description, proc_dt
FROM procedureevents, d_codeditems
WHERE procedureevents.itemid = d_codeditems.itemid
AND description LIKE '%extracorpor%';

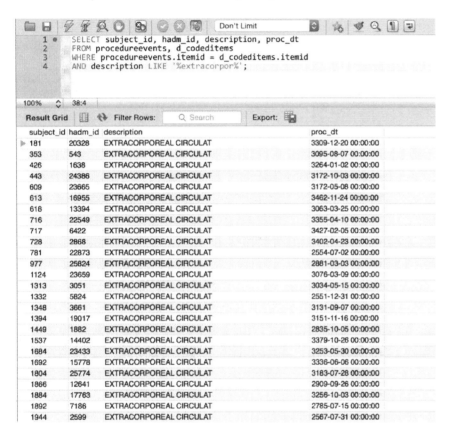

 Question 67

Calculate the mortality rate of the patients that underwent extra-corporeal circulation.

Volumes by procedure

We summarize the volumes of patients and admissions by grouping on the procedure:

SELECT description, COUNT(DISTINCT hadm_id) AS NumAdmit,
COUNT(DISTINCT subject_id) AS NumPts
FROM procedureevents, d_codeditems
WHERE procedureevents.itemid = d_codeditems.itemid
GROUP BY code
ORDER BY NumPts DESC;

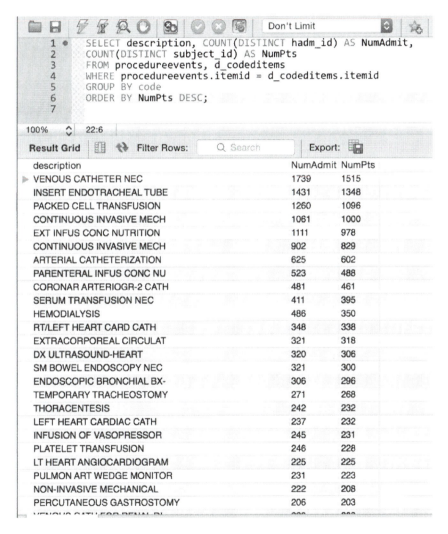

description	NumAdmit	NumPts
VENOUS CATHETER NEC	1739	1515
INSERT ENDOTRACHEAL TUBE	1431	1348
PACKED CELL TRANSFUSION	1260	1096
CONTINUOUS INVASIVE MECH	1061	1000
EXT INFUS CONC NUTRITION	1111	978
CONTINUOUS INVASIVE MECH	902	829
ARTERIAL CATHETERIZATION	625	602
PARENTERAL INFUS CONC NU	523	488
CORONAR ARTERIOGR-2 CATH	481	461
SERUM TRANSFUSION NEC	411	395
HEMODIALYSIS	486	350
RT/LEFT HEART CARD CATH	348	338
EXTRACORPOREAL CIRCULAT	321	318
DX ULTRASOUND-HEART	320	306
SM BOWEL ENDOSCOPY NEC	321	300
ENDOSCOPIC BRONCHIAL BX-	306	296
TEMPORARY TRACHEOSTOMY	271	268
THORACENTESIS	242	232
LEFT HEART CARDIAC CATH	237	232
INFUSION OF VASOPRESSOR	245	231
PLATELET TRANSFUSION	246	228
LT HEART ANGIOCARDIOGRAM	225	225
PULMON ART WEDGE MONITOR	231	223
NON-INVASIVE MECHANICAL	222	208
PERCUTANEOUS GASTROSTOMY	206	203

Mortality by procedure

Using the mortality flag in the **d_patients** table we can calculate mortality for all procedures. The query strategy is to use two temporary tables:

- **AllPts** - all the patients grouped by procedure
- **Died** - all the patients that have died, grouped by procedure

We are going to link between the two tables with the procedure unique identifier – **itemid**:

```
SELECT description, NumDied, NumPts, ROUND(100* NumDied / NumPts,1) AS Mortality FROM

(SELECT description, d_codeditems.itemid AS ItemDied, COUNT(DISTINCT
d_patients.subject_id) AS NumDied
FROM procedureevents, d_codeditems, d_patients
WHERE d_patients.subject_id = procedureevents.subject_id
AND procedureevents.itemid = d_codeditems.itemid
AND hospital_expire_flg = 'Y'
GROUP BY code) AS Died,

(SELECT d_codeditems.itemid AS Item All, COUNT(DISTINCT d_patients.subject_id) AS
NumPts
FROM procedureevents, d_codeditems, d_patients
WHERE d_patients.subject_id = procedureevents.subject_id
AND procedureevents.itemid = d_codeditems.itemid
GROUP BY code) AS AllPts

WHERE ItemAll = ItemDied
ORDER BY NumDied DESC;
```

Medical Information Extraction and Analysis

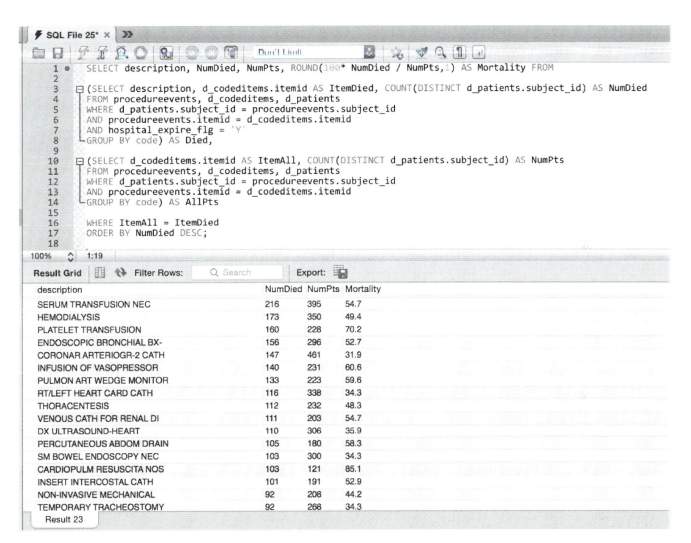

LOS by procedure

Using the column **hospital_los** in the **icustay_detail** table, we can calculate the LOS for all the procedures. The link between the **icustay_detail** and **procedureevents** tables is the unique admission **hadm_id**:

```
SELECT description, ROUND(AVG(hospital_los/60/24),1) AS AVGLOSdays,
COUNT(DISTINCT icustay_detail.hadm_id) as NumAdmis
FROM procedureevents, d_codeditems, icustay_detail
WHERE icustay_detail.hadm_id = procedureevents.hadm_id
AND procedureevents.itemid = d_codeditems.itemid
GROUP BY code
ORDER BY AVGLOSdays DESC, NumAdmis DESC;
```

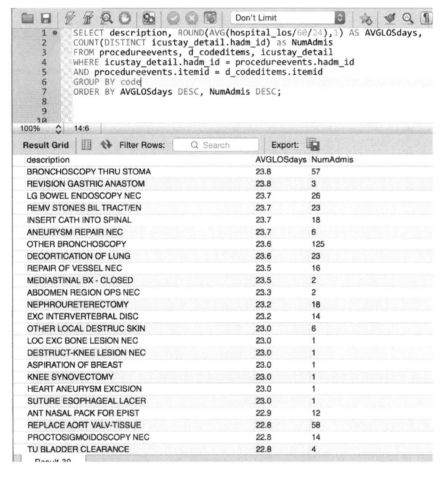

Readmissions by procedure

The technique to calculate the readmission rate was detailed in the chapter devoted solely to this subject. We'll use two temporary tables:

- **AllPts** for the number of admissions by procedure
- **Readmit** for the number of readmissions by procedure

The link between the two tables is the procedure description:

```
SELECT Readmit.description, NumReadmit, NumAdmit,
ROUND((100 * NumReadmit / NumAdmit),1) AS ReadmitRate
FROM

(SELECT description, COUNT(DISTINCT hadm_id) AS NumAdmit
FROM procedureevents, d_codeditems
WHERE procedureevents.itemid = d_codeditems.itemid
GROUP BY code) AS AllPts,

(SELECT description, COUNT(X.admit_dt) AS NumReadmit
FROM procedureevents, d_codeditems, admissions X, admissions Y
WHERE X.hadm_id = procedureevents.hadm_id
AND procedureevents.itemid = d_codeditems.itemid
AND X.subject_id = Y.subject_id
AND X.hadm_id <> Y.hadm_id
AND TIMESTAMPDIFF(DAY, X.disch_dt, Y.admit_dt) BETWEEN 0 AND 30
GROUP BY description) AS Readmit

WHERE AllPts.description = Readmit.description
ORDER BY NumReadmit DESC;
```

```sql
SELECT Readmit.description, NumReadmit, NumAdmit,
ROUND((100 * NumReadmit / NumAdmit),1) AS ReadmitRate
FROM

(SELECT description, COUNT(DISTINCT hadm_id) AS NumAdmit
 FROM procedureevents, d_codeditems
 WHERE procedureevents.itemid = d_codeditems.itemid
 GROUP BY code) AS AllPts,

(SELECT description, COUNT(X.admit_dt) AS NumReadmit
 FROM procedureevents, d_codeditems, admissions X, admissions Y
 WHERE X.hadm_id = procedureevents.hadm_id
 AND procedureevents.itemid = d_codeditems.itemid
 AND X.subject_id = Y.subject_id
 AND X.hadm_id <> Y.hadm_id
 AND TIMESTAMPDIFF(DAY, X.disch_dt, Y.admit_dt) BETWEEN 0 AND 30
 GROUP BY description) AS Readmit

WHERE AllPts.description = Readmit.description
ORDER BY NumReadmit DESC;
```

description	NumReadmit	NumAdmit	ReadmitRate
CONTINUOUS INVASIVE MECH	144	902	16.0
PACKED CELL TRANSFUSION	124	1260	9.8
EXT INFUS CONC NUTRITION	102	1111	9.2
INSERT ENDOTRACHEAL TUBE	93	1431	6.5
HEMODIALYSIS	52	486	10.7
ARTERIAL CATHETERIZATION	49	625	7.8
TEMPORARY TRACHEOSTOMY	41	271	15.1
PARENTERAL INFUS CONC NU	39	523	7.5
THORACENTESIS	36	242	14.9
PERCUTANEOUS GASTROSTOMY	35	206	17.0
CORONAR ARTERIOGR-2 CATH	33	481	6.9
DX ULTRASOUND-HEART	32	320	10.0
SERUM TRANSFUSION NEC	32	411	7.8
EXTRACORPOREAL CIRCULAT	32	321	10.0
ENDOSCOPIC BRONCHIAL BX	30	306	9.8

18. Chart, note and much more

- Patient chart: labs, drugs, vitals etc.
- One patient: all chart instances
- One ICU stay: respiratory parameters
- Discharge, imaging report and MD notes
- One patient: all free text notes

Patient chart: labs, drugs, vitals, etc.

The MIMIC2 ERD displays the following relationships:

MIMIC2V26.A_CHARTDURATIONS

PF	* SUBJECT_ID	NUMBER (7)
F	ICUSTAY_ID	NUMBER (7)
PF	* ITEMID	NUMBER (7)
P	* ELEMID	NUMBER (7)
P	* STARTTIME	TIMESTAMP WITH TIME ZONE
	* STARTREALTIME	TIMESTAMP WITH TIME ZONE
	ENDTIME	TIMESTAMP WITH TIME ZONE
F	CUID	NUMBER (7)
	DURATION	NUMBER

A_CHARTDURATIONS_PK (SUBJECT_ID, ITEMID, ELEMID, STARTTIM

MIMIC2V26.D_CHARTITEMS

P	* ITEMID	NUMBER (7)
	LABEL	VARCHAR2 (110 BYTE)
	CATEGORY	VARCHAR2 (50 BYTE)
	DESCRIPTION	VARCHAR2 (255 BYTE)

D_CHARTITEMS_PK (ITEMID)

MIMIC2V26.CHARTEVENTS

PF	* SUBJECT_ID	NUMBER (7)
F	ICUSTAY_ID	NUMBER (7)
PF	* ITEMID	NUMBER (7)
P	* CHARTTIME	TIMESTAMP WITH TIME ZONE
P	* ELEMID	NUMBER (7)
	* REALTIME	TIMESTAMP WITH TIME ZONE
F	CGID	NUMBER (7)
F	CUID	NUMBER (7)
	VALUE1	VARCHAR2 (110 BYTE)
	VALUE1NUM	NUMBER
	VALUE1UOM	VARCHAR2 (20 BYTE)
	VALUE2	VARCHAR2 (110 BYTE)
	VALUE2NUM	NUMBER
	VALUE2UOM	VARCHAR2 (20 BYTE)
	RESULTSTATUS	VARCHAR2 (20 BYTE)
	STOPPED	VARCHAR2 (20 BYTE)
	ANNOTATION	VARCHAR2 (500 BYTE)

CHARTEVENTS_PK (SUBJECT_ID, ITEMID, CHARTTIME, ELEMID)

Let's review the items in the dictionary table **d_chartitems**:

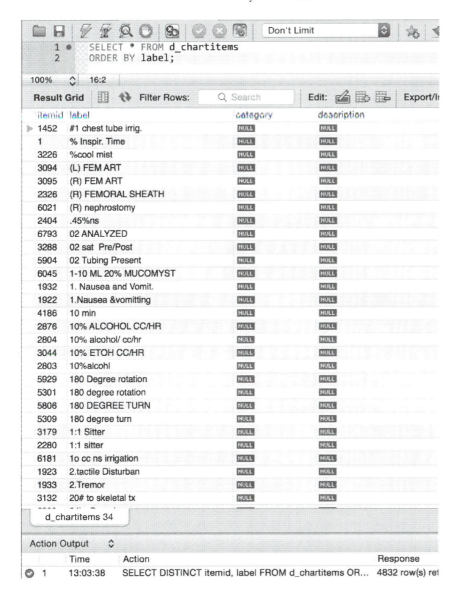

There are 4,832 items in this dictionary tables including: labs, drugs, procedures, vital signs, ventilation settings, cardiac output measurements, nursing findings and interventions, physical exams, scoring values and much more.

The actual values of these parameters are stored in the **chartevents** table and their durations in the **a_chartdurations** table.

The table **chartevents** has more than 30 million rows, so queries using this table will take longer than usual and may cause errors like: **"Lost connection to MySQL server"** or **"Query was cancelled"** if the run time is more than 60 seconds. Try to limit the queries on this table with restrictions on the time frame set to several years instead of the whole millenium.

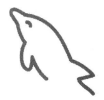

One patient: all chart instances

Using the MIMIC2 ERD we can retrieve all chart instances for a patient:

SELECT subject_id, icustay_id, realtime, label, value1
FROM chartevents, d_chartitems
WHERE chartevents.itemid = d_chartitems.itemid
AND subject_id = 9331
ORDER BY realtime;

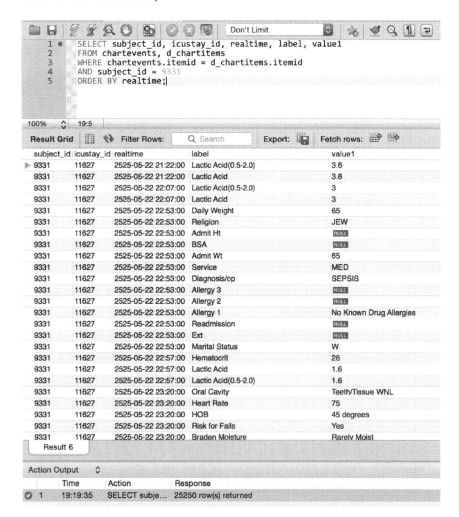

Obviously some of these items may be found in other tables, such as lab results or meds administered, but many other chart events are not replicated in any other table in MIMIC2. We will revisit the **chartevents** table in the next chapters on vital signs and scoring.

One ICU stay: respiratory parameters

As the vital signs are dispersed within the dictionary table **d_chartitems** together with drugs, wound dressings, lab results, ventilator settings and etc., and since the category column in this table is null – there is no simple way to query all the vital signs of a patient.

Instead, let's focus on a limited set of parameters related to the respiratory status of a single patient during a single ICU stay: mechanical ventilator mode, inspired oxygen (FiO2), positive end expiratory pressure (PEEP) and the resulting oxygenation status as reflected in the saturated hemoglobin – SpO2.

We need to query the same table several times and consolidate results in a chronological order with **UNION**:

```
(SELECT charttime, label, value1
FROM d_chartitems, chartevents
WHERE d_chartitems.itemid = chartevents.itemid
AND icustay_id = 17234
AND value1 IS NOT NULL
AND label LIKE '%vent%mode%')
UNION
(SELECT charttime, label, value1
FROM d_chartitems, chartevents
WHERE d_chartitems.itemid = chartevents.itemid
AND icustay_id = 17234
AND value1 IS NOT NULL
AND label LIKE '%SpO2%')
UNION
(SELECT charttime, label, ROUND(value1,1)
FROM d_chartitems, chartevents
WHERE d_chartitems.itemid = chartevents.itemid
AND icustay_id = 17234
AND value1 IS NOT NULL
AND label LIKE '%FiO2%')
UNION
(SELECT charttime, label, ROUND(value1,0)
FROM d_chartitems, chartevents
WHERE d_chartitems.itemid = chartevents.itemid
AND icustay_id = 17234
AND value1 IS NOT NULL
AND label LIKE '%PEEP%')
ORDER BY charttime;
```

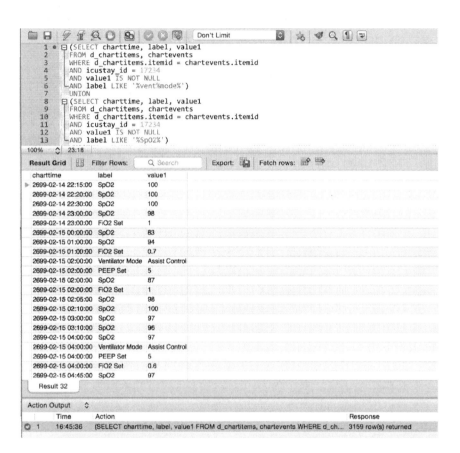

Discharge, imaging report and MD note

Most of the free-text notes related to a patient can be found in the **noteevents** table. From the MIMIC2 User Guide:

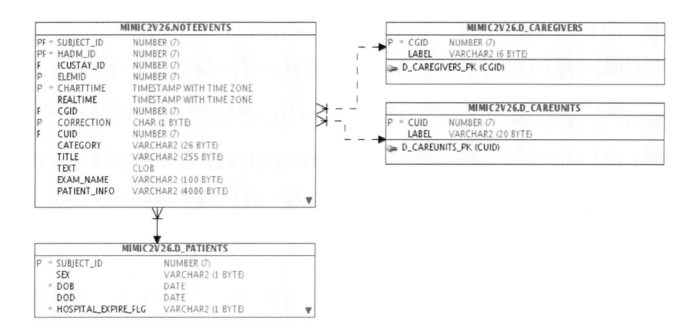

Checking the categories in the **noteevents** table:

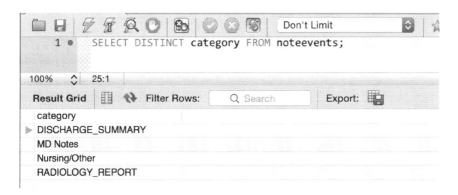

In this chapter, we are going to discuss the MD Notes, Discharge summary and Radiology reports. The Nursing notes are being detailed in another chapter.

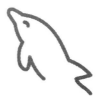

One patient: all notes

Retrieving from the **noteevents** table one patient's discharge summaries, radiology reports and MD notes (everything that is not 'Nursing/Other'):

SELECT subject_id, hadm_id, charttime, category, text
FROM noteevents
WHERE category <> 'Nursing/Other'
AND subject_id = 4655
ORDER BY charttime;

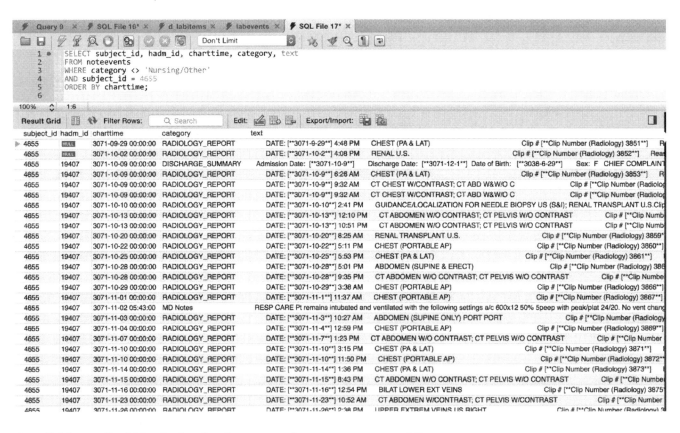

One field or cell within the **text** column, may have many pages of free text.
You can view the content of the discharge summary for example, by copying the field to a text editor such as MS Word or you can export the results table to a spreadsheet.

One page (out of 8) from the discharge summary of the above **subject_id = 4655**:

Admission Date: [**3071-10-9**]   Discharge Date: [**3071-12-1**]

Date of Birth: [**3038-6-29**]   Sex: F

CHIEF COMPLAINT: Post-transplant lymphoproliferative disorder.

HISTORY OF PRESENT ILLNESS: The patient is a 33 year old [**4-/3070**] at another institution. The patient had no immediate postoperative transplant complications there, but prior to admission here, the patient had been diagnosed with PTLD (post-transplant lymphoproliferative disorder). The patient is currently off Immuno-suppressant medications except for Prednisone. Following the cessation of immunosuppressant medications, the patient developed acute rejection. The patient's initial fever associated with the rejection subsided when she received treatments for the acute rejection with Solu-Medrol 500 times four and then her baseline Prednisone dose increased to 20 mg per day from 10 mg. The patient was initially discharged home within a week of this admission and was doing relatively well.

Just prior to admission, the patient developed abdominal pain which was predominantly in the lower back and described as continuous pain in the moderate to severe range. The patient also had some nausea but denied urinary symptoms or diarrhea. The patient also complained of chills and rigor.

PAST MEDICAL HISTORY:
1. Bipolar disorder.
2. End-stage renal disease secondary to Lithium toxicity.
3. Increased cholesterol.
4. Post-transplant lymphoproliferative disorder diagnosed in [**8-/3071**] from a biopsy during a colonoscopy. At that time, the Prograf, Rapamycin was discontinued but the patient was continued on low dose Prednisone.

PAST SURGICAL HISTORY:
1. Renal transplant 06/2001.
2. Appendectomy.

MEDICATIONS:
1. Prednisone 20 mg p.o. q. day.
2. Depakote 1000/500.
3. Zoloft 75 p.o. q. day.
4. Atenolol 25 p.o. q. day.
5. Norvasc 2.5 p.o. q. day.
6. Lamictal 50 mg p.o. q. day.
7. Seroquel 125 mg p.o. q. day.
8. Lipitor 20 mg p.o. q. day.

19. Provider and care unit

- Care giver, care unit and their relationships
- One patient: all care givers
- One patient: all care units
- One care giver: all ICU stays related
- One care unit: all ICU stays related

Care giver, care unit and their relationships

The MIMIC2 User Guide offers the following ERD related to clinicians, providers or care givers:

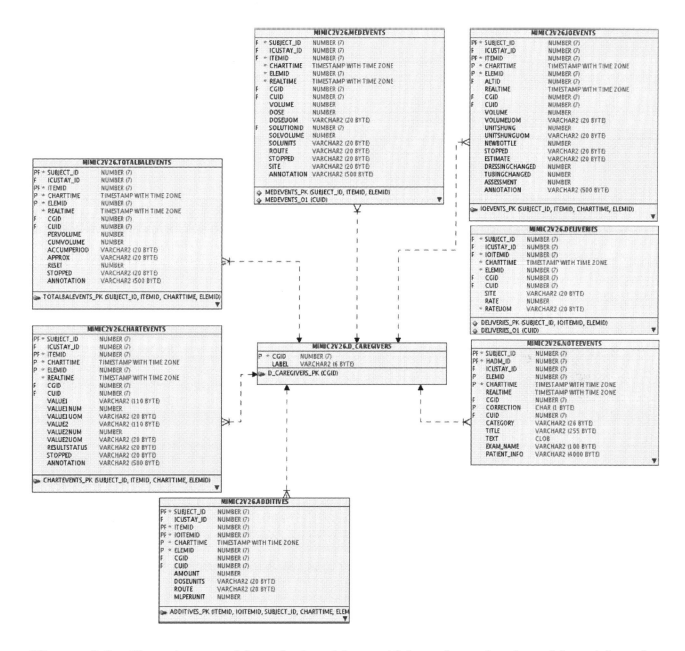

Figure 2.3: Caregivers table relationships. Although a simple table with only 2 columns, the caregivers table is related to many other tables in the database. Caregivers are assigned to *inter alia* medical events, problems and notes.

Similarly, the ERD on care units:

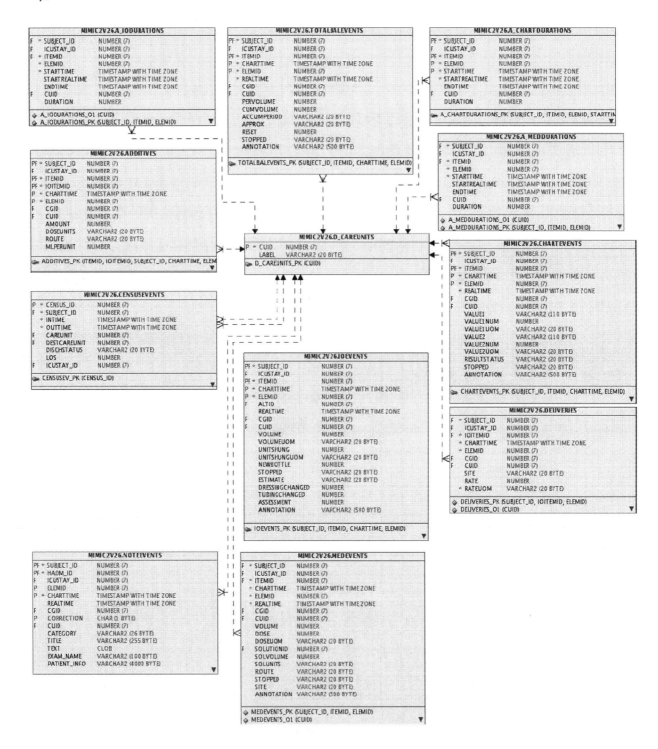

Figure 2.4: Careunits table and relationships. The careunits table is related to many other tables and contains information about the particular care unit where an event occurred.

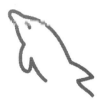

One patient: all care givers

The care givers are related to patients via events as reflected in the following 7 tables in the ERD:

- chartevents
- medevents
- totalbalevents
- ioevents
- noteevents
- deliveries
- additives

Note: in the ERD there is no direct relationship between a care giver and a patient or admission.

If we'd like to retrieve all the care givers of a patient from one of the tables above - **chartevents**:

```
SELECT d_caregivers.cgid AS CareGiver,
icustay_id, d_caregivers.label AS ProvTitle
FROM chartevents, d_caregivers
WHERE d_caregivers.cgid = chartevents.cgid
AND subject_id = 4655
GROUP BY d_caregivers.cgid;
```

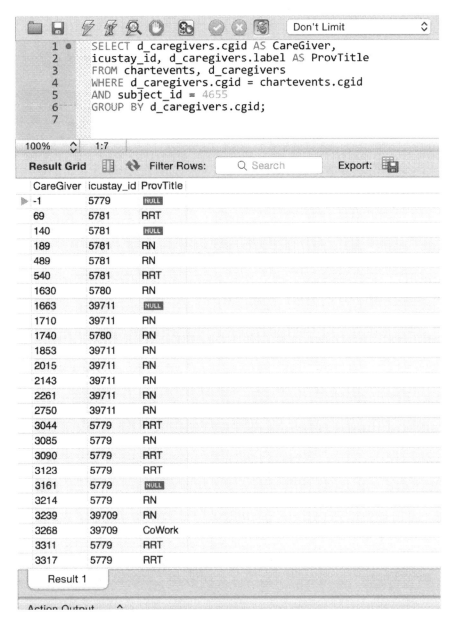

 # Question 68

Add to the above query the number of hours a provider was related to the patient, calculated as the difference between the first and last charted events by the provider.

This query is on a single table that **d_caregivers** has relationships with. If we repeat a similar query on **noteevents**:

SELECT d_caregivers.cgid AS CareGiver,
icustay_id, d_caregivers.label AS ProvTitle
FROM noteevents, d_caregivers
WHERE d_caregivers.cgid = noteevents.cgid
AND subject_id = 4655
GROUP BY d_caregivers.cgid;

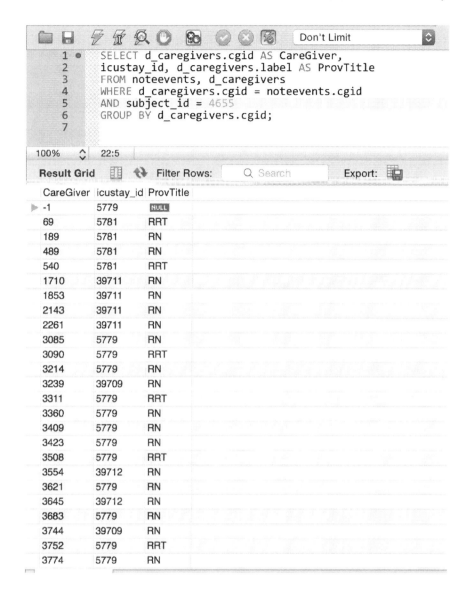

As the results of the last two queries are in a similar format, we can use the **UNION** to consolidate the two sets into one:

(SELECT 'chartevents' AS OrigTable,
d_caregivers.cgid AS CareGiver,
icustay_id, d_caregivers.label AS ProvTitle
FROM chartevents, d_caregivers
WHERE d_caregivers.cgid = chartevents.cgid
AND subject_id = 4655
GROUP BY d_caregivers.cgid)
UNION
(SELECT 'noteevents' AS OrigTable,
d_caregivers.cgid AS CareGiver,
icustay_id, d_caregivers.label AS ProvTitle
FROM noteevents, d_caregivers
WHERE d_caregivers.cgid = noteevents.cgid
AND subject_id = 4655
GROUP BY d_caregivers.cgid);

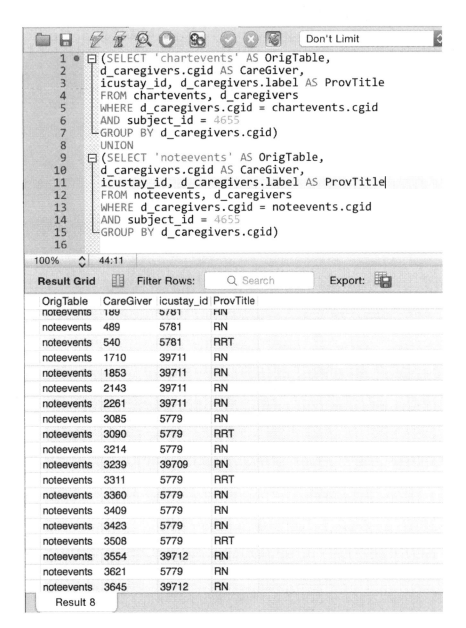

Question 69

Add to the this last query the results from the **medevents** and **ioevents** tables.

One patient: all care units

The care units are related to patients via events, as reflected in the following 11 tables in the ERD:

- chartevents
- censusevents
- medevents
- totalbalevents
- ioevents
- noteevents
- deliveries
- additives
- a_iodurations
- a_meddurations
- a_chartdurations

Note that in the ERD there is no direct relationship between a care unit and a patient or admission.

Retrieving all the care units for one patient, using one table (out of 11 related tables) - **chartevents**:

SELECT d_careunits.label AS CareUnit, icustay_id
FROM chartevents, d_careunits
WHERE d_careunits.cuid = chartevents.cuid
AND subject_id = 4655
AND charttime BETWEEN '3071-01-01' AND '3077-12-31'
GROUP BY CareUnit;

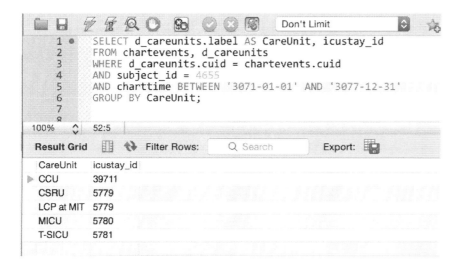

Note the time limit between the years 3071 and 3077: without this restriction and since the **chartevents** table has more than 30 million rows – the query will not be done before the 60 seconds limit and will cause a lost connection to server error.

Question 70

Add to the last query the results from the **medevents** and **noteevents** tables.

 Question 71

Using the **chartevents** table, find the care units and the hours patient 4655 spent in each unit of care. Restrict your limit to the years 3071-3077 so you will not experience a "lost connection to server" error

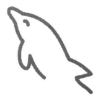

One care giver: all ICU stays related

Let's retrieve from the **chartevents** table all the ICU stays, that care giver 3891 was involved with:

SELECT COUNT(DISTINCT icustay_id) AS ICUadmit
FROM chartevents, d_caregivers
WHERE d_caregivers.cgid = chartevents.cgid
AND d_caregivers.cgid = 3891;

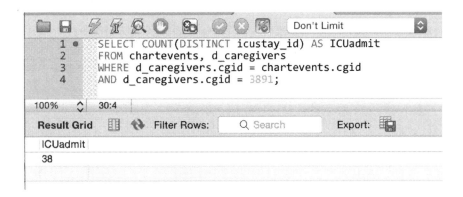

We can add another table to the same query and consolidate the two results with UNION:

(SELECT 'chartevents' AS OrigTable, COUNT(DISTINCT icustay_id) AS ICUadmit
FROM chartevents, d_caregivers
WHERE d_caregivers.cgid = chartevents.cgid
AND d_caregivers.cgid = 3891)
UNION
(SELECT 'noteevents' AS OrigTable, COUNT(DISTINCT icustay_id) AS ICUadmit
FROM noteevents, d_caregivers
WHERE d_caregivers.cgid = noteevents.cgid

AND d_caregivers.cgid = 3891);

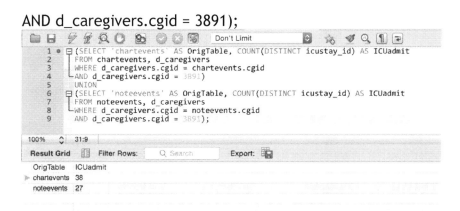

Question 72

Count all the ICU stays for caregiver 3891 from all the related tables and consolidate the results into one set.

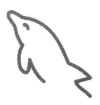

One care unit: all ICU stays related

Similarly to the previous query on care giver, we can retrieve from the **chartevents** table all the ICU stays, that care unit 1 (CCU) was involved with:

SELECT COUNT(DISTINCT icustay_id) AS ICUadmit
FROM chartevents, d_careunits
WHERE d_careunits.cuid = chartevents.cuid
AND d_careunits.cuid = 1;

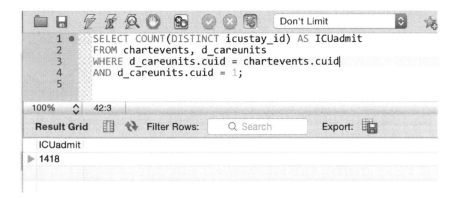

Question 73

Count the number of ICU stays for care unit 1 from the **chartevents, noteevents, medevents** tables and consolidate the results into one set.

20. Nursing

- One patient: all nursing events
- Restraints utilization
- Braden score

One patient: all nursing events

We have previously identified the following tables as containers of nursing information:

- chartevents
- medevents
- totalbalevents
- ioevents
- noteevents
- deliveries
- additives

Extracting all the nursing information on one patient from **chartevents**:

```
SELECT icustay_id, d_caregivers.cgid AS CareGiver,
d_caregivers.label AS ProvTitle, d_chartitems.label, value1
FROM chartevents, d_caregivers, d_chartitems
WHERE d_caregivers.cgid = chartevents.cgid
AND d_chartitems.itemid = chartevents.itemid
AND subject_id = 4655
AND d_caregivers.label = 'RN'
GROUP BY d_caregivers.cgid
ORDER BY realtime;
```

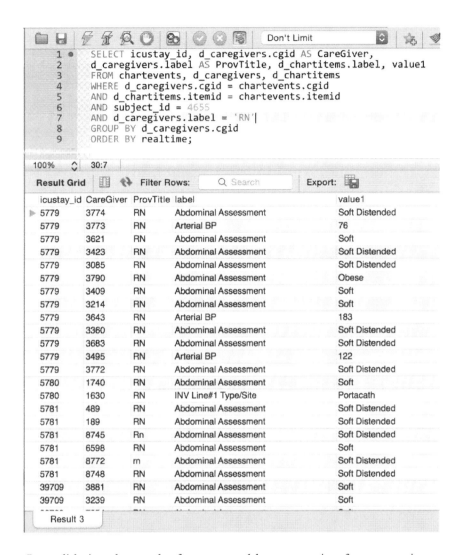

Consolidating the results from two tables on nursing for one patient:

(SELECT 'chartevents' AS OrigTable, icustay_id, d_caregivers.cgid AS CareGiver, realtime
FROM chartevents, d_caregivers
WHERE d_caregivers.cgid = chartevents.cgid
AND subject_id = 4655
AND d_caregivers.label = 'RN'
GROUP BY d_caregivers.cgid)
UNION
(SELECT 'totalbalevents' AS OrigTable, icustay_id, d_caregivers.cgid AS CareGiver, realtime
FROM totalbalevents, d_caregivers
WHERE d_caregivers.cgid = totalbalevents.cgid
AND subject_id = 4655
AND d_caregivers.label = 'RN'
GROUP BY d_caregivers.cgid)
ORDER BY realtime;

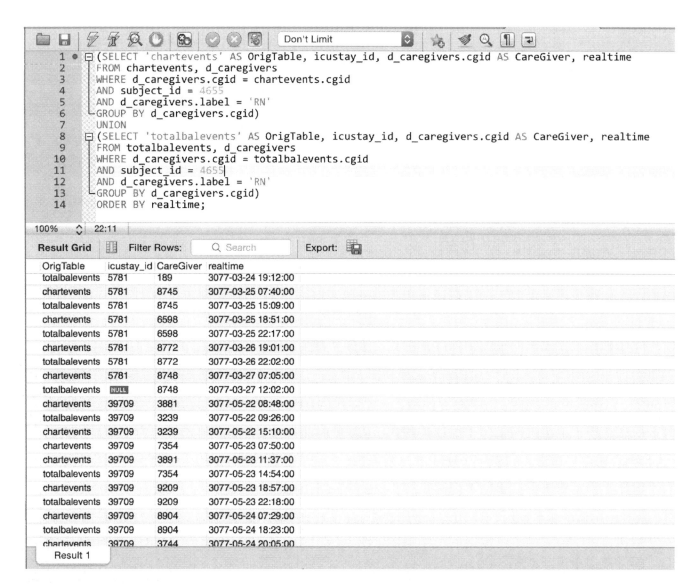

Question 74

Retrieve all the RN care givers, charting date and time, icustay_id related to patient 4655 from the seven relevant tables in the ERD on care givers. Consolidate all the query results into one set.

One patient: all nursing notes

From noteevents table we can retrieve all the nursing notes on a single patient:

```
SELECT icustay_id, charttime, d_caregivers.cgid, title, text
FROM noteevents, d_caregivers
WHERE d_caregivers.cgid = noteevents.cgid
AND subject_id = 4655
AND d_caregivers.label = 'RN'
ORDER BY charttime;
```

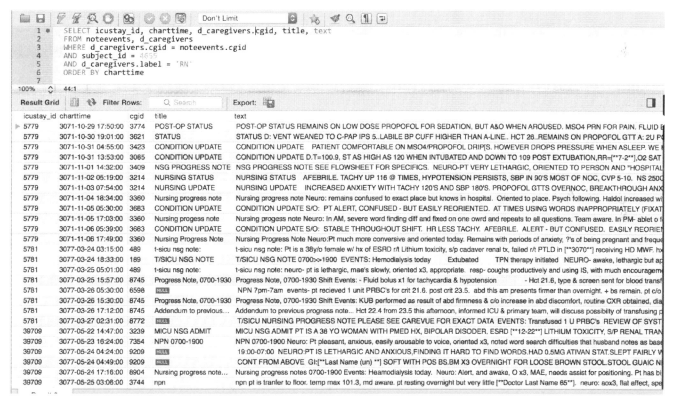

Restraints utilization

One of the nursing quality metrics is the utilization of physical restraints. The documentation of restraints use may be found in the **chartevents** table:

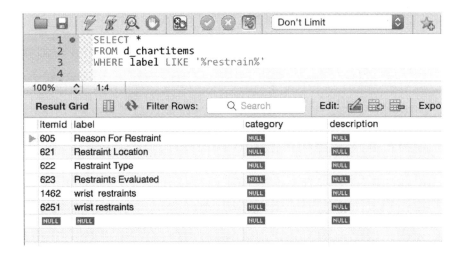

First, let's count the number of unique **icustay_id**, as the denominator:

SELECT COUNT(DISTINCT icustay_id) AS AllICUstays
FROM chartevents;

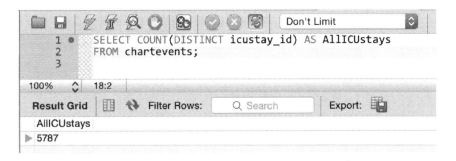

Now let's count the number of unique **icustay_id** where a restraint was used, as the numerator:

SELECT COUNT(DISTINCT icustay_id) AS RestrainedICUstays
FROM chartevents, d_chartitems
WHERE label LIKE '%restrain%'
AND d_chartitems.itemid = chartevents.itemid;

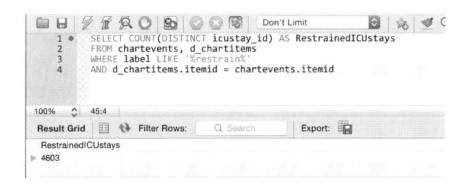

Restraints were used in (4,603 / 5,787 =) **79.5%** of ICU stays.

Question 75

Out of the 4,603 ICU stays where restraints have been used, how many had a documentation on the reason for the restraint ?

Question 76

Retrieve the number of patients that have been restrained by century.

Braden score

Another nursing quality indicator is the Braden Scale for predicting pressure ulcer risk. A score of 9 or less means a very high risk of developing a pressure ulcer.

Let's count the number of ICU stays where the Braden score was used, the denominator:

```
SELECT COUNT(DISTINCT icustay_id) AS BradenPts
FROM chartevents, d_chartitems
WHERE label = 'Braden Score'
AND d_chartitems.itemid = chartevents.itemid;
```

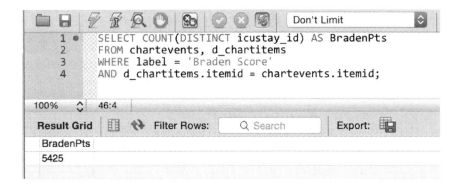

The numerator is the number of ICU stays with a Braden score of 9 or less:

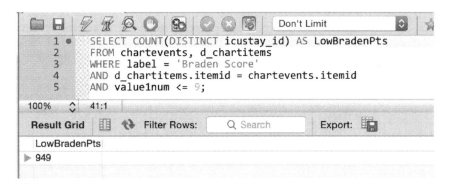

Percentage of ICU stays with a Braden score of 9 or less: 949 / 5,425 = **17.5%**

Question 77

Calculate the percentage of ICU stays with a Braden <=9 by century.

21. Fluid

- Fluids ERD
- One patient: all fluids
- One patient: all hourly fluid balances
- Hemoglobin level before blood is transfused

Fluids ERD

The MIMIC2 User Guide provides the following ERD related to fluids:

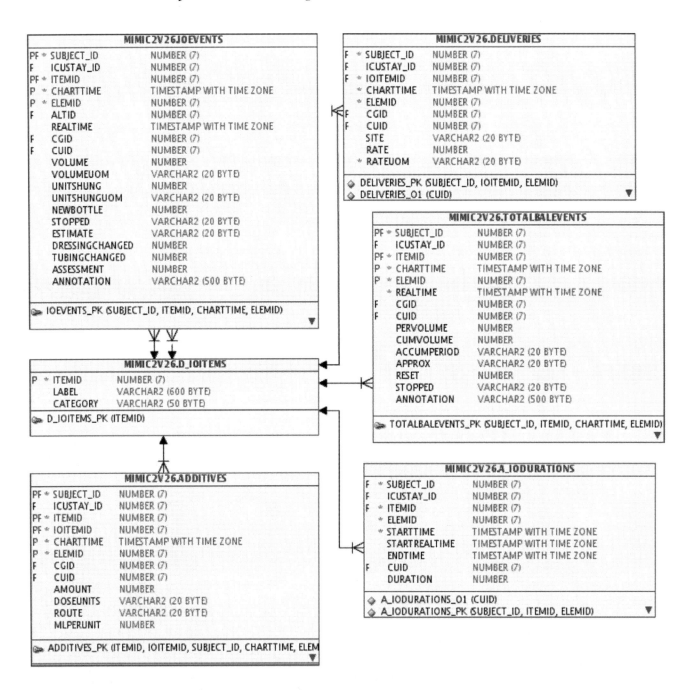

Figure 2.11: Patient IO data is stored in 6 tables. The ioevents, d_ioitems, a_iodurations, deliveries, totalbalevents and additives tables record all data related to patient charts.

One patient: all fluids

Using the last ERD, we can retrieve all the information about **subject_id = 4655** fluids from the table **ioevents**:

SELECT icustay_id, charttime, category, label, volume, volumeuom
FROM ioevents, d_ioitems
WHERE ioevents.itemid = d_ioitems.itemid
AND subject_id = 4655
ORDER BY charttime, category;

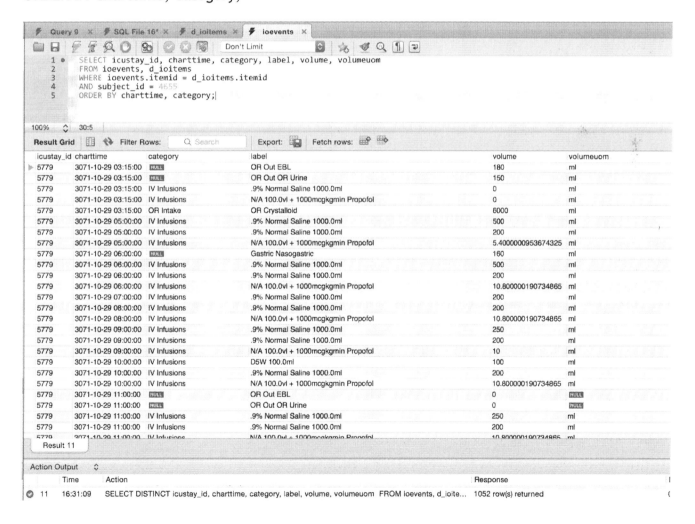

Question 78

The last query, retrieves information from only one table – **ioevents**. Retrieve all the information on fluids from the tables in the above ERD and order them by charttime, table and category.
Note the PK / FK mechanism is different between these tables.

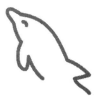

One patient: all hourly fluid balances

 Question 79

Retrieve all the net hourly fluid balances for patient **subject_id** = 12613 and display them in chronographic order.

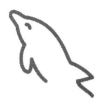

Hemoglobin level before blood is transfused

"Red blood cell (RBC) transfusions in most hospitalized patients should be performed based on "restrictive," rather than "liberal," **hemoglobin levels (7 - 8 g/dL)**, *according to new clinical guidelines from the* **American Association of Blood Banks (AABB)."* ... *Mar 26, 2012*

With the above recommendation in mind, let's identify the patients that have received RBC with a Hemoglobin (Hgb) level above 8 g/dL.

The query strategy:
- Identify the patients with a Hgb higher than 8
- Identify the patients that have received blood products
- Consolidate the two result sets into one, based on the **icustay_id**
- Limit the results to those with the Hgb date and time prior to the initiation of the blood transfusion
- Additionally we'll restrict the results to those with non-zero volumes of transfusions

Identify the patients with a Hgb higher than 8:

SELECT icustay_id, valuenum AS HbValue, charttime AS HbDT
FROM labevents, d_labitems
WHERE labevents.itemid = d_labitems.itemid
AND test_name = 'HGB'
AND valuenum > 8
GROUP BY icustay_id;

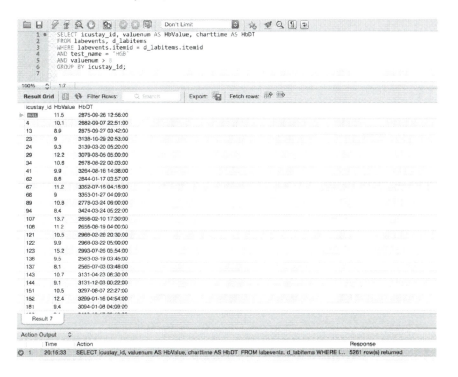

5,261 patients with at least one Hgb > 8 lab result.

Identify the patients that have received blood products:

We'll retrieve the earliest time that blood was transfused during an ICU stay, so we'll be able to compare the time of that blood transfusion with the time of the prior Hgb lab result:

SELECT icustay_id, MIN(realtime) AS BloodDT, label, cumvolume
FROM totalbalevents, d_ioitems
WHERE totalbalevents.itemid = d_ioitems.itemid
AND label = 'Blood Products Total'
GROUP BY icustay_id;

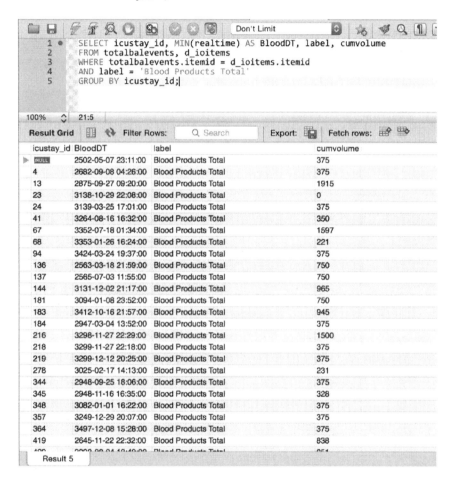

Consolidating the above two results:

SELECT PtsBlood.icustay_id, HbDT, HbValue, BloodDT, label, cumvolume
FROM

(SELECT icustay_id, valuenum AS HbValue, charttime AS HbDT
FROM labevents, d_labitems
WHERE labevents.itemid = d_labitems.itemid
AND test_name = 'HGB'
AND valuenum > 8
GROUP BY icustay_id) AS PtsHb,

```
(SELECT icustay_id, MIN(realtime) AS BloodDT, label, cumvolume
FROM totalbalevents, d_ioitems
WHERE totalbalevents.itemid = d_ioitems.itemid
AND label = 'Blood Products Total'
GROUP BY icustay_id) AS PtsBlood

WHERE PtsBlood.icustay_id = PtsHb.icustay_id
AND HbDT < BloodDT
AND cumvolume > 0
ORDER BY PtsBlood.icustay_id;
```

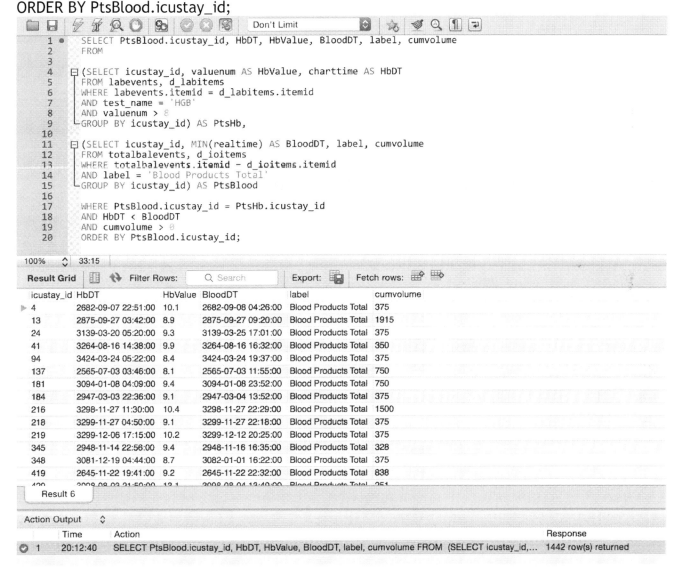

1,442 / 5,261 = 27% of ICU stays, patients have received blood products, while their pre-transfusion Hgb was higher than 8 g/dL

22. Score and scale

- Score and scale in MIMIC2
- One patient: all scores and scales
- SOFA and mortality
- SOFA and LOS
- SOFA and readmissions

Score and scale in MIMIC2

There are numerous scoring systems used in ICU.
Querying the Information Schema on columns related to score or scale will reveal only the SAPS-I (Simplified Acute Physiology Score) and SOFA (Sequential Organ Failure Assessment):

```
SELECT * FROM INFORMATION_SCHEMA.COLUMNS
WHERE TABLE_SCHEMA = 'mimic2'
AND (COLUMN_NAME LIKE '%scor%'
OR COLUMN_NAME LIKE '%scale%'
OR COLUMN_NAME LIKE '%SAPS%'
OR COLUMN_NAME LIKE '%SOFA%'
OR COLUMN_NAME LIKE '%GCS%'
OR COLUMN_NAME LIKE '%apache%');
```

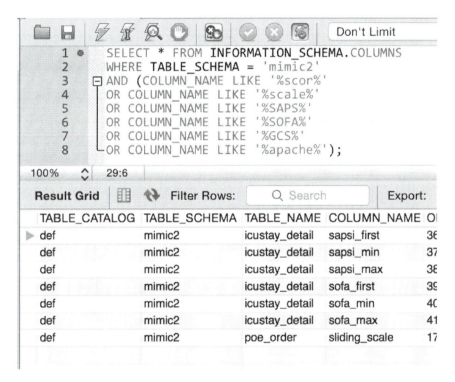

The sliding scale in the **poe_order** table is the Insulin dosing scale and has nothing to do with the score and scale at hand.
In the chapter on Nursing we have already retrieved information about the Braden score, from the **chartevents** table, which in turn is serviced by the dictionary table **d_chartitems**,. Thus, Braden score is not repeated in the **icustay_detail** table.
Let's check what other scores and scales are in the dictionary table **d_chartitems**:

```
SELECT * FROM d_chartitems
WHERE label LIKE '%scor%'
OR label LIKE '%GCS%'
OR label LIKE '%apache%'
OR label LIKE '%SAPS%'
```

OR label LIKE '%ramsey%'
OR label LIKE '%scale%';

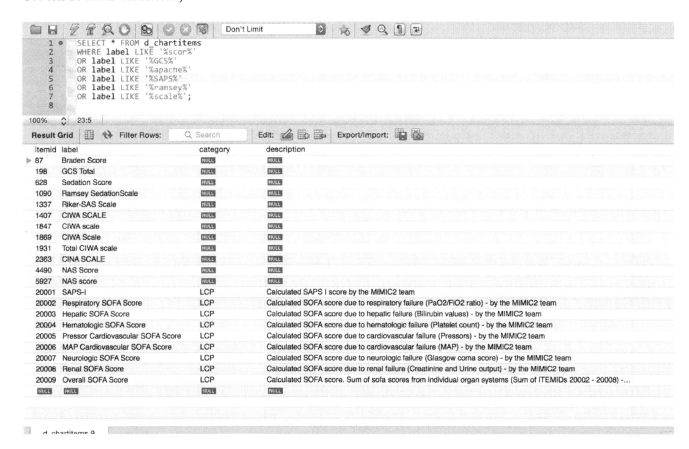

One patient: all scores and scales

It becomes clear that in order to retrieve all scores and scales of a patient we need search both the **chartvents** and the **icustay_detail** tables.

From the **chartvents** table, all the scores and scales documented for patient 1313:

SELECT icustay_id, label, charttime, value1
FROM d_chartitems, chartevents
WHERE d_chartitems.itemid = chartevents.itemid
AND (label = 'GCS Total'
OR label = 'Sedation Score'
OR label = 'NAS Score'
OR label = 'SAPS-I'
OR label = 'Overall SOFA Score')

AND subject_id = 1313
ORDER BY charttime;

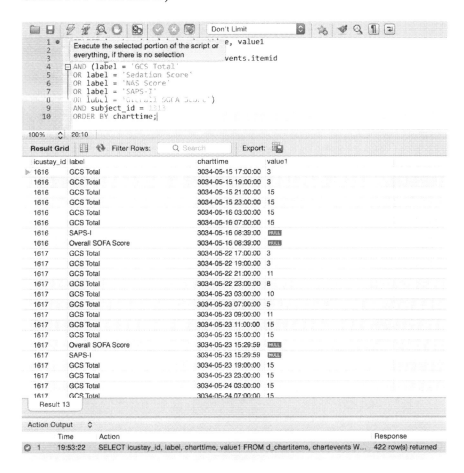

For the same patient, from the **icustay_detail** table, the SAPS-I and SOFA documented:

SELECT icustay_id, sapsi_first, sapsi_max, sapsi_min,
sofa_first, sofa_max, sofa_min
FROM mimic2.icustay_detail
WHERE subject_id = 1313;

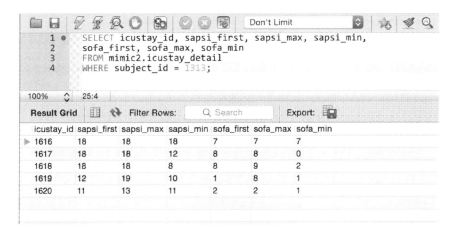

SOFA score and mortality

The SOFA score has predicting capabilities in terms of mortality and there are numerous articles on this subject. Let's compare the mortality vs. the SOFA score in MIMIC2. As there are three types of SOFA scores – first, min and max – we'll need to create 3 charts and see which one fits best.

First, let's find the denominator, the number of ICU stays with information on mortality, for each SOFA score:

SELECT sofa_first, COUNT(hospital_expire_flg)
FROM icustay_detail
GROUP BY sofa_first;

sofa_first	COUNT(hospital_expire_flg)
NULL	203
0	136
1	382
2	478
3	472
4	461
5	505
6	469
7	460
8	377
9	324
10	240
11	212
12	170
13	153
14	116
15	72
16	56
17	38
18	27
19	10
20	9
21	7
22	6
24	1

Export the above results to your favorite spreadsheet.

The numerator is the number of patients that have died, for each SOFA score:

SELECT sofa_first, COUNT(hospital_expire_flg)
FROM icustay_detail
WHERE hospital_expire_flg = 'Y'
GROUP BY sofa_first;

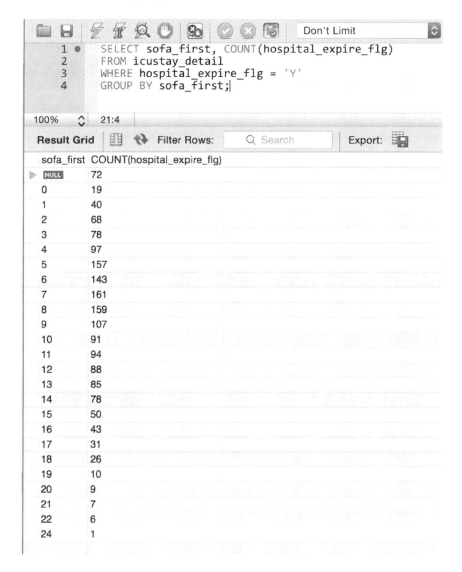

sofa_first	COUNT(hospital_expire_flg)
NULL	72
0	19
1	40
2	68
3	78
4	97
5	157
6	143
7	161
8	159
9	107
10	91
11	94
12	88
13	85
14	78
15	50
16	43
17	31
18	26
19	10
20	9
21	7
22	6
24	1

Export these results to a spreadsheet as well.
Eliminating the null values and consolidating the results into one chart:

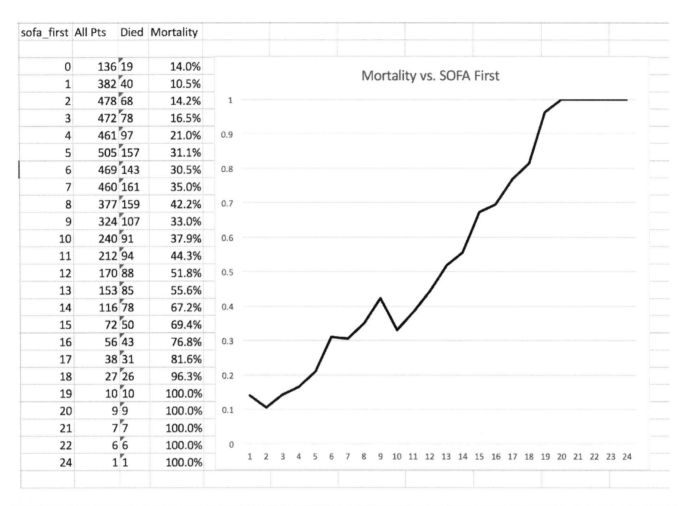

sofa_first	All Pts	Died	Mortality
0	136	19	14.0%
1	382	40	10.5%
2	478	68	14.2%
3	472	78	16.5%
4	461	97	21.0%
5	505	157	31.1%
6	469	143	30.5%
7	460	161	35.0%
8	377	159	42.2%
9	324	107	33.0%
10	240	91	37.9%
11	212	94	44.3%
12	170	88	51.8%
13	153	85	55.6%
14	116	78	67.2%
15	72	50	69.4%
16	56	43	76.8%
17	38	31	81.6%
18	27	26	96.3%
19	10	10	100.0%
20	9	9	100.0%
21	7	7	100.0%
22	6	6	100.0%
24	1	1	100.0%

Question 80

Repeat the above for SOFA min and SOFA max and plot their charts – mortality vs SOFA.

SOFA score and LOS

Let's chart the LOS in days vs the SOFA score. For this exercise, we are going to use only the SOFA First score. As both the SOFA score and the LOS are in the same table, we only need calculate average LOS for each score, by grouping on the SOFA score:

```
SELECT sofa_first, ROUND(AVG(hospital_los/60/24),1)
FROM icustay_detail
GROUP BY sofa_first;
```

sofa_first	AVG LOS
0	13.1
1	12
2	10.5
3	12.5
4	11.3
5	12.9
6	13.4
7	15.1
8	16.1
9	16
10	16.2
11	16.3
12	17.2
13	19.5
14	14.6
15	16.8
16	15.4
17	11.8
18	13
19	8.6
20	9.3
21	14.6
22	13.3
24	2

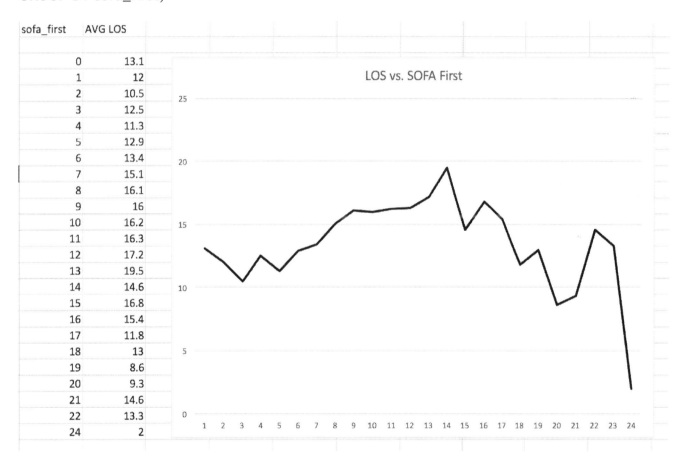

SOFA score and readmissions

Please review the chapter on readmissions, as the query mechanism is detailed there. Basically, we are going to compare the **icustay_detail** table to itself: once to get the admission dates, and the second time to identify the readmissions within 30 days.

First, let's identify the patients that have been readmitted and have a SOFA First score:

```
SELECT X.subject_id, X.hadm_id, X.hospital_admit_dt, X.hospital_disch_dt AS DISCHdate,
Y.hadm_id, Y.hospital_admit_dt AS READMITdate,
TIMESTAMPDIFF(DAY, X.hospital_disch_dt, Y.hospital_admit_dt) AS Time2Readmit,
X.sofa_first
FROM icustay_detail X, icustay_detail Y
WHERE X.subject_id = Y.subject_id
AND X.hadm_id <> Y.hadm_id
AND TIMESTAMPDIFF(DAY, X.hospital_disch_dt, Y.hospital_admit_dt) BETWEEN 0 AND 30;
```

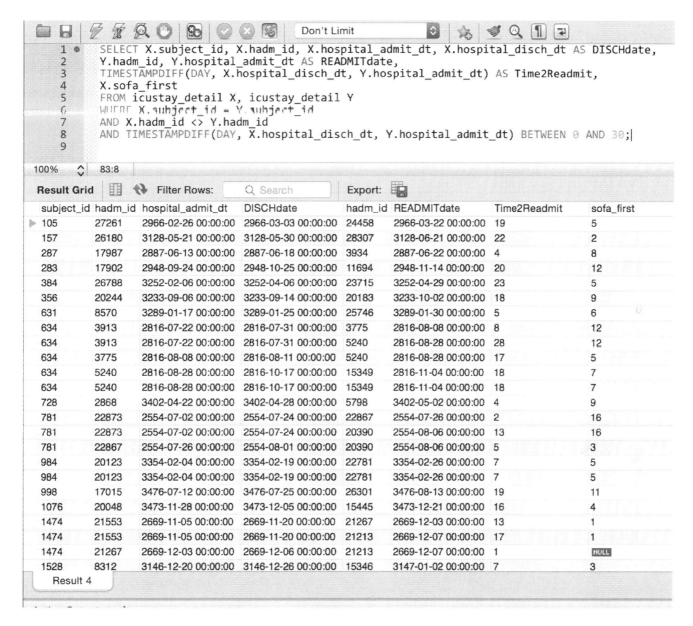

Now we can group the last results on **sofa_first**:

SELECT X.sofa_first, COUNT(X.hadm_id) AS Readmit
FROM icustay_detail X, icustay_detail Y
WHERE X.subject_id = Y.subject_id
AND X.hadm_id <> Y.hadm_id
AND TIMESTAMPDIFF(DAY, X.hospital_disch_dt, Y.hospital_admit_dt) BETWEEN 0 AND 30
GROUP BY X.sofa_first;

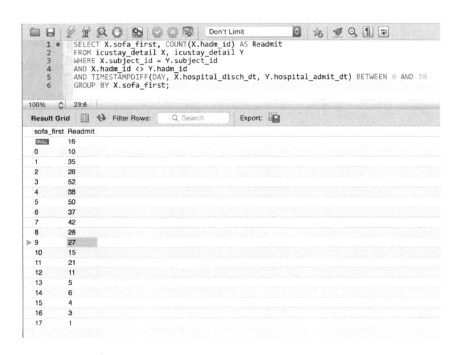

The above is the numerator –the number of patients readmitted, grouped by their SOFA First score. The denominator, the number of overall admissions by SOFA First:

SELECT sofa_first, COUNT(hadm_id) AS Admit
FROM icustay_detail
GROUP BY sofa_first;

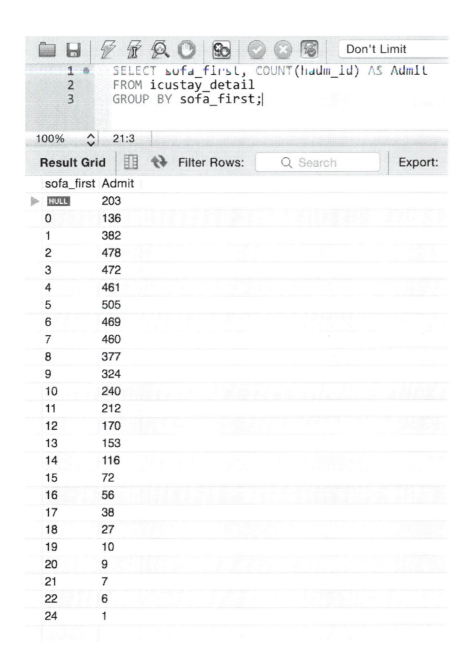

The numerator and denominator nicely arranged and charted in a spreadsheet:

sofa_first	Readmit	Admit	ReadmitRatio
0	10	136	7.4%
1	35	382	9.2%
2	28	478	5.9%
3	52	472	11.0%
4	38	461	8.2%
5	50	505	9.9%
6	37	469	7.9%
7	42	460	9.1%
8	28	377	7.4%
9	27	324	8.3%
10	15	240	6.3%
11	21	212	9.9%
12	11	170	6.5%
13	5	153	3.3%
14	6	116	5.2%
15	4	72	5.6%
16	3	56	5.4%
17	1	38	2.6%

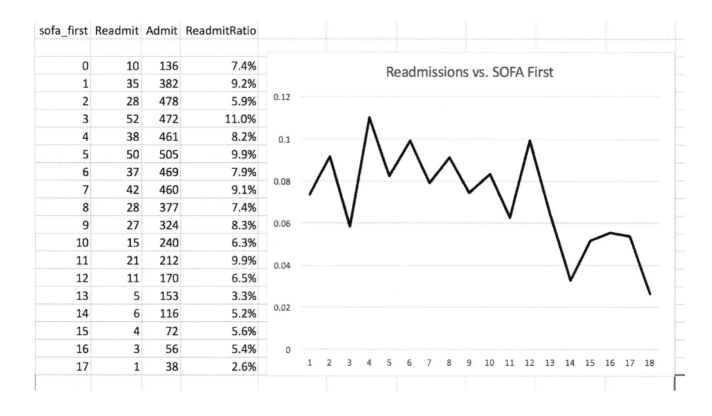

Appendix A. Answers to Questions

Answer 1

SELECT * FROM admissions;

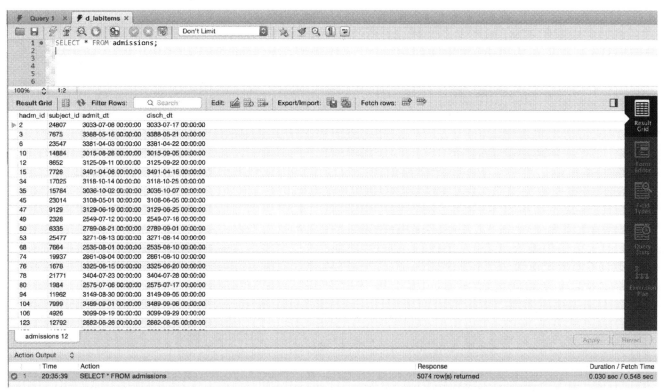

Answer 2

SELECT gender AS PatientGender, dob AS BirthDate, dod AS DeathDate

FROM icustay_detail;

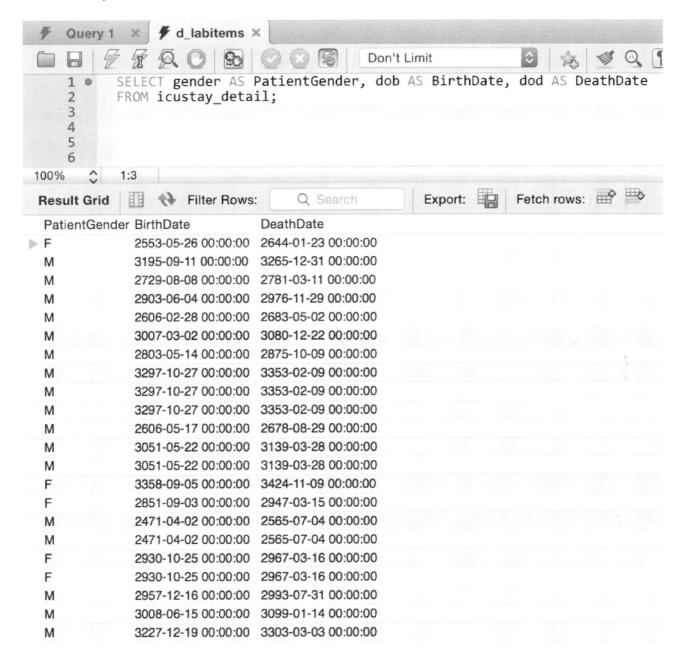

Answer 3

SELECT DISTINCT category

FROM noteevents;

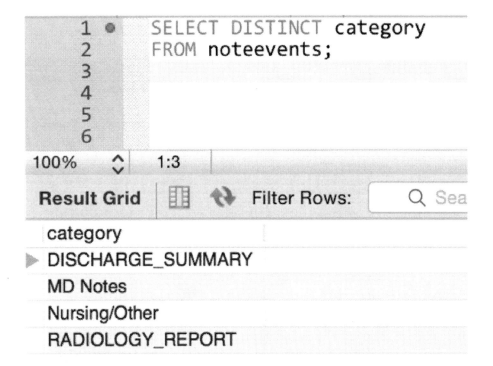

Answer 4

SELECT DISTINCT medication, doses_per_24hrs
FROM poe_order
ORDER BY medication, doses_per_24hrs;

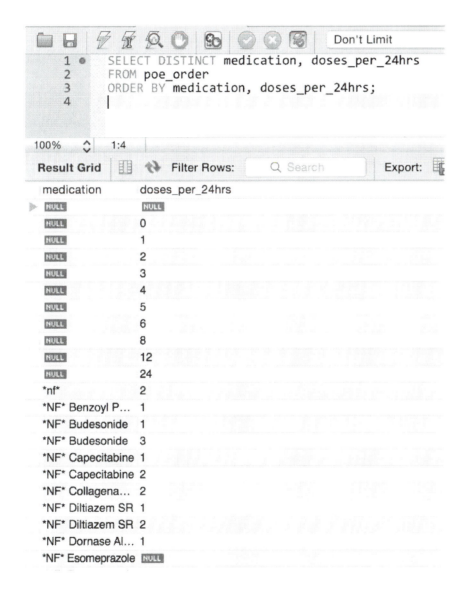

Answer 5

SELECT * FROM poe_order
WHERE medication = 'Diazepam'
AND route <> 'PO';

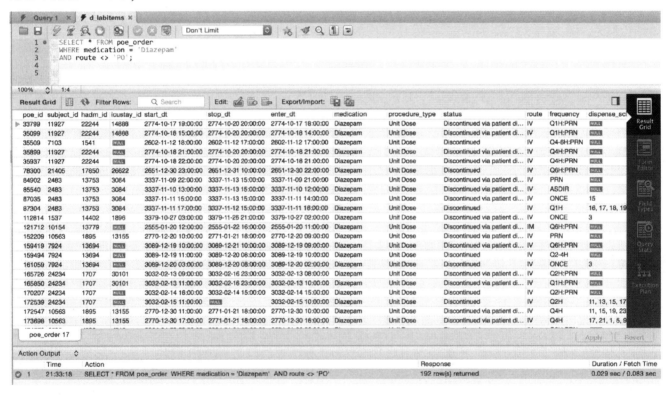

Answer 6

```
SELECT * FROM admissions
WHERE admit_dt BETWEEN '3000-01-01' AND '3100-12-31'
ORDER BY admit_dt;
```

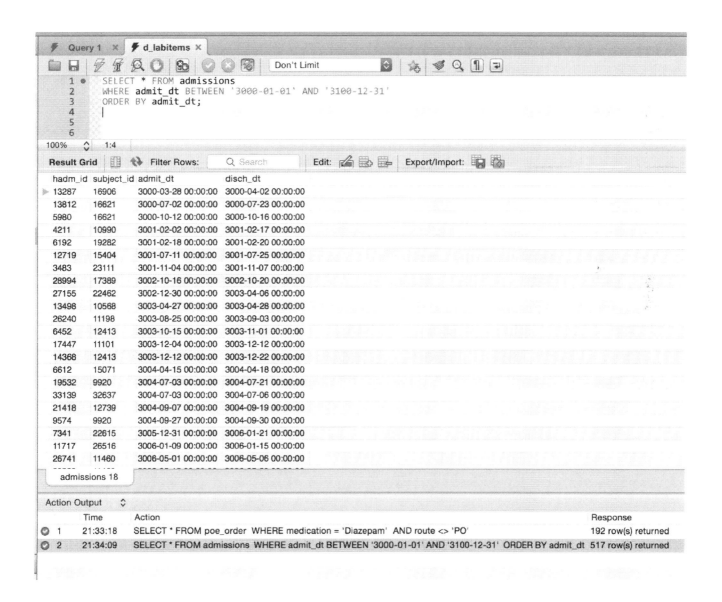

Answer 7

SELECT DISTINCT drug_name

FROM poe_med

WHERE drug_name LIKE '%azolam';

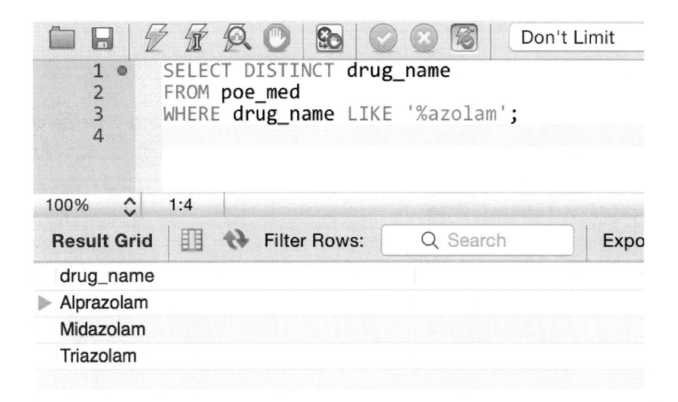

Answer 8

SELECT * FROM poe_order
WHERE medication LIKE '%ephrine%'
AND route NOT IN ('IV', 'IV drip', 'IM', 'SC')
AND start_dt BETWEEN '3000-01-01' AND '3500-01-01';

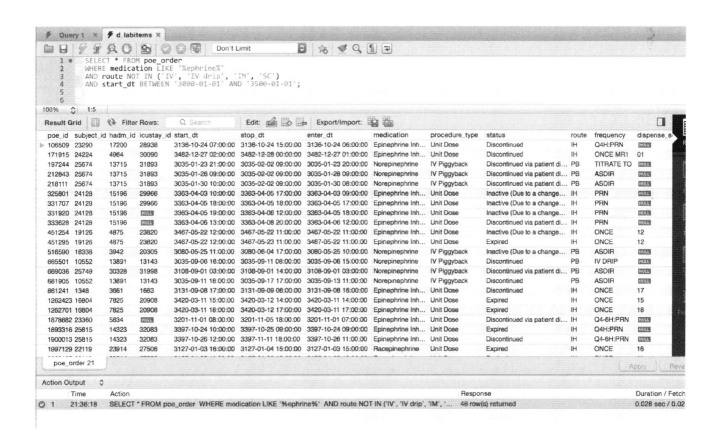

Answer 9

SELECT medication, start_dt, stop_dt, TIMESTAMPDIFF(HOUR, start_dt, stop_dt) AS PropofolInfusionHours
FROM poe_order
WHERE medication LIKE 'Propofol%'
AND TIMESTAMPDIFF(HOUR, start_dt, stop_dt) > 24;

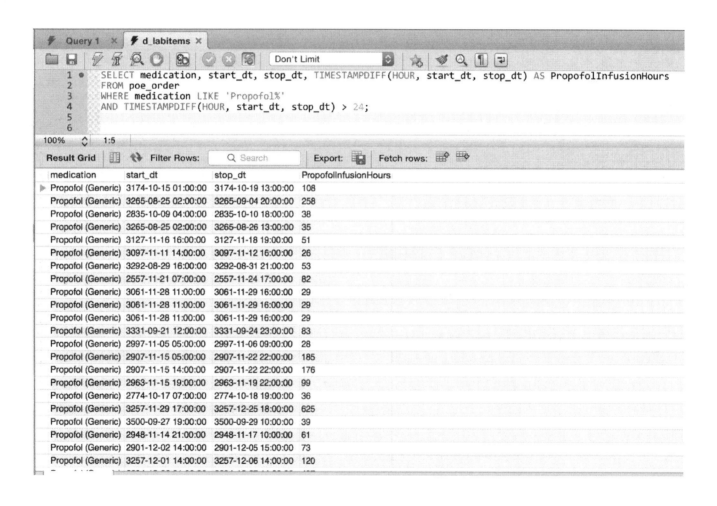

Answer 10

SELECT * FROM icustay_detail
WHERE height IS NOT NULL
AND weight_max IS NOT NULL;

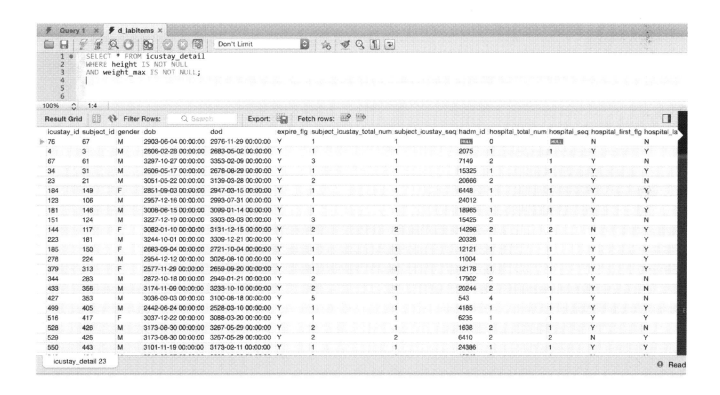

Answer 11

SELECT COUNT(DISTINCT drug_name)

FROM poe_med;

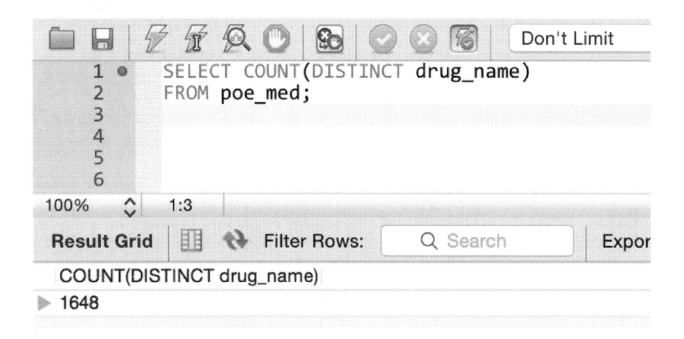

Answer 12

SELECT drug_name, AVG(dose_val_disp) AS Average, STD(dose_val_disp) AS StandDev
FROM poe_med
WHERE drug_name LIKE '%morphine%';

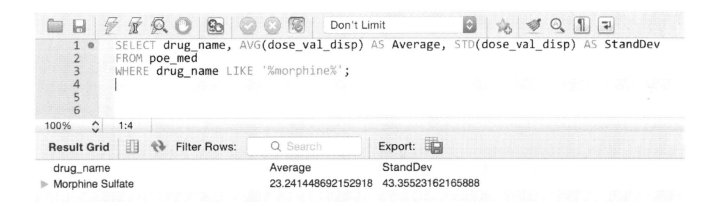

Answer 13

SELECT drug_name, AVG(dose_val_disp) AS Average

FROM poe_med

WHERE dose_val_disp IS NOT NULL

GROUP BY drug_name;

drug_name	Average
nf	600
NF Benzoyl Peroxide 5% Wash	10
NF Caspofungin Acetate	43.75
NF Collagenase Oint	1
NF Diltiazem SR	105
NF Fenoldopam Mesylate	20
NF Guaifenesin LA	600
NF Imatinib	100
NF Irbesartan	150
NF Levocarnitine	200
NF Lidocaine Patch 5%	1
NF Naltrexone	50
NF Ofloxacin 0.3% Ophth Soln	75
NF Phenytoin Sodium **Brand Name ONLY**	100
NF Sodium Chloride 5% (Hypertonic)	150
NF Sumatriptan	25
NF Tacrolimus Suspension	0.75
NF TIMOLOL HEMIHYDRATE (BETIMOL)	100
NF Tobramycin Soln	300
NF Valacyclovir	500
*NF*ESOMEPRAZOLE	20
1/2 NS	1

Answer 14

SELECT subject_id, COUNT(DISTINCT medication) AS Counter
FROM poe_order
GROUP BY subject_id, start_dt
HAVING Counter > 20;

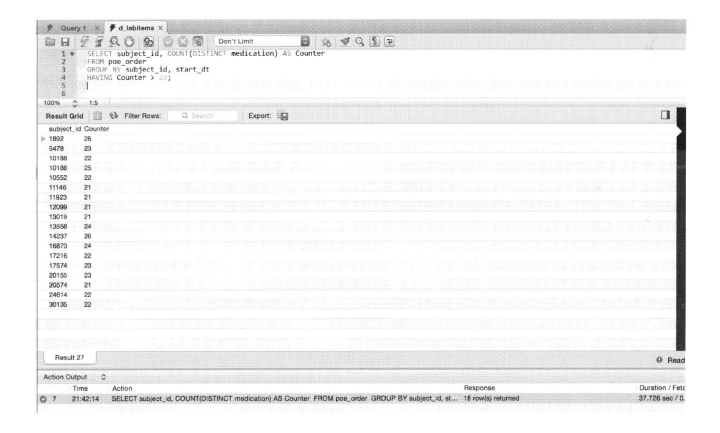

Answer 15

```
SELECT AVG(MedCounter) FROM
(
SELECT subject_id, COUNT(medication) AS MedCounter
FROM poe_order
GROUP BY subject_id, DATE(start_dt)
) AS MyTable;
```

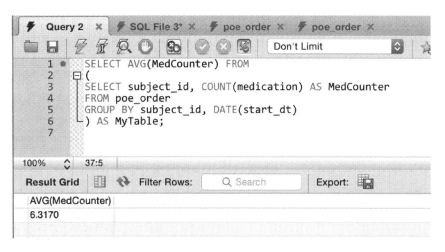

```
SELECT subject_id, start_dt, COUNT(medication) AS MedCounter
FROM poe_order
GROUP BY subject_id, DATE(start_dt)
HAVING MedCounter > 5 * 6.317
ORDER BY MedCounter DESC;
```

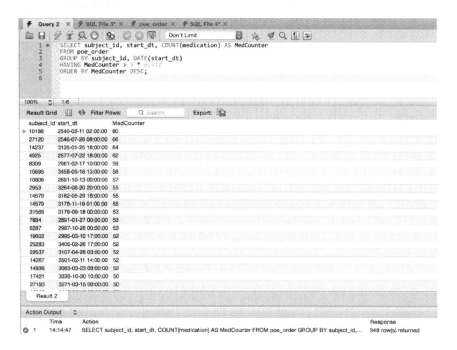

Answer 16

SELECT *
FROM d_labitems, d_meditems
WHERE test_name = label;

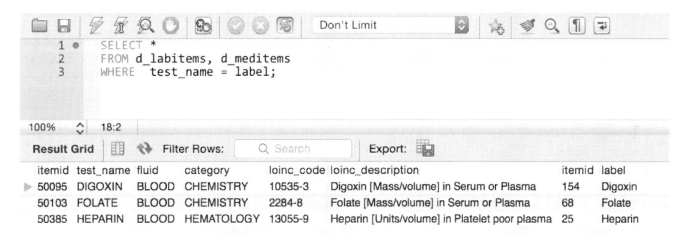

Answer 17

SELECT YEAR(datefield), MONTH(datefield), COUNT(dischstatus)
FROM calendar LEFT JOIN censusevents
ON DATE(datefield) = DATE(outtime)
WHERE datefield BETWEEN '2501-01-01' AND '2600-01-01'
GROUP BY YEAR(datefield), MONTH(datefield)
ORDER BY YEAR(datefield), MONTH(datefield);

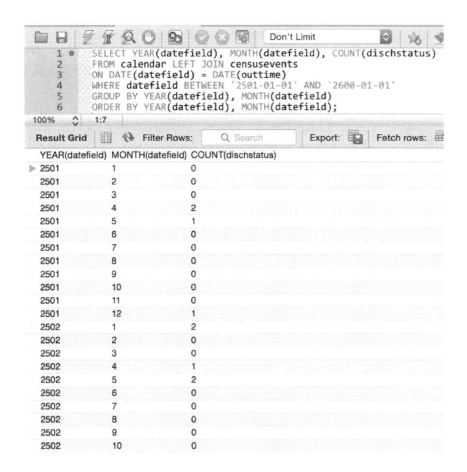

Answer 18

SELECT DISTINCT A.subject_id, A.medication, A.start_dt, B.medication, B.start_dt,
TIMESTAMPDIFF(HOUR, A.start_dt, B.start_dt)
FROM poe_order A, poe_order B
WHERE A.subject_id = B.subject_id
AND A.medication LIKE 'Morphine%'
AND B.medication LIKE 'Naloxone%'
AND TIMESTAMPDIFF(HOUR, A.start_dt, B.start_dt) BETWEEN 0 AND 24;

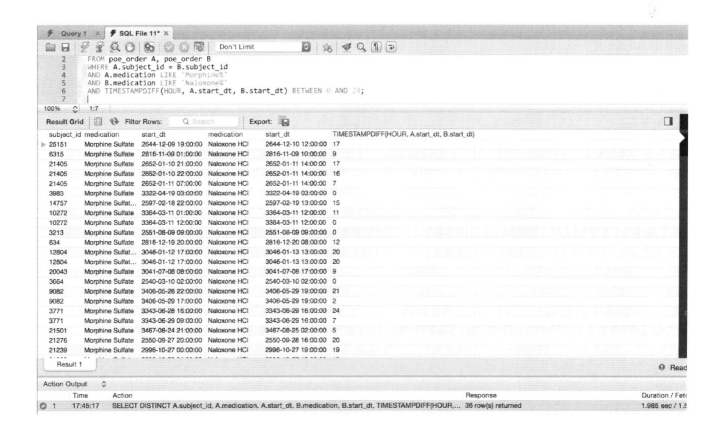

Answer 19

SELECT DISTINCT type FROM d_codeditems;

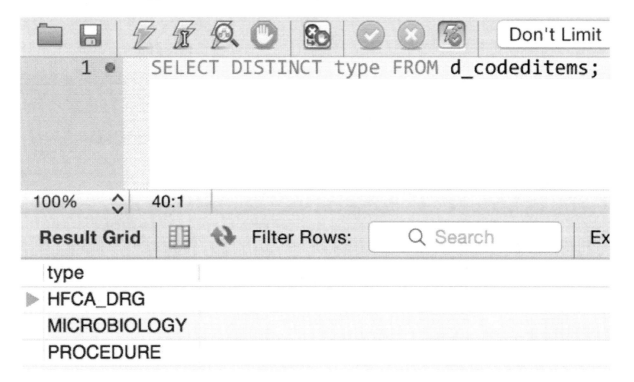

Answer 20

SELECT type, COUNT(*)

FROM d_codeditems

GROUP BY type;

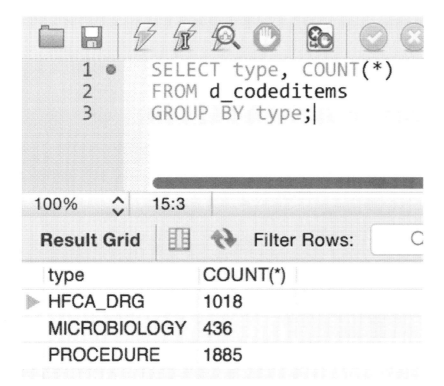

Answer 21

```
SELECT Description, COUNT(icd9.subject_id)
FROM d_patients, ICD9
WHERE d_patients.subject_id = ICD9.subject_id
GROUP BY Description
Order BY COUNT(icd9.subject_id) DESC;
```

Description	COUNT(icd9.subject_id)
UNSPECIFIED ESSENTIAL HYPERTENSION	1441
CONGESTIVE HEART FAILURE UNSPECIFIED	1330
ATRIAL FIBRILLATION	1197
ACUTE RESPIRATORY FAILURE	890
ACUTE RENAL FAILURE UNSPECIFIED	852
CORONARY ATHEROSCLEROSIS OF NATIVE...	816
DIABETES MELLITUS WITHOUT COMPLICATI...	681
URINARY TRACT INFECTION SITE NOT SPE...	606
CONGESTIVE HEART FAILURE	515
PNEUMONIA ORGANISM UNSPECIFIED	487
CHRONIC AIRWAY OBSTRUCTION NOT ELS...	465
PNEUMONITIS DUE TO INHALATION OF FOO...	463
NULL	461
SYSTEMIC INFLAMMATORY RESPONSE SY...	456
UNSPECIFIED SEPTICEMIA	443
PURE HYPERCHOLESTEROLEMIA	412
ACIDOSIS	399
SUBENDOCARDIAL INFARCTION INITIAL EPI...	381
ATRIAL FIBRILLATION	357
HYPERTENSION NOS	336
ANEMIA UNSPECIFIED	321
UNSPECIFIED ACQUIRED HYPOTHYROIDISM	316

Answer 22

SELECT Description, COUNT(drgevents.subject_id)
FROM drgevents, d_codeditems
WHERE drgevents.itemid = d_codeditems.itemid
GROUP BY Description
ORDER BY COUNT(drgevents.subject_id) DESC;

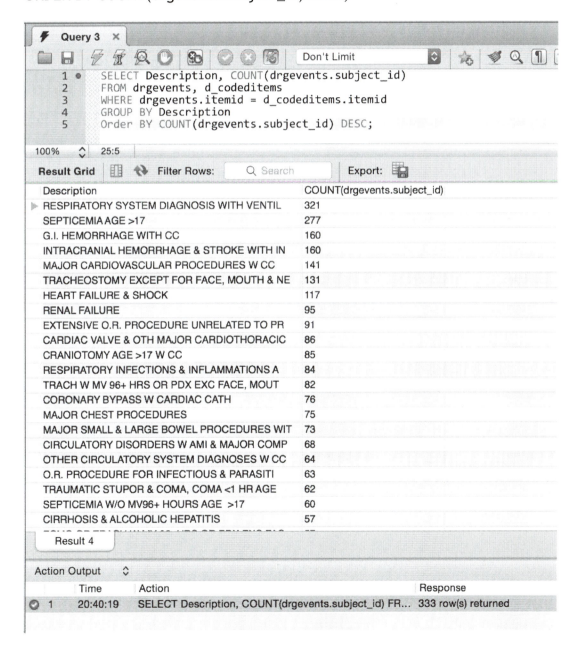

Answer 23

labevents is an intersection / junction entity that resolves multiple M:M relationships, such as one patient may have many labs and one lab may be used for many patients.

As such, it has the PK from the tables it connects, as FK:

itemid connects **labevents** to **d_labitems** table
subject_id connects **labevents** to **d_patients** table
hadm_id connects **labevents** to **admissions** table
icustay_id connects **labevents** to **icustay_detail** table

Answer 24

SELECT d_patients.subject_id, admit_dt, dob, TIMESTAMPDIFF(YEAR, dob, admit_dt) AS AgeAtAdmit
FROM admissions, d_patients
WHERE d_patients.subject_id = admissions.subject_id
ORDER BY d_patients.subject_id

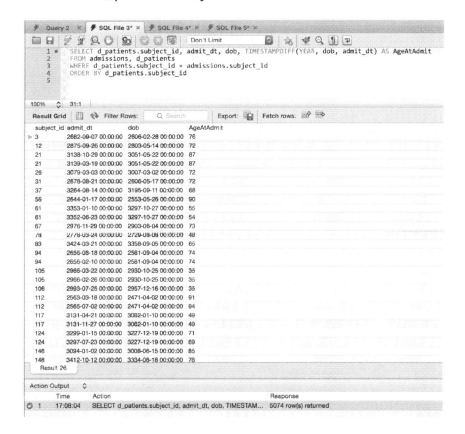

SELECT MIN(TIMESTAMPDIFF(YEAR, dob, admit_dt))AS MinAgeAtAdmit,
MAX(TIMESTAMPDIFF(YEAR, dob, admit_dt))AS MaxAgeAtAdmit,
AVG(TIMESTAMPDIFF(YEAR, dob, admit_dt))AS AVGAgeAtAdmit
FROM admissions, d_patients
WHERE d_patients.subject_id = admissions.subject_id

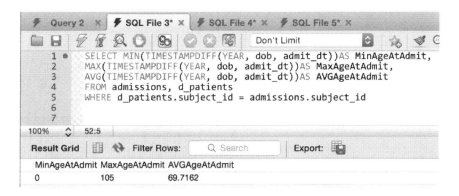

Answer 25

SELECT MIN(icustay_admit_age),
MAX(icustay_admit_age),
AVG(icustay_admit_age)
FROM icustay_detail;

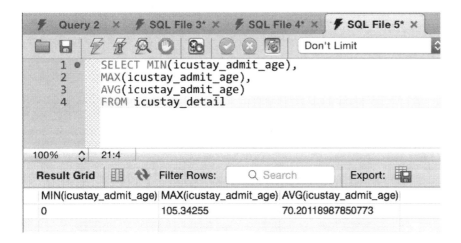

The reason there is a slight difference between results, is that the **icustay_admit_age** is at the decimal point precision, while the calculated values are based on integers, as the age is represented in whole years by the function TIMESTAMPDIFF (YEAR, etc).

Answer 26

SELECT FLOOR(icustay_admit_age/10) +1 AS Decade, COUNT(subject_id)
FROM icustay_detail
GROUP BY Decade;

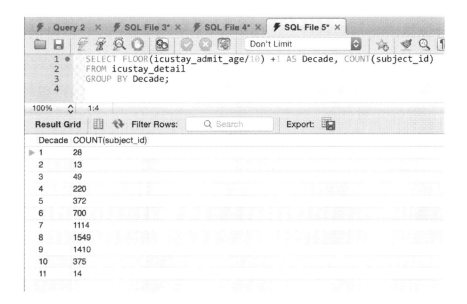

Answer 27

SELECT *
FROM admissions
WHERE subject_id = 25030;

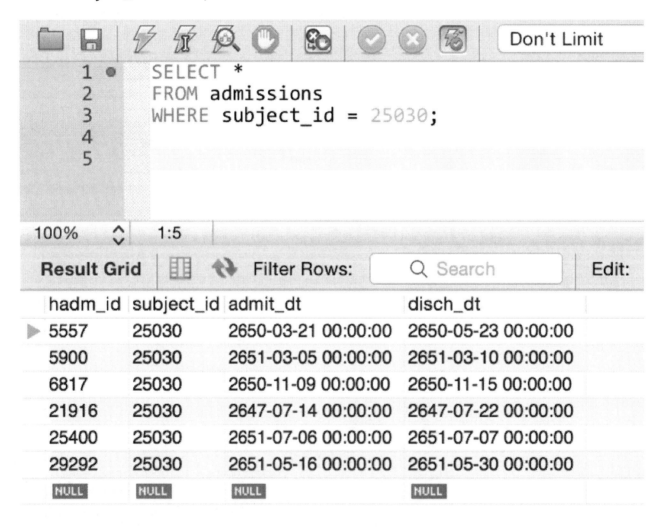

Answer 28

```
SELECT d_patients.subject_id, COUNT(hadm_id)
FROM d_patients LEFT JOIN admissions
ON d_patients.subject_id = admissions.subject_id
GROUP BY d_patients.subject_id
ORDER BY COUNT(hadm_id) DESC;
```

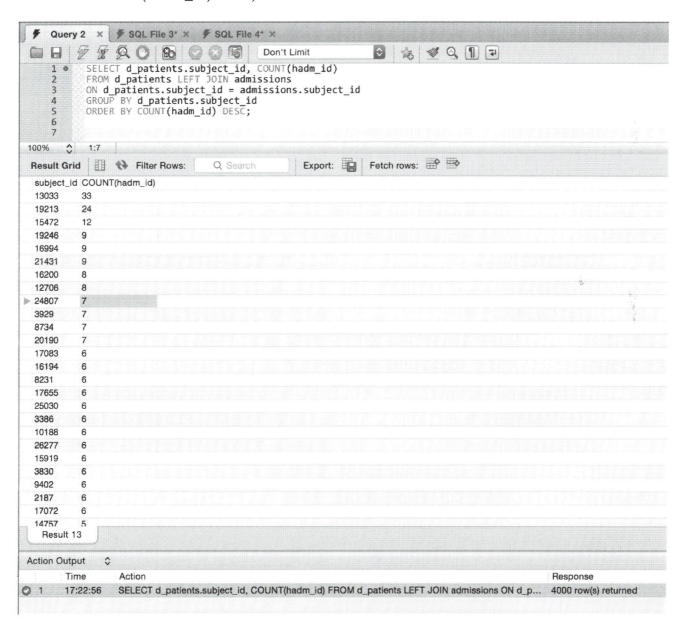

Answer 29

SELECT d_patients.subject_id, COUNT(hadm_id)
FROM d_patients LEFT JOIN admissions
ON d_patients.subject_id = admissions.subject_id
GROUP BY d_patients.subject_id
HAVING COUNT(hadm_id) = 0;

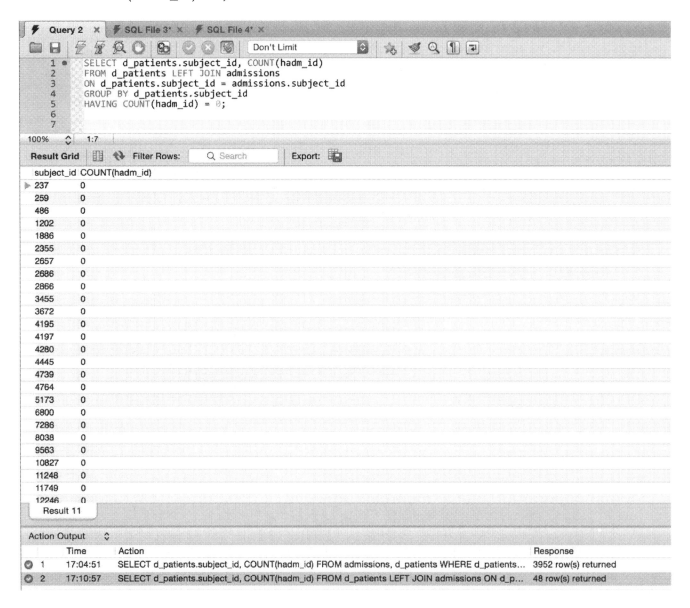

Answer 30

```sql
SELECT ROUND(MIN(weight_first), 1) AS MinW,
ROUND(MAX(weight_first),1 ) AS MaxW,
ROUND(AVG(weight_first),1) AS AvgW,
ROUND(STD(weight_first),1) AS StdW
FROM icustay_detail;
```

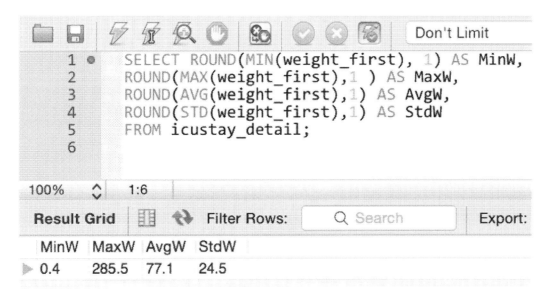

Answer 31

```sql
SELECT ROUND(MIN(height), 1) AS MinH,
ROUND(MAX(height),1 ) AS MaxH,
ROUND(AVG(height),1) AS AvgH,
ROUND(STD(height),1) AS StdH
FROM icustay_detail;
```

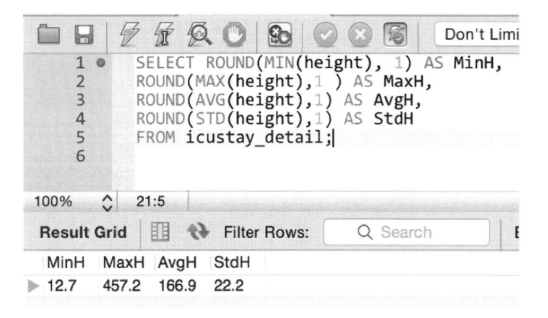

Answer 32

```sql
SELECT ROUND(MIN(height), 1) AS MinH,
ROUND(MAX(height),1 ) AS MaxH,
ROUND(AVG(height),1) AS AvgH,
ROUND(STD(height),1) AS StdH
FROM icustay_detail
WHERE height <= 208.28;
```

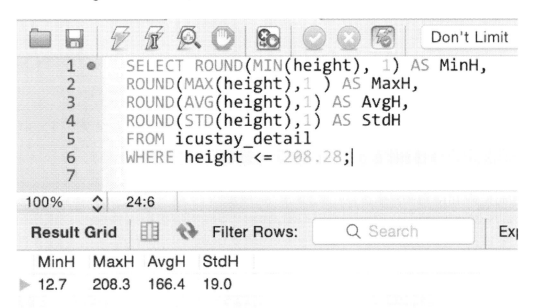

Answer 33

SELECT ROUND(AVG(weight_first/POWER((height/100),2)),2) AS BMI
FROM icustay_detail
WHERE weight_first/POWER((height/100),2) BETWEEN 10 AND 100;

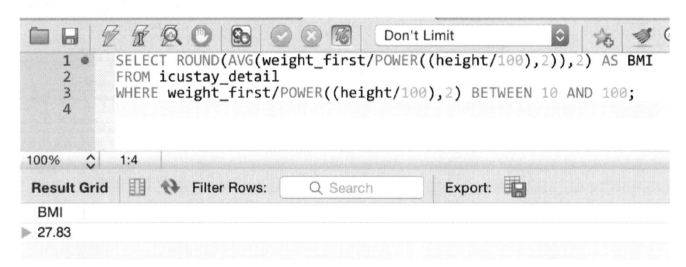

Answer 34

SELECT admission_source_descr, COUNT(DISTINCT subject_id) AS Counter
FROM demographic_detail
GROUP BY admission_source_descr
ORDER BY COUNT(DISTINCT subject_id) DESC;

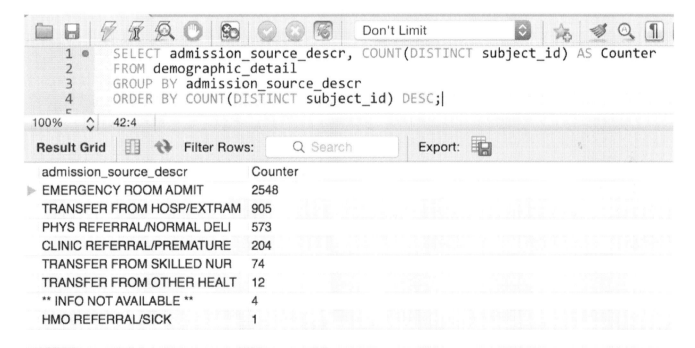

Answer 35

SELECT religion_descr, COUNT(DISTINCT subject_id) AS Counter
FROM demographic_detail
GROUP BY religion_descr
ORDER BY COUNT(DISTINCT subject_id) DESC;

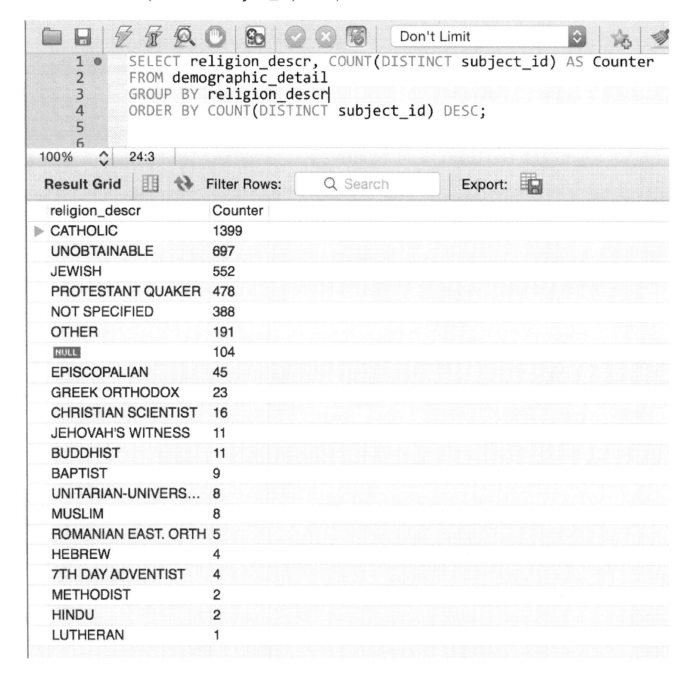

Answer 36

SELECT ethnicity_descr, overall_payor_group_descr, COUNT(subject_id) AS Counter
FROM demographic_detail
GROUP BY ethnicity_descr, overall_payor_group_descr
ORDER BY ethnicity_descr, Counter DESC;

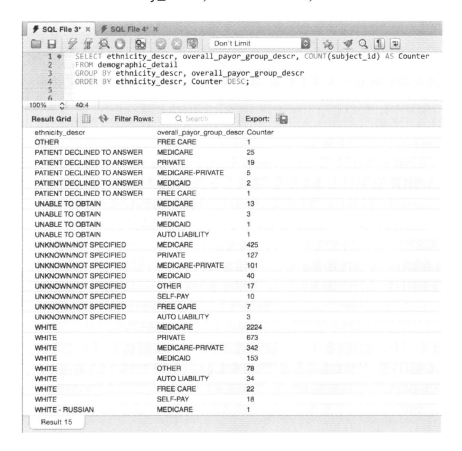

Answer 37

SELECT gender, COUNT(DISTINCT hadm_id), icustay_expire_flg
FROM icustay_detail
GROUP BY gender, icustay_expire_flg;

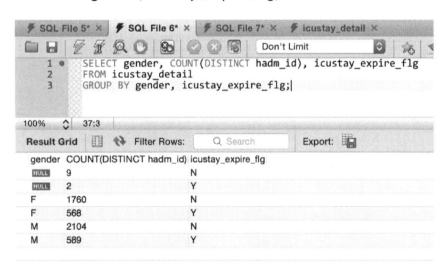

Female ICU mortality: 568 /(1760+568) = 24.4%
Male ICU mortality: 589 /(2104+589) = 21.9%

Answer 38

SELECT admission_type_descr, hospital_expire_flg, COUNT(icustay_detail.hadm_id) AS NumAdmissions
FROM demographic_detail, icustay_detail
WHERE demographic_detail.hadm_id = icustay_detail.hadm_id
GROUP BY admission_type_descr, hospital_expire_flg;

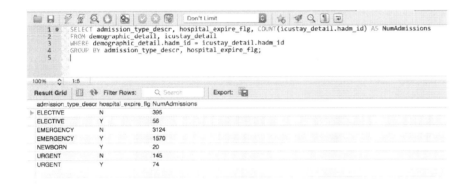

admission_type_descr	hospital_expire_flg	NumAdmissions	Total	Mortality
ELECTIVE	N	395		
ELECTIVE	Y	56	451	12.4%
EMERGENCY	N	3124		
EMERGENCY	Y	1570	4694	33.4%
NewBORN	N	0		
NEWBORN	Y	20	20	100.0%
URGENT	N	145		
URGENT	Y	74	219	33.8%
Total		5384	5384	

Answer 39

SELECT hospital_expire_flg, YEAR(datefield) AS YearAdmit,
COUNT(hospital_admit_dt) AS NumAdmissions
FROM calendar LEFT JOIN icustay_detail
ON datefield = hospital_admit_dt
WHERE hospital_expire_flg IS NOT NULL
GROUP BY hospital_expire_flg, YEAR(datefield)
ORDER BY YEAR(datefield);

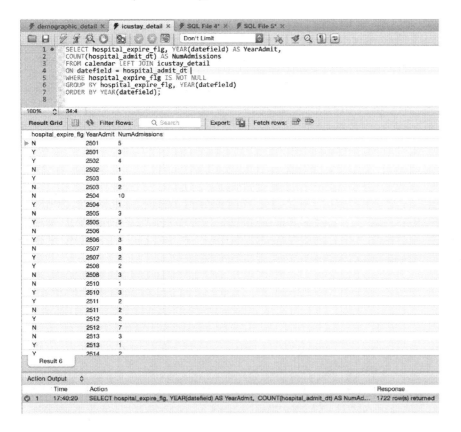

Answer 40

SELECT ROUND(AVG(hospital_los/60/24),2) AS AvgLOSdays
FROM icustay_detail;

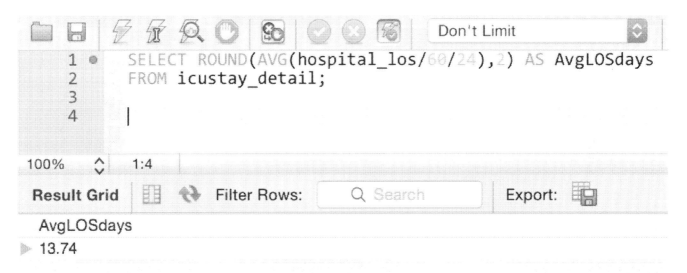

AvgLOSdays
13.74

Answer 41

SELECT gender,
ROUND(AVG(hospital_los/60/24),1) AvgLOSdays,
COUNT(hadm_id) AS NumAdmissions
FROM icustay_detail
GROUP BY gender;

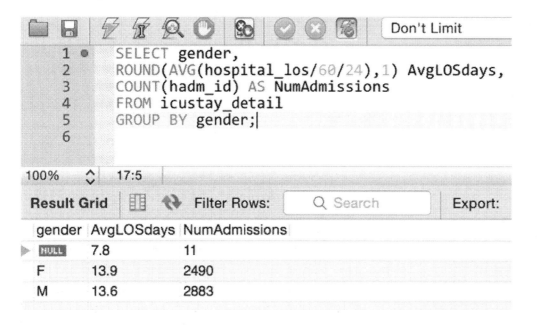

Answer 42

```
SELECT ROUND(AVG(weight_first/POWER((height/100),2)),1) AS AvgLOS,
COUNT(hadm_id) AS NumAdmissions
FROM icustay_detail
WHERE weight_first/POWER((height/100),2) BETWEEN 10 AND 18.5
AND hospital_los IS NOT NULL;

SELECT ROUND(AVG(weight_first/POWER((height/100),2)),1) AS AvgLOS,
COUNT(hadm_id) AS NumAdmissions
FROM icustay_detail
WHERE weight_first/POWER((height/100),2) BETWEEN 18.6 AND 24.9
AND hospital_los IS NOT NULL;

SELECT ROUND(AVG(weight_first/POWER((height/100),2)),1) AS AvgLOS,
COUNT(hadm_id) AS NumAdmissions
FROM icustay_detail
WHERE weight_first/POWER((height/100),2) BETWEEN 25.0 AND 29.9
AND hospital_los IS NOT NULL;

SELECT ROUND(AVG(weight_first/POWER((height/100),2)),1) AS AvgLOS,
COUNT(hadm_id) AS NumAdmissions
FROM icustay_detail
WHERE weight_first/POWER((height/100),2) BETWEEN 30 AND 100
AND hospital_los IS NOT NULL;
```

BMI	LOS	Admissions
Underweight	16.8	104
Normal	22.2	733
Overweight	27.4	610
Obese	37.1	608
Total		2055

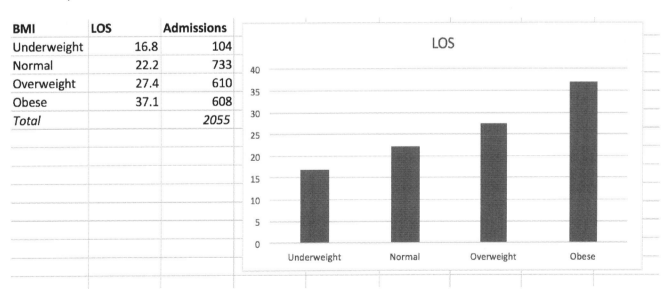

Answer 43

SELECT admission_type_descr,
ROUND(AVG(hospital_los/60/24),1) AS AvgLOSdays,
COUNT(icustay_detail.hadm_id) AS NumAdmissions
FROM demographic_detail, icustay_detail
WHERE demographic_detail.hadm_id = icustay_detail.hadm_id
GROUP BY admission_type_descr;

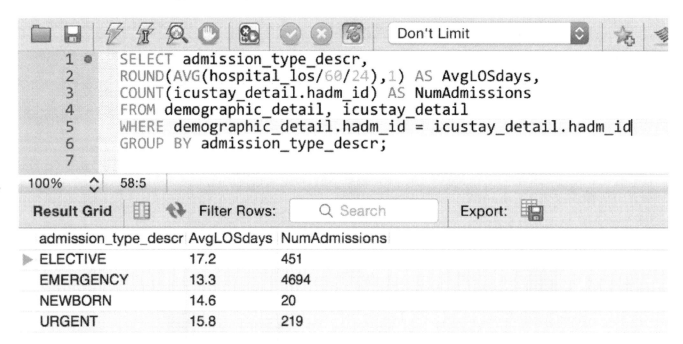

Answer 44

SELECT FLOOR(YEAR(hospital_admit_dt)/100) AS CenturyAdmit,
ROUND(AVG(hospital_los/60/24),1) AS CenturyAVGLOS
FROM icustay_detail
WHERE hospital_expire_flg IS NOT NULL
GROUP BY CenturyAdmit;

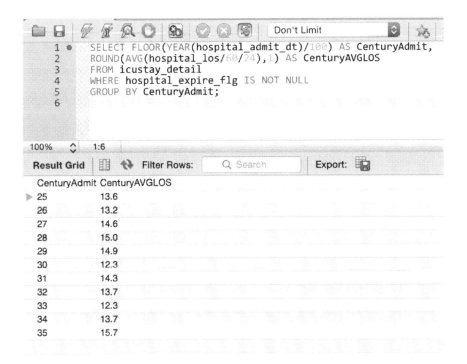

Answer 45

SELECT FLOOR(YEAR(hospital_admit_dt)/100) AS CenturyAdmit,
COUNT(hadm_id) as NumAdmissions
FROM icustay_detail
GROUP by CenturyAdmit;

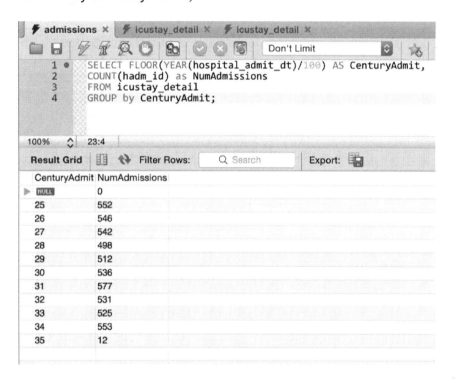

CenturyAdmit	NumPtsReadmit	Admissions	Readmit Rate
25	52	552	9.4%
26	43	546	7.9%
27	40	542	7.4%
28	28	498	5.6%
29	39	512	7.6%
30	44	536	8.2%
31	64	577	11.1%
32	25	531	4.7%
33	43	525	8.2%
34	51	553	9.2%
35	0	12	0.0%
Total	429	5384	8.0%

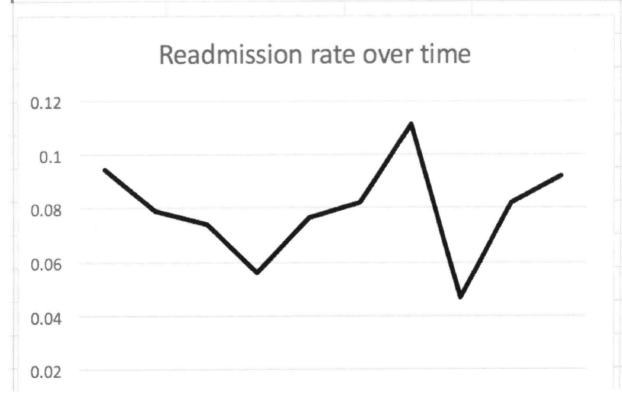

Readmission rate over time

Answer 46

```sql
SELECT TotPts.code, TotPts.description,
NumPts, IFNULL(Died,0) AS Died,
IFNULL(ROUND((((Died / NumPts) * 100),1),0) AS MortalityByDiagnosis

FROM (
SELECT code, description, COUNT(DISTINCT icustay_detail.subject_id) AS NumPts
FROM icustay_detail, icd9
WHERE icustay_detail.subject_id = icd9.subject_id
AND hospital_expire_flg IS NOT NULL
GROUP BY code) AS TotPts

LEFT JOIN

(SELECT code, description, COUNT(DISTINCT icustay_detail.subject_id) AS Died
FROM icustay_detail, icd9
WHERE icustay_detail.subject_id = icd9.subject_id
AND hospital_expire_flg ='Y'
GROUP BY code) AS DeadPts

ON TotPts.code = DeadPts.code

ORDER BY MortalityByDiagnosis;
```

```sql
SELECT TotPts.code, TotPts.description,
NumPts, IFNULL(Died,0) AS Died,
IFNULL(ROUND(((Died / NumPts) * 100),1),0) AS MortalityByDiagnosis

FROM (
    SELECT code, description, COUNT(DISTINCT icustay_detail.subject_id) AS NumPts
    FROM icustay_detail, icd9
    WHERE icustay_detail.subject_id = icd9.subject_id
    AND hospital_expire_flg IS NOT NULL
    GROUP BY code) AS TotPts

LEFT JOIN

(SELECT code, description, COUNT(DISTINCT icustay_detail.subject_id) AS Died
    FROM icustay_detail, icd9
    WHERE icustay_detail.subject_id = icd9.subject_id
    AND hospital_expire_flg ='Y'
    GROUP BY code) AS DeadPts

ON TotPts.code = DeadPts.code

ORDER BY MortalityByDiagnosis;
```

code	description	NumPts	Died	MortalityByDiagnosis
110.9	DERMATOPHYTOSIS OF UNSPECIFIED SITE	1	0	0.0
E950.4	SUICIDE AND SELF-INFLICTED POISONING BY OTHER SPEC	1	0	0.0
482.32	PNEUMONIA DUE TO STREPTOCOCCUS GROUP B	1	0	0.0
252.02	SECONDARY HYPERPARATHYRO	1	0	0.0
202.81	LYMPHOMAS NEC HEAD	2	0	0.0
969.8	POISONING BY OTHER SPECIFIED PSYCHOTROPIC AGENTS	2	0	0.0
V58.43	AFTRCRE FOLW SURG/TRAUMA	1	0	0.0
277.4	DISORDERS OF BILIRUBIN EXCRETION	1	0	0.0
709.9	SKIN DISORDER NOS	2	0	0.0
423.1	ADHESIVE PERICARDITIS	3	0	0.0
V12.71	PERS HIST PEPTIC ULC DIS	1	0	0.0
244.0	POSTSURGICAL HYPOTHYROIDISM	8	0	0.0
724.3	SCIATICA	4	0	0.0

Answer 47

SELECT TotPts.code, TotPts.description,
NumPts, Died,
ROUND(((Died / NumPts) * 100),1) AS MortalityByDRG

FROM (
SELECT code, description, COUNT(hospital_expire_flg) AS NumPts
FROM drgevents, d_codeditems, icustay_detail
WHERE drgevents.itemid = d_codeditems.itemid
AND icustay_detail.hadm_id = drgevents.hadm_id
GROUP BY code) AS TotPts

LEFT JOIN

(SELECT code, description, COUNT(hospital_expire_flg) AS Died
FROM drgevents, d_codeditems, icustay_detail
WHERE drgevents.itemid = d_codeditems.itemid
AND icustay_detail.hadm_id = drgevents.hadm_id
AND hospital_expire_flg = 'Y'
GROUP BY code) AS DeadPts

ON TotPts.code = DeadPts.code
ORDER BY MortalityByDRG DESC;

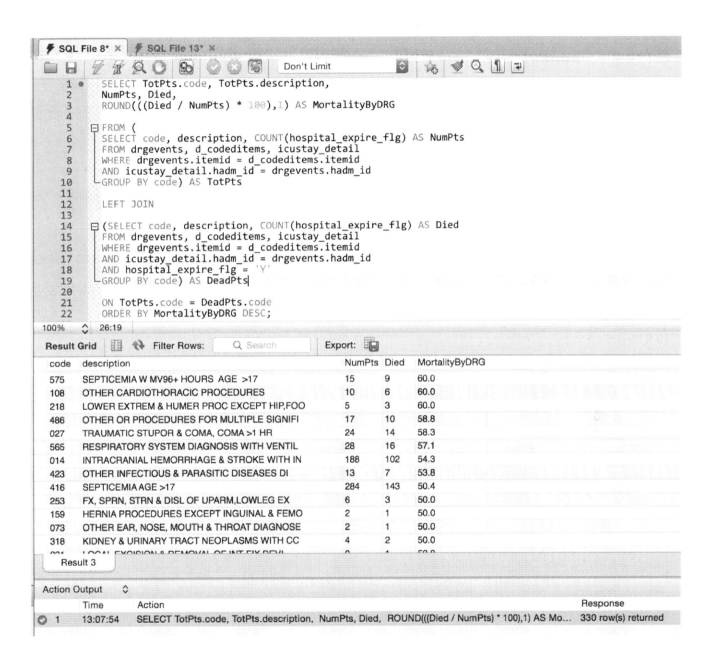

Answer 48

SELECT code, description,
ROUND(AVG(hospital_los/60/24),1) AS AvgLOSdays, COUNT(icustay_detail.hadm_id) AS NumAdmit
FROM icustay_detail, drgevents, d_codeditems
WHERE icustay_detail.hadm_id = drgevents.hadm_id
AND drgevents.itemid = d_codeditems.itemid
GROUP BY code
ORDER BY NumAdmit DESC;

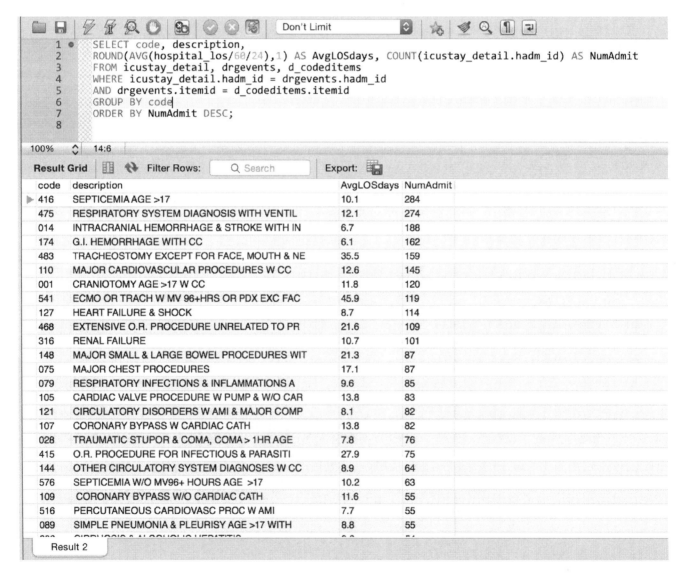

code	description	AvgLOSdays	NumAdmit
416	SEPTICEMIA AGE >17	10.1	284
475	RESPIRATORY SYSTEM DIAGNOSIS WITH VENTIL	12.1	274
014	INTRACRANIAL HEMORRHAGE & STROKE WITH IN	6.7	188
174	G.I. HEMORRHAGE WITH CC	6.1	162
483	TRACHEOSTOMY EXCEPT FOR FACE, MOUTH & NE	35.5	159
110	MAJOR CARDIOVASCULAR PROCEDURES W CC	12.6	145
001	CRANIOTOMY AGE >17 W CC	11.8	120
541	ECMO OR TRACH W MV 96+HRS OR PDX EXC FAC	45.9	119
127	HEART FAILURE & SHOCK	8.7	114
468	EXTENSIVE O.R. PROCEDURE UNRELATED TO PR	21.6	109
316	RENAL FAILURE	10.7	101
148	MAJOR SMALL & LARGE BOWEL PROCEDURES WIT	21.3	87
075	MAJOR CHEST PROCEDURES	17.1	87
079	RESPIRATORY INFECTIONS & INFLAMMATIONS A	9.6	85
105	CARDIAC VALVE PROCEDURE W PUMP & W/O CAR	13.8	83
121	CIRCULATORY DISORDERS W AMI & MAJOR COMP	8.1	82
107	CORONARY BYPASS W CARDIAC CATH	13.8	82
028	TRAUMATIC STUPOR & COMA, COMA > 1HR AGE	7.8	76
415	O.R. PROCEDURE FOR INFECTIOUS & PARASITI	27.9	75
144	OTHER CIRCULATORY SYSTEM DIAGNOSES W CC	8.9	64
576	SEPTICEMIA W/O MV96+ HOURS AGE >17	10.2	63
109	CORONARY BYPASS W/O CARDIAC CATH	11.6	55
516	PERCUTANEOUS CARDIOVASC PROC W AMI	7.7	55
089	SIMPLE PNEUMONIA & PLEURISY AGE >17 WITH	8.8	55

Answer 49

```sql
SELECT code, description,
AVG(TIMESTAMPDIFF(DAY, X.disch_dt, Y.admit_dt)) AS AvgDays2Readmit,
COUNT(Y.hadm_id) AS NumAdmit
FROM admissions X, admissions Y, icd9
WHERE X.subject_id = Y.subject_id
AND X.hadm_id <> Y.hadm_id
AND TIMESTAMPDIFF(DAY, X.disch_dt, Y.admit_dt) BETWEEN 0 AND 30
AND Y.hadm_id = icd9.hadm_id
GROUP BY code
ORDER by NumAdmit DESC, AvgDays2Readmit ASC;
```

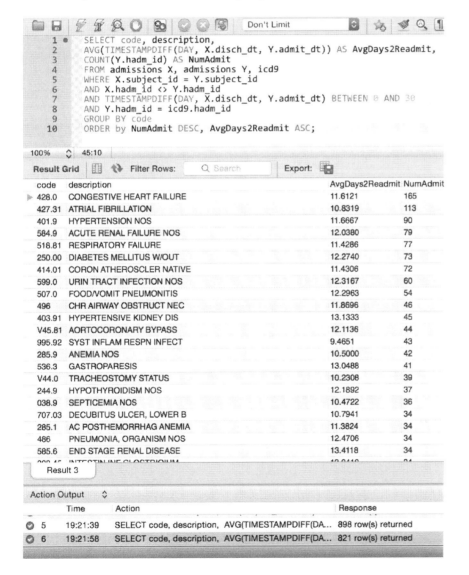

Answer 50

SELECT code, description,
ROUND(AVG(TIMESTAMPDIFF(DAY, X.disch_dt, Y.admit_dt)),1) AS AvgDays2Readmit,
COUNT(Y.hadm_id) AS NumAdmit
FROM admissions X, admissions Y, drgevents, d_codeditems
WHERE X.subject_id = Y.subject_id
AND X.hadm_id <> Y.hadm_id
AND Y.hadm_id = drgevents.hadm_id
AND drgevents.itemid = d_codeditems.itemid
AND TIMESTAMPDIFF(DAY, X.disch_dt, Y.admit_dt) BETWEEN 0 AND 30
GROUP BY code
ORDER by NumAdmit DESC, AvgDays2Readmit ASC;

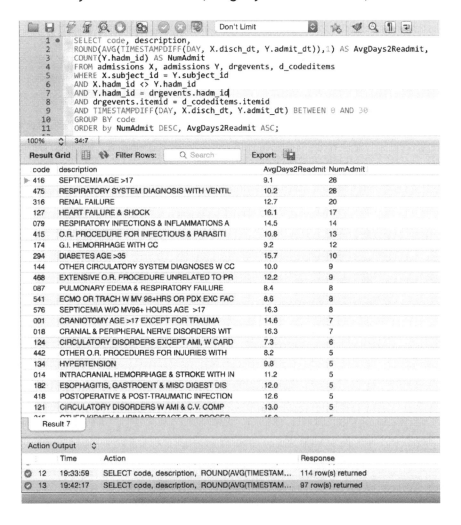

Answer 51

```
SELECT admit_dt, code, type, description
FROM drgevents, d_codeditems, admissions
WHERE d_codeditems.itemid = drgevents.itemid
AND admissions.hadm_id =drgevents.hadm_id
AND admissions.subject_id = 4410
ORDER BY admit_dt DESC;
```

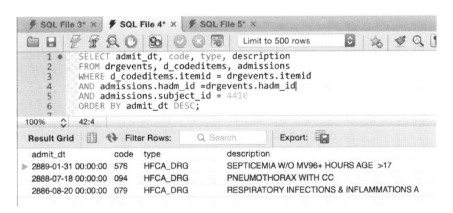

Answer 52

```
SELECT FLOOR(YEAR(admit_dt)) AS YearAdmit, Month(admit_dt) AS MonthAdmit,
COUNT(DISTINCT subject_id) AS NumPts,
COUNT(DISTINCT hadm_id) AS NumAdmit
FROM admissions
GROUP BY YearAdmit, MonthAdmit
ORDER BY YearAdmit, MonthAdmit;
```

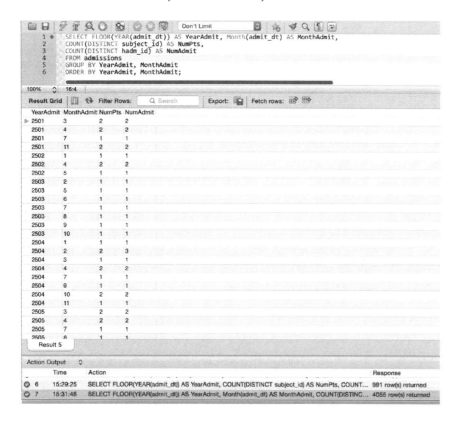

Answer 53

SELECT gender, COUNT(DISTINCT icustay_detail.hadm_id)
FROM icustay_detail, icd9
WHERE icustay_detail.hadm_id = icd9.hadm_id
AND description LIKE '%sep%'
AND description NOT LIKE '%septal%'
AND description NOT LIKE '%aseptic%'
AND description NOT LIKE '%sept def%'
AND description NOT LIKE '%separation%'
GROUP BY gender;

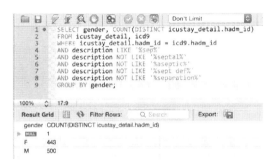

SELECT gender, COUNT(DISTINCT icustay_detail.hadm_id)
FROM icustay_detail
WHERE icustay_detail.hadm_id NOT IN
(SELECT DISTINCT icustay_detail.hadm_id
FROM icustay_detail, icd9
WHERE icustay_detail.hadm_id = icd9.hadm_id
AND description LIKE '%sep%'
AND description NOT LIKE '%septal%'
AND description NOT LIKE '%aseptic%'
AND description NOT LIKE '%sept def%'
AND description NOT LIKE '%separation%')
GROUP BY gender;

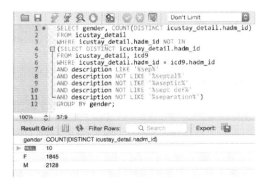

Answer 54

```sql
SELECT ROUND(AVG(hospital_los/60/24),1) AS AvgLOS
FROM icustay_detail, icd9
WHERE icustay_detail.hadm_id = icd9.hadm_id
AND icustay_detail.hadm_id NOT IN
(SELECT DISTINCT icustay_detail.hadm_id
FROM icustay_detail, icd9
WHERE icustay_detail.hadm_id = icd9.hadm_id
AND description LIKE '%sep%'
AND description NOT LIKE '%septal%'
AND description NOT LIKE '%aseptic%'
AND description NOT LIKE '%sept def%'
AND description NOT LIKE '%separation%');
```

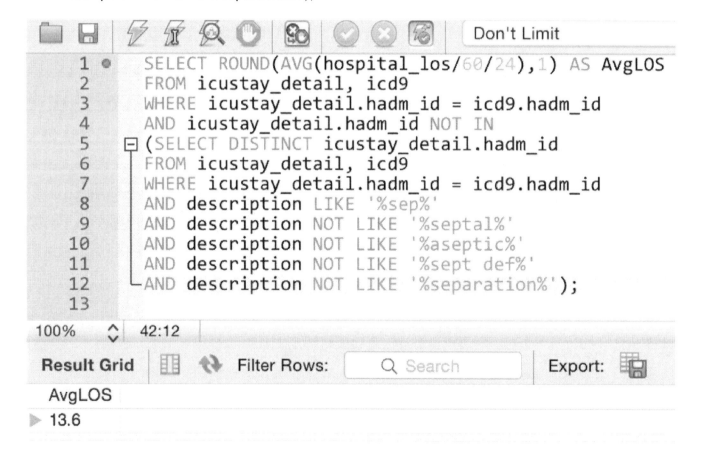

AvgLOS
▶ 13.6

Answer 55

```sql
SELECT FLOOR(YEAR(hospital_admit_dt)/100) AS CenturyAdmit,
ROUND(AVG(hospital_los/60/24),1) AS AvgLOS
FROM icustay_detail, icd9
WHERE icustay_detail.hadm_id = icd9.hadm_id
AND icustay_detail.hadm_id NOT IN
(SELECT DISTINCT icustay_detail.hadm_id
FROM icustay_detail, icd9
WHERE icustay_detail.hadm_id = icd9.hadm_id
AND description LIKE '%sep%'
AND description NOT LIKE '%septal%'
AND description NOT LIKE '%aseptic%'
AND description NOT LIKE '%sept def%'
AND description NOT LIKE '%separation%')
GROUP BY CenturyAdmit;
```

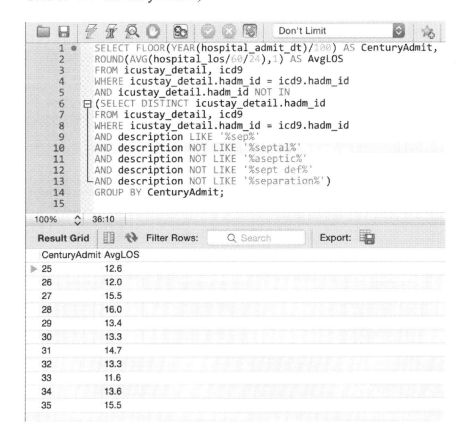

CenturyAdmit	AvgLOS
25	12.6
26	12.0
27	15.5
28	16.0
29	13.4
30	13.3
31	14.7
32	13.3
33	11.6
34	13.6
35	15.5

Answer 56

Sepsis related:

SELECT COUNT(DISTINCT X.hadm_id) as NumPtsAdmit
FROM icustay_detail X, icd9
WHERE X.hadm_id = icd9.hadm_id
AND description LIKE '%sep%'
AND description NOT LIKE '%septal%'
AND description NOT LIKE '%aseptic%'
AND description NOT LIKE '%sept def%'
AND description NOT LIKE '%separation%';

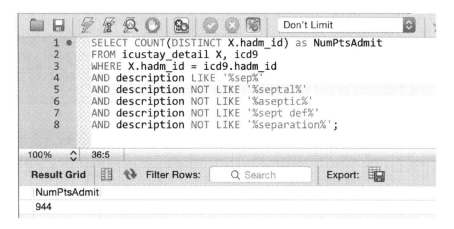

SELECT COUNT(DISTINCT X.hadm_id) as NumPtsReadmit
FROM icustay_detail X, icustay_detail Y, icd9
WHERE X.subject_id = Y.subject_id
AND X.hadm_id <> Y.hadm_id
AND TIMESTAMPDIFF(DAY, X.hospital_disch_dt, Y.hospital_admit_dt) BETWEEN 0 AND 30
AND X.hadm_id = icd9.hadm_id
AND description LIKE '%sep%'
AND description NOT LIKE '%septal%'
AND description NOT LIKE '%aseptic%'
AND description NOT LIKE '%sept def%'
AND description NOT LIKE '%separation%';

Sepsis average readmission rate = 49 / 944 = **5.2%**

Sepsis unrelated:

SELECT COUNT(DISTINCT X.hadm_id) AS NumPtsAdmit
FROM icustay_detail X, icd9
WHERE X.hadm_id = icd9.hadm_id
AND X.hadm_id NOT IN
(SELECT DISTINCT icustay_detail.hadm_id
FROM icustay_detail, icd9
WHERE icustay_detail.hadm_id = icd9.hadm_id
AND description LIKE '%sep%'
AND description NOT LIKE '%septal%'
AND description NOT LIKE '%aseptic%'
AND description NOT LIKE '%sept def%'
AND description NOT LIKE '%separation%');

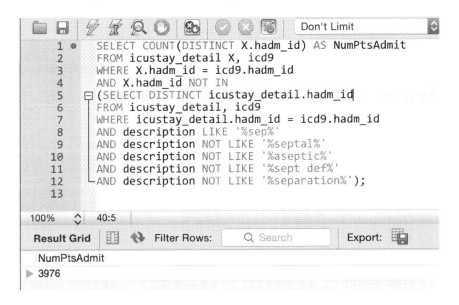

SELECT COUNT(DISTINCT X.hadm_id) as NumPtsReadmit
FROM icustay_detail X, icustay_detail Y, icd9
WHERE X.subject_id = Y.subject_id
AND X.hadm_id <> Y.hadm_id
AND TIMESTAMPDIFF(DAY, X.hospital_disch_dt, Y.hospital_admit_dt) BETWEEN 0 AND 30
AND X.hadm_id = icd9.hadm_id
AND X.hadm_id NOT IN
(SELECT DISTINCT icustay_detail.hadm_id
FROM icustay_detail, icd9
WHERE icustay_detail.hadm_id = icd9.hadm_id
AND description LIKE '%sep%'
AND description NOT LIKE '%septal%'
AND description NOT LIKE '%aseptic%'
AND description NOT LIKE '%sept def%'
AND description NOT LIKE '%separation%');

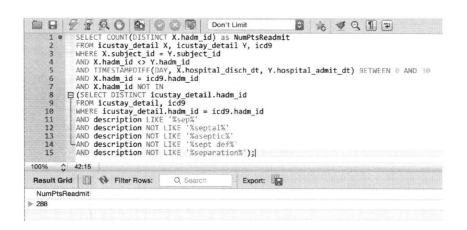

Sepsis unrelated average readmission rate = 288 / 3,976 = **7.2 %**

Answer 57

Denominator:

```sql
SELECT FLOOR(YEAR(X.hospital_admit_dt)/100) AS CenturyAdmit,
COUNT(DISTINCT X.hadm_id) as NumPtsAdmit
FROM icustay_detail X, icd9
WHERE X.hadm_id = icd9.hadm_id
AND X.hadm_id NOT IN
(SELECT DISTINCT icustay_detail.hadm_id
FROM icustay_detail, icd9
WHERE icustay_detail.hadm_id = icd9.hadm_id
AND description LIKE '%sep%'
AND description NOT LIKE '%septal%'
AND description NOT LIKE '%aseptic%'
AND description NOT LIKE '%sept def%'
AND description NOT LIKE '%separation%')
GROUP BY CenturyAdmit;
```

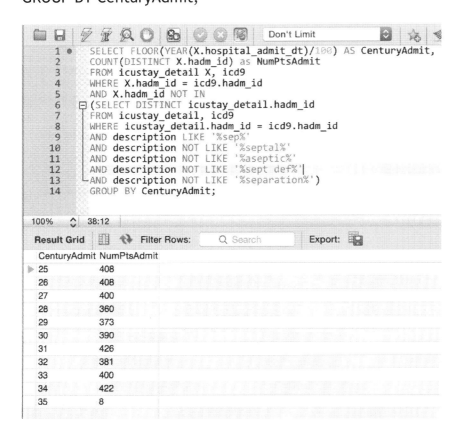

CenturyAdmit	NumPtsAdmit
25	408
26	408
27	400
28	360
29	373
30	390
31	426
32	381
33	400
34	422
35	8

Numerator:

```
SELECT FLOOR(YEAR(X.hospital_admit_dt)/100) AS CenturyAdmit,
COUNT(DISTINCT X.hadm_id) as NumPtsReadmit
FROM icustay_detail X, icustay_detail Y, icd9
WHERE X.subject_id = Y.subject_id
AND X.hadm_id <> Y.hadm_id
AND TIMESTAMPDIFF(DAY, X.hospital_disch_dt, Y.hospital_admit_dt) BETWEEN 0 AND 30
AND X.hadm_id = icd9.hadm_id
AND X.hadm_id NOT IN
(SELECT DISTINCT icustay_detail.hadm_id
FROM icustay_detail, icd9
WHERE icustay_detail.hadm_id = icd9.hadm_id
AND description LIKE '%sep%'
AND description NOT LIKE '%septal%'
AND description NOT LIKE '%aseptic%'
AND description NOT LIKE '%sept def%'
AND description NOT LIKE '%separation%')
GROUP BY CenturyAdmit;
```

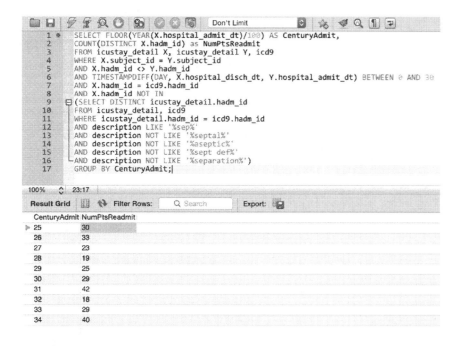

Answer 58

```
SELECT d_codeditems.code, d_codeditems.description, cost_weight,
COUNT(DISTINCT drgevents.hadm_id) AS NumAdmit
FROM d_codeditems, drgevents, icd9
WHERE d_codeditems.itemid = drgevents.itemid
AND drgevents.hadm_id = icd9.hadm_id
AND icd9.description LIKE '%sep%'
AND icd9.description NOT LIKE '%septal%'
AND icd9.description NOT LIKE '%aseptic%'
AND icd9.description NOT LIKE '%sept def%'
AND icd9.description NOT LIKE '%separation%'
GROUP BY d_codeditems.code
ORDER BY NumAdmit DESC;
```

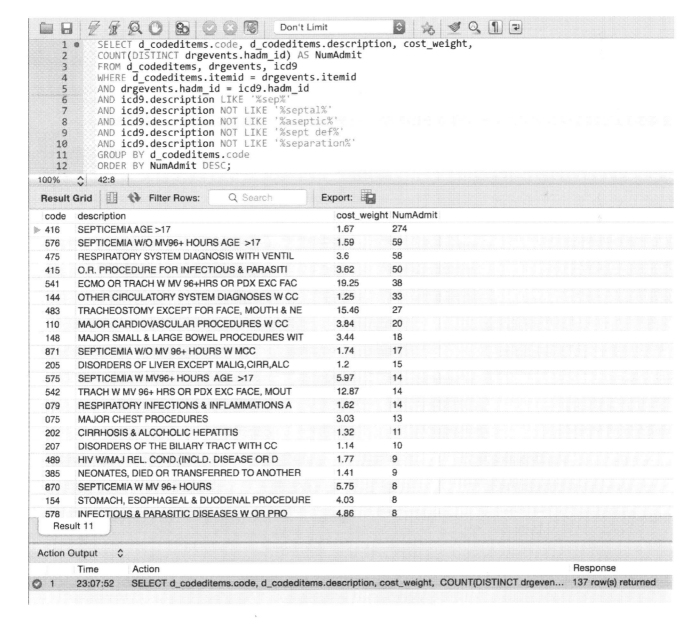

Answer 59

```
SELECT * FROM labevents, d_labitems
WHERE subject_id = 61
AND labevents.itemid = d_labitems.itemid
AND flag = 'abnormal'
ORDER BY charttime DESC;
```

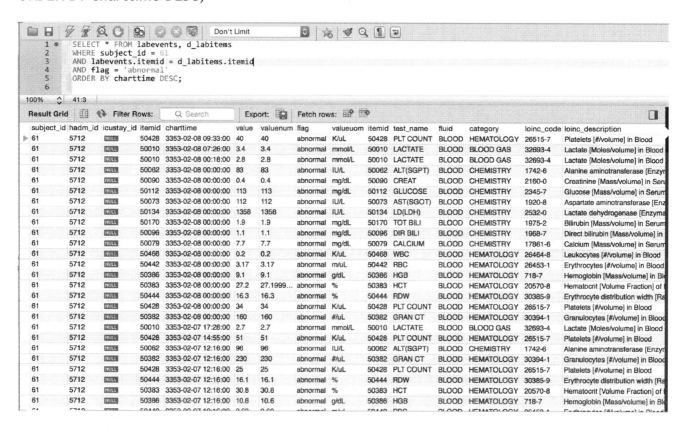

Answer 60

```
SELECT * FROM
(SELECT charttime, subject_id, hadm_id, spec_itemid, org_itemid, ab_itemid FROM microbiologyevents) AS Patient,
(SELECT itemid, label AS Specimen FROM d_codeditems) AS Specimen,
(SELECT itemid, label AS Organism FROM d_codeditems WHERE label LIKE '%DIFF%') AS Organism,
(SELECT itemid, label AS Antibiotic FROM d_codeditems) AS Ab
WHERE Specimen.itemid = spec_itemid
AND Organism.itemid = org_itemid
AND Ab.itemid = ab_itemid
ORDER BY charttime DESC;
```

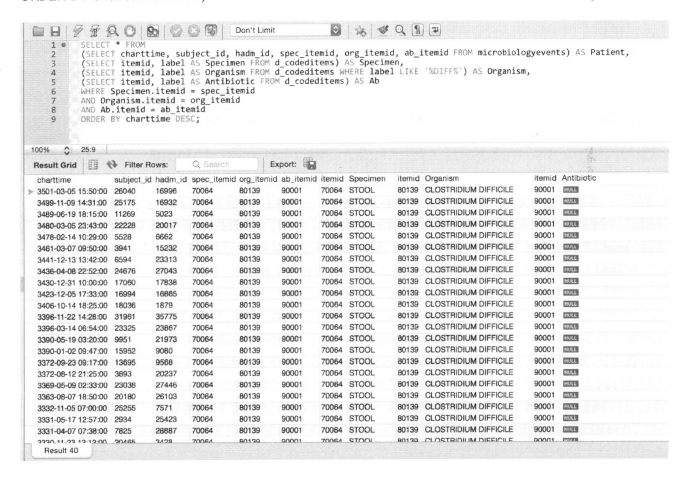

Answer 61

```sql
SELECT ROUND(AVG(HypoValue),0) AS AVGHypo,
ROUND(AVG(TIMESTAMPDIFF(HOUR, HypoDT, NextDT)),0) AS AVGHrsBetweenLabs,
ROUND(AVG(NextValue),0) AS AVGNextGluc
FROM

(SELECT DISTINCT icd9.hadm_id, value AS HypoValue, charttime AS HypoDT
FROM icd9, d_labitems, labevents
WHERE icd9.hadm_id = labevents.hadm_id
AND d_labitems.itemid = labevents.itemid
AND description LIKE '%DIABETES%'
AND description NOT LIKE '%INSIPIDUS%'
AND description NOT LIKE '%FAM%'
AND loinc_description LIKE '%glucose %'
AND fluid = 'BLOOD'
AND value < 60) AS HypoEvents,

(SELECT DISTINCT icd9.hadm_id, value AS NextValue, charttime AS NextDT
FROM icd9, d_labitems, labevents
WHERE icd9.hadm_id = labevents.hadm_id
AND d_labitems.itemid = labevents.itemid
AND description LIKE '%DIABETES%'
AND description NOT LIKE '%INSIPIDUS%'
AND description NOT LIKE '%FAM%'
AND loinc_description LIKE '%glucose %'
AND fluid = 'BLOOD') AS GlucEvents

WHERE HypoEvents.hadm_id = GlucEvents.hadm_id
AND GlucEvents.NextDT > HypoEvents.HypoDT;
```

```sql
SELECT ROUND(AVG(HypoValue),0) AS AVGHypo,
    ROUND(AVG(TIMESTAMPDIFF(HOUR, HypoDT, NextDT)),0) AS AVGHrsBetweenLabs,
    ROUND(AVG(NextValue),0) AS AVGNextGluc
FROM

(SELECT DISTINCT icd9.hadm_id, value AS HypoValue, charttime AS HypoDT
 FROM icd9, d_labitems, labevents
 WHERE icd9.hadm_id = labevents.hadm_id
 AND d_labitems.itemid = labevents.itemid
 AND description LIKE '%DIABETES%'
 AND description NOT LIKE '%INSIPIDUS%'
 AND description NOT LIKE '%FAM%'
 AND loinc_description LIKE '%glucose %'
 AND fluid = 'BLOOD'
 AND value < 60) AS HypoEvents,

(SELECT DISTINCT icd9.hadm_id, value AS NextValue, charttime AS NextDT
 FROM icd9, d_labitems, labevents
 WHERE icd9.hadm_id = labevents.hadm_id
 AND d_labitems.itemid = labevents.itemid
 AND description LIKE '%DIABETES%'
 AND description NOT LIKE '%INSIPIDUS%'
 AND description NOT LIKE '%FAM%'
 AND loinc_description LIKE '%glucose %'
 AND fluid = 'BLOOD') AS GlucEvents

WHERE HypoEvents.hadm_id = GlucEvents.hadm_id
AND GlucEvents.NextDT > HypoEvents.HypoDT;
```

AVGHypo	AVGHrsBetweenLabs	AVGNextGluc
47	310	142

Answer 62

The relationship between **poe_order** and **poe_med** is 1:M.
The column **poe_id** connects between the two tables.

Answer 63

```
SELECT DISTINCT medevents.icustay_id, medevents.itemid, d_meditems.label AS DrugName,
realtime, dose, doseuom, d_ioitems.label AS SolnName, solvolume, solunits,
medevents.route
FROM medevents, d_meditems, additives, d_ioitems
WHERE medevents.itemid = d_meditems.itemid
AND additives.itemid = medevents.itemid
AND additives.icustay_id = medevents.icustay_id
AND d_ioitems.itemid = ioitemid
AND medevents.subject_id = 11710
and stopped IS NULL
ORDER BY realtime;
```

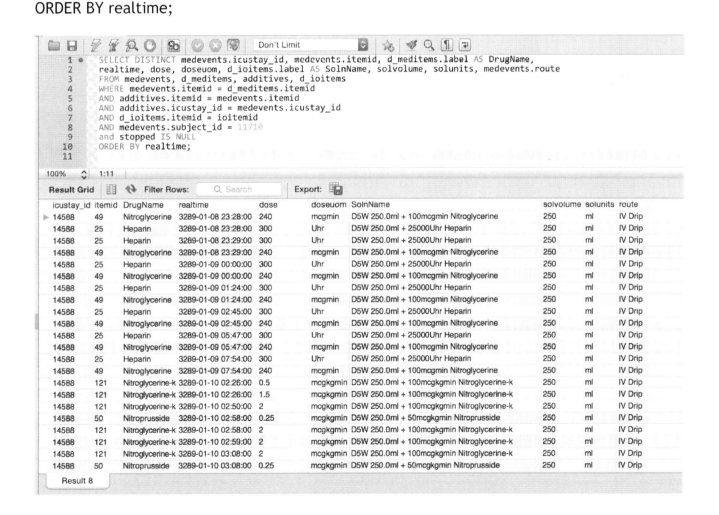

Answer 64

SELECT drug_name, COUNT(DISTINCT subject_id) AS Patients, COUNT(DISTINCT hadm_id) AS Admissions
FROM poe_med, poe_order
WHERE poe_med.poe_id = poe_order.poe_id
GROUP BY drug_name
ORDER BY Admissions DESC;

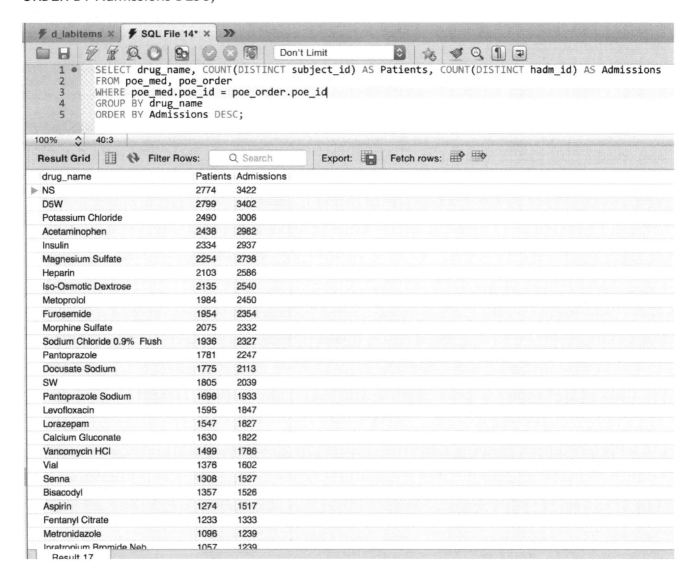

Answer 65

```
SELECT route, ROUND(AVG(TIMESTAMPDIFF(MINUTE, enter_dt, start_dt)),0) AS AVGTime2Exec,
COUNT(DISTINCT hadm_id) AS Admissions
FROM poe_order
GROUP BY route
ORDER BY route;
```

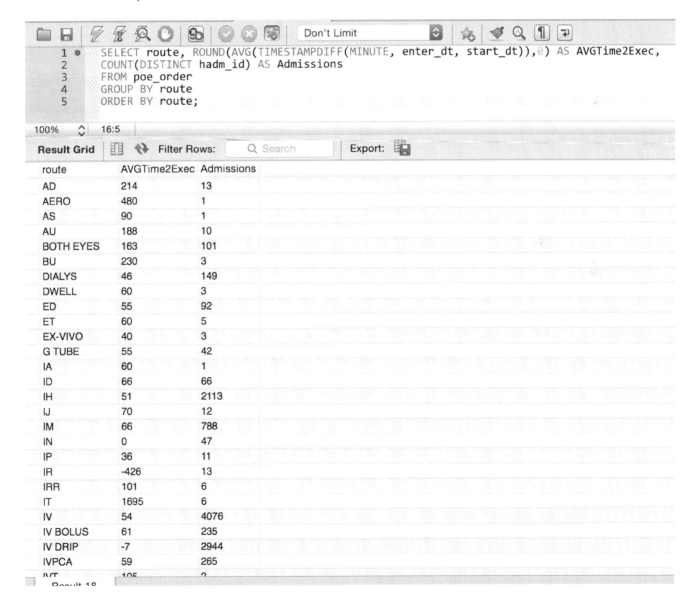

route	AVGTime2Exec	Admissions
AD	214	13
AERO	480	1
AS	90	1
AU	188	10
BOTH EYES	163	101
BU	230	3
DIALYS	46	149
DWELL	60	3
ED	55	92
ET	60	5
EX-VIVO	40	3
G TUBE	55	42
IA	60	1
ID	66	66
IH	51	2113
IJ	70	12
IM	66	788
IN	0	47
IP	36	11
IR	-426	13
IRR	101	6
IT	1695	6
IV	54	4076
IV BOLUS	61	235
IV DRIP	-7	2944
IVPCA	59	265

Answer 66

```sql
SELECT subject_id, hadm_id, description, proc_dt
FROM procedureevents,d_codeditems
WHERE procedureevents.itemid = d_codeditems.itemid
AND subject_id = 11710
ORDER BY proc_dt;
```

subject_id	hadm_id	description	proc_dt
11710	17408	LEFT HEART CARDIAC CATH	3289-01-06 00:00:00
11710	17408	CORONAR ARTERIOGR-2 CATH	3289-01-06 00:00:00
11710	17408	1 INT MAM-COR ART BYPASS	3289-01-08 00:00:00
11710	17408	(AORTO)CORONARY BYPASS T	3289-01-08 00:00:00
11710	17408	EXTRACORPOREAL CIRCULAT	3289-01-08 00:00:00
11710	17408	CATHETER BASED INVASIVE	3289-01-13 00:00:00
11710	17408	HEART COUNTERSHOCK NEC	3289-01-13 00:00:00
11710	17408	EXCISION OR DESTRUCT OTH	3289-01-13 00:00:00
11710	17408	CARDIAC MAPPING	3289-01-13 00:00:00
11710	17449	VENOUS CATHETER NEC	3289-02-08 00:00:00
11710	17449	PARENTERAL INFUS CONC NU	3289-02-09 00:00:00
11710	17449	EXC CHEST CAGE BONE LES	3289-02-09 00:00:00
11710	17449	MUSCLE OR FASCIA GRAFT	3289-02-11 00:00:00
11710	17449	EXT INFUS CONC NUTRITION	3289-02-16 00:00:00
11710	17449	CONTINUOUS INVASIVE MECH	3289-02-16 00:00:00
11710	17449	INSERT ENDOTRACHEAL TUBE	3289-02-16 00:00:00
11710	17144	OTH AND OPEN REPAIR OTH	3289-06-27 00:00:00
11710	17144	INSERT ENDOTRACHEAL TUBE	3289-06-28 00:00:00
11710	17144	CONTINUOUS INVASIVE MECH	3289-06-28 00:00:00
11710	17144	CONTINUOUS INVASIVE MECH	3289-06-29 00:00:00
11710	17144	INSER TEMP TRANSVEN PACE	3289-06-29 00:00:00
11710	17144	LEFT HEART CARDIAC CATH	3289-06-29 00:00:00
11710	17144	CORONAR ARTERIOGR-2 CATH	3289-06-29 00:00:00
11710	17144	PTCA-MULTIPLE VESSEL	3289-06-29 00:00:00
11710	17144	INSERT CORON ARTER STENT	3289-06-29 00:00:00

Answer 67

SELECT COUNT(hospital_expire_flg) AS Died
FROM procedureevents, d_codeditems, d_patients
WHERE d_patients.subject_id = procedureevents.subject_id
AND procedureevents.itemid = d_codeditems.itemid
AND hospital_expire_flg = 'Y'
AND description LIKE '%extracorpor%';

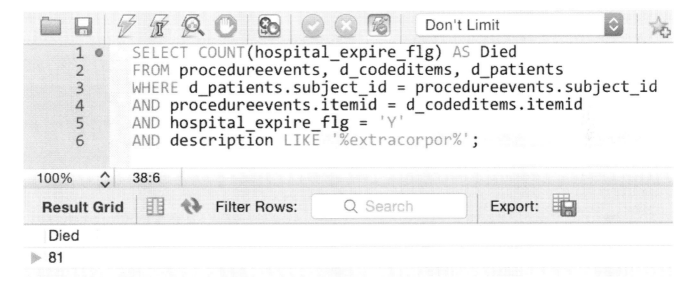

81 / 329 = 24.6% mortality rate for extra-corporeal circulation

Answer 68

SELECT d_caregivers.cgid AS CareGiver,
icustay_id,
d_caregivers.label AS ProvTitle,
MIN(realtime) AS MINtime,
MAX(realtime) AS MAXtime,
TIMESTAMPDIFF(HOUR, MIN(realtime), MAX(realtime)) AS HoursRelated
FROM chartevents, d_caregivers
WHERE d_caregivers.cgid = chartevents.cgid
AND subject_id = 4655
GROUP BY d_caregivers.cgid
ORDER BY icustay_id;

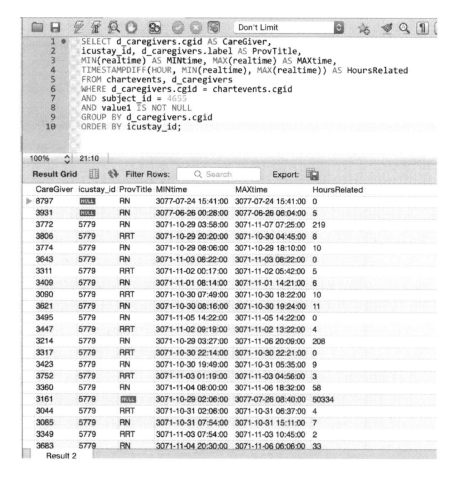

Answer 69

```sql
(SELECT 'chartevents' AS OrigTable,
d_caregivers.cgid AS CareGiver,
icustay_id, d_caregivers.label AS ProvTitle
FROM chartevents, d_caregivers
WHERE d_caregivers.cgid = chartevents.cgid
AND subject_id = 4655
GROUP BY d_caregivers.cgid)
UNION
(SELECT 'noteevents' AS OrigTable,
d_caregivers.cgid AS CareGiver,
icustay_id, d_caregivers.label AS ProvTitle
FROM noteevents, d_caregivers
WHERE d_caregivers.cgid = noteevents.cgid
AND subject_id = 4655
GROUP BY d_caregivers.cgid)
UNION
(SELECT 'medevents' AS OrigTable,
d_caregivers.cgid AS CareGiver,
icustay_id, d_caregivers.label AS ProvTitle
FROM medevents, d_caregivers
WHERE d_caregivers.cgid = medevents.cgid
AND subject_id = 4655
GROUP BY d_caregivers.cgid)
UNION
(SELECT 'ioevents' AS OrigTable,
d_caregivers.cgid AS CareGiver,
icustay_id, d_caregivers.label AS ProvTitle
FROM ioevents, d_caregivers
WHERE d_caregivers.cgid = ioevents.cgid
AND subject_id = 4655
GROUP BY d_caregivers.cgid);
```

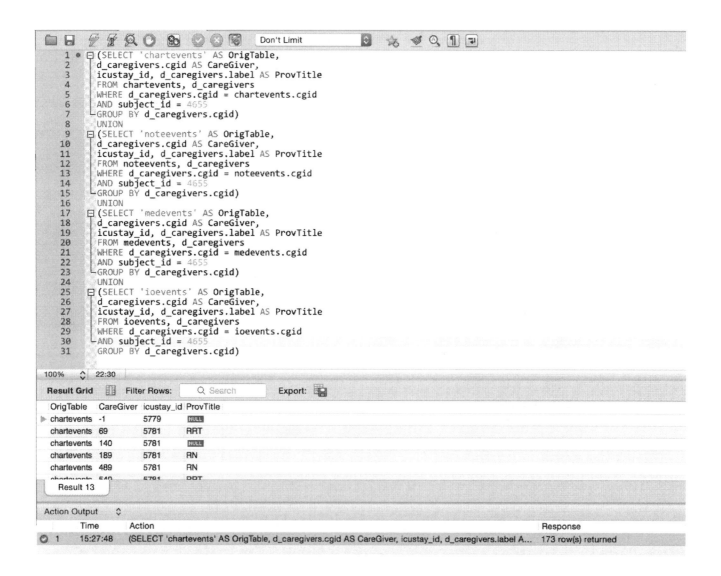

Answer 70

(SELECT 'chartevents' AS OrigTable, d_careunits.label AS CareUnit, icustay_id
FROM chartevents, d_careunits
WHERE d_careunits.cuid = chartevents.cuid
AND subject_id = 4655
GROUP BY CareUnit)
UNION
(SELECT 'noteevents' AS OrigTable, d_careunits.label AS CareUnit, icustay_id
FROM noteevents, d_careunits
WHERE d_careunits.cuid = noteevents.cuid
AND subject_id = 4655
GROUP BY CareUnit)
UNION
(SELECT 'medevents' AS OrigTable, d_careunits.label AS CareUnit, icustay_id
FROM medevents, d_careunits
WHERE d_careunits.cuid = medevents.cuid
AND subject_id = 4655
GROUP BY CareUnit)
ORDER BY icustay_id;

```sql
1  (SELECT 'chartevents' AS OrigTable, d_careunits.label AS CareUnit, icustay_id
2   FROM chartevents, d_careunits
3   WHERE d_careunits.cuid = chartevents.cuid
4   AND subject_id = 4655
5   GROUP BY CareUnit)
6  UNION
7  (SELECT 'noteevents' AS OrigTable, d_careunits.label AS CareUnit, icustay_id
8   FROM noteevents, d_careunits
9   WHERE d_careunits.cuid = noteevents.cuid
10  AND subject_id = 4655
11  GROUP BY CareUnit)
12 UNION
13 (SELECT 'medevents' AS OrigTable, d_careunits.label AS CareUnit, icustay_id
14  FROM medevents, d_careunits
15  WHERE d_careunits.cuid = medevents.cuid
16  AND subject_id = 4655
17  GROUP BY CareUnit)
18  ORDER BY icustay_id
19
```

OrigTable	CareUnit	icustay_id
chartevents	LCP at MIT	5779
chartevents	CSRU	5779
noteevents	CSRU	5779
noteevents	MICU	5780
chartevents	MICU	5780
chartevents	T-SICU	5781
noteevents	T-SICU	5781
medevents	T-SICU	5781
medevents	CSRU	39709
medevents	CCU	39711
chartevents	CCU	39711
noteevents	CCU	39711

Answer 71

SELECT d_careunits.label AS CareUnit, chartevents.icustay_id,
TIMESTAMPDIFF(HOUR,MIN(charttime), MAX(charttime)) AS ICUstayHours
FROM chartevents, d_careunits, icustay_detail
WHERE d_careunits.cuid = chartevents.cuid
AND chartevents.subject_id = 4655
AND icustay_detail.icustay_id = chartevents.icustay_id
AND charttime BETWEEN '3071-01-01' AND '3077-12-31'
GROUP BY CareUnit, icustay_id;

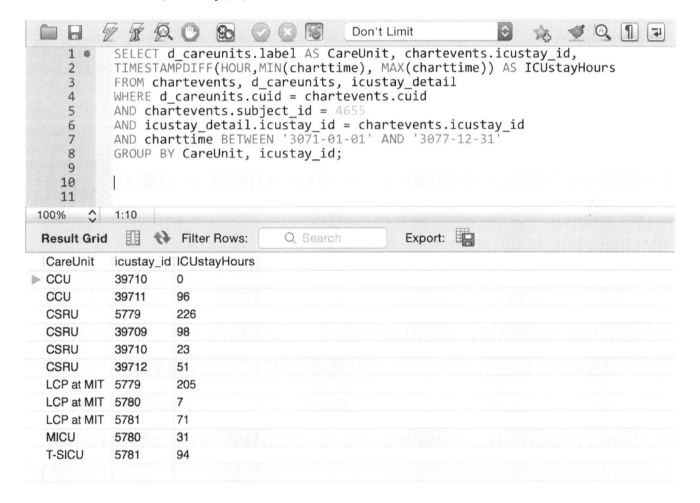

CareUnit	icustay_id	ICUstayHours
CCU	39710	0
CCU	39711	96
CSRU	5779	226
CSRU	39709	98
CSRU	39710	23
CSRU	39712	51
LCP at MIT	5779	205
LCP at MIT	5780	7
LCP at MIT	5781	71
MICU	5780	31
T-SICU	5781	94

Answer 72

(SELECT 'chartevents' AS OrigTable, COUNT(DISTINCT icustay_id) AS ICUadmit
FROM chartevents, d_caregivers
WHERE d_caregivers.cgid = chartevents.cgid
AND d_caregivers.cgid = 3891)
UNION
(SELECT 'noteevents' AS OrigTable, COUNT(DISTINCT icustay_id) AS ICUadmit
FROM noteevents, d_caregivers
WHERE d_caregivers.cgid = noteevents.cgid
AND d_caregivers.cgid = 3891)
UNION
(SELECT 'medevents' AS OrigTable, COUNT(DISTINCT icustay_id) AS ICUadmit
FROM medevents, d_caregivers
WHERE d_caregivers.cgid = medevents.cgid
AND d_caregivers.cgid = 3891)
UNION
(SELECT 'ioevents' AS OrigTable, COUNT(DISTINCT icustay_id) AS ICUadmit
FROM ioevents, d_caregivers
WHERE d_caregivers.cgid = ioevents.cgid
AND d_caregivers.cgid = 3891)
UNION
(SELECT 'totalbalevents' AS OrigTable, COUNT(DISTINCT icustay_id) AS ICUadmit
FROM totalbalevents, d_caregivers
WHERE d_caregivers.cgid = totalbalevents.cgid
AND d_caregivers.cgid = 3891)
UNION
(SELECT 'additives' AS OrigTable, COUNT(DISTINCT icustay_id) AS ICUadmit
FROM additives, d_caregivers
WHERE d_caregivers.cgid = additives.cgid
AND d_caregivers.cgid = 3891)
UNION
(SELECT 'deliveries' AS OrigTable, COUNT(DISTINCT icustay_id) AS ICUadmit
FROM deliveries, d_caregivers
WHERE d_caregivers.cgid = deliveries.cgid
AND d_caregivers.cgid = 3891);

```sql
  6  (SELECT 'noteevents' AS OrigTable, COUNT(DISTINCT icustay_id) AS ICUadmit
  7   FROM noteevents, d_caregivers
  8   WHERE d_caregivers.cgid = noteevents.cgid
  9   AND d_caregivers.cgid = 3891)
 10  UNION
 11  (SELECT 'medevents' AS OrigTable, COUNT(DISTINCT icustay_id) AS ICUadmit
 12   FROM medevents, d_caregivers
 13   WHERE d_caregivers.cgid = medevents.cgid
 14   AND d_caregivers.cgid = 3891)
 15  UNION
 16  (SELECT 'ioevents' AS OrigTable, COUNT(DISTINCT icustay_id) AS ICUadmit
 17   FROM ioevents, d_caregivers
 18   WHERE d_caregivers.cgid = ioevents.cgid
 19   AND d_caregivers.cgid = 3891)
 20  UNION
 21  (SELECT 'totalbalevents' AS OrigTable, COUNT(DISTINCT icustay_id) AS ICUadmit
 22   FROM totalbalevents, d_caregivers
 23   WHERE d_caregivers.cgid = totalbalevents.cgid
 24   AND d_caregivers.cgid = 3891)
 25  UNION
 26  (SELECT 'additives' AS OrigTable, COUNT(DISTINCT icustay_id) AS ICUadmit
 27   FROM additives, d_caregivers
 28   WHERE d_caregivers.cgid = additives.cgid
 29   AND d_caregivers.cgid = 3891)
 30  UNION
 31  (SELECT 'deliveries' AS OrigTable, COUNT(DISTINCT icustay_id) AS ICUadmit
 32   FROM deliveries, d_caregivers
 33   WHERE d_caregivers.cgid = deliveries.cgid
 34   AND d_caregivers.cgid = 3891);
```

OrigTable	ICUadmit
chartevents	38
noteevents	27
medevents	19
ioevents	36
totalbalevents	20
additives	9
deliveries	7

Answer 73

(SELECT 'chartevents' AS OrigTable, COUNT(DISTINCT icustay_id) AS ICUadmit
FROM chartevents, d_careunits
WHERE d_careunits.cuid = chartevents.cuid
AND d_careunits.cuid = 1)
UNION
(SELECT 'noteevents' AS OrigTable, COUNT(DISTINCT icustay_id) AS ICUadmit
FROM noteevents, d_careunits
WHERE d_careunits.cuid = noteevents.cuid
AND d_careunits.cuid = 1)
UNION
(SELECT 'medevents' AS OrigTable, COUNT(DISTINCT icustay_id) AS ICUadmit
FROM medevents, d_careunits
WHERE d_careunits.cuid = medevents.cuid
AND d_careunits.cuid = 1);

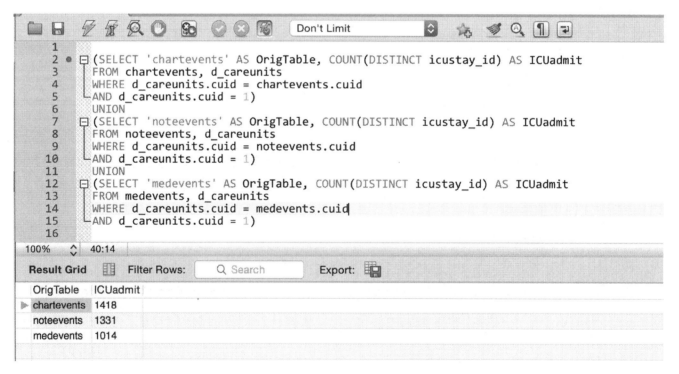

Answer 74

```sql
(SELECT 'chartevents' AS OrigTable, icustay_id, d_caregivers.cgid AS CareGiver, charttime
FROM chartevents, d_caregivers
WHERE d_caregivers.cgid = chartevents.cgid
AND subject_id = 4655
AND d_caregivers.label = 'RN'
GROUP BY d_caregivers.cgid)
UNION
(SELECT 'totalbalevents' AS OrigTable, icustay_id, d_caregivers.cgid AS CareGiver, charttime
FROM totalbalevents, d_caregivers
WHERE d_caregivers.cgid = totalbalevents.cgid
AND subject_id = 4655
AND d_caregivers.label = 'RN'
GROUP BY d_caregivers.cgid)
UNION
(SELECT 'medevents' AS OrigTable, icustay_id, d_caregivers.cgid AS CareGiver, charttime
FROM medevents, d_caregivers
WHERE d_caregivers.cgid = medevents.cgid
AND subject_id = 4655
AND d_caregivers.label = 'RN'
GROUP BY d_caregivers.cgid)
UNION
(SELECT 'ioevents' AS OrigTable, icustay_id, d_caregivers.cgid AS CareGiver, charttime
FROM ioevents, d_caregivers
WHERE d_caregivers.cgid = ioevents.cgid
AND subject_id = 4655
AND d_caregivers.label = 'RN'
GROUP BY d_caregivers.cgid)
UNION
(SELECT 'deliveries' AS OrigTable, icustay_id, d_caregivers.cgid AS CareGiver, charttime
FROM deliveries, d_caregivers
WHERE d_caregivers.cgid = deliveries.cgid
AND subject_id = 4655
AND d_caregivers.label = 'RN'
GROUP BY d_caregivers.cgid)
UNION
(SELECT 'additives' AS OrigTable, icustay_id, d_caregivers.cgid AS CareGiver, charttime
FROM additives, d_caregivers
WHERE d_caregivers.cgid = additives.cgid
AND subject_id = 4655
AND d_caregivers.label = 'RN'
GROUP BY d_caregivers.cgid)
UNION
(SELECT 'noteevents' AS OrigTable, icustay_id, d_caregivers.cgid AS CareGiver, charttime
FROM noteevents, d_caregivers
WHERE d_caregivers.cgid = noteevents.cgid
```

```
AND subject_id = 4655
AND d_caregivers.label = 'RN'
GROUP BY d_caregivers.cgid)
ORDER BY charttime;
```

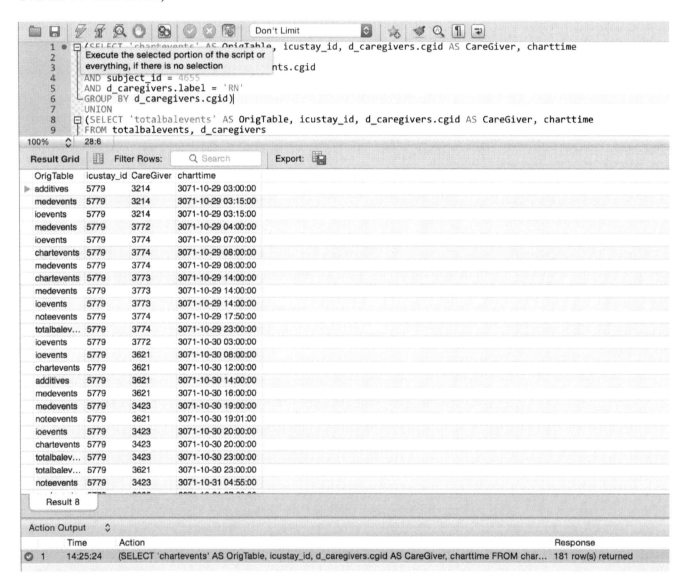

Answer 75

SELECT COUNT(DISTINCT icustay_id) AS RestrainedICUstays
FROM chartevents, d_chartitems
WHERE label LIKE '%reason%restrain%'
AND d_chartitems.itemid = chartevents.itemid;

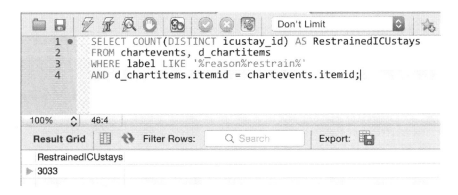

Answer 76

SELECT FLOOR(YEAR(charttime)/100) AS CenturyICUstay,
COUNT(DISTINCT icustay_id) AS RestrainedICUstays
FROM chartevents, d_chartitems
WHERE label LIKE '%restrain%'
AND d_chartitems.itemid = chartevents.itemid
GROUP BY CenturyICUstay;

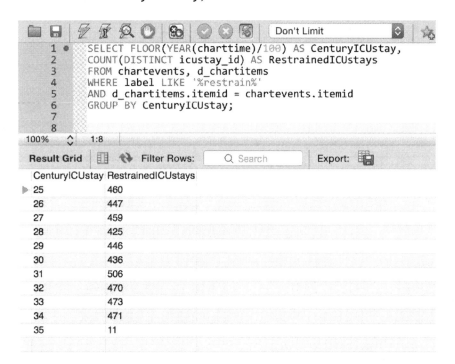

CenturyICUstay	RestrainedICUstays
25	460
26	447
27	459
28	425
29	446
30	436
31	506
32	470
33	473
34	471
35	11

Answer 77

SELECT FLOOR(YEAR(charttime)/100) AS CenturyICUstay,
COUNT(DISTINCT icustay_id) AS BradenPts
FROM chartevents, d_chartitems
WHERE label = 'Braden Score'
AND d_chartitems.itemid = chartevents.itemid
GROUP BY CenturyICUstay;

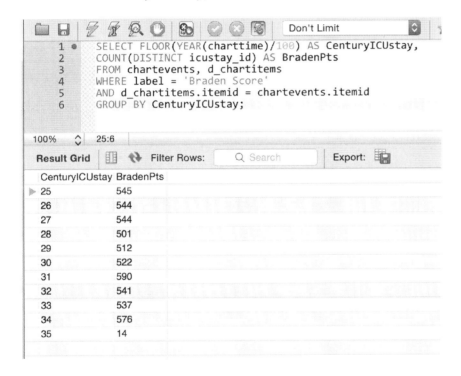

SELECT FLOOR(YEAR(charttime)/100) AS CenturyICUstay,
COUNT(DISTINCT icustay_id) AS BradenPts
FROM chartevents, d_chartitems
WHERE label = 'Braden Score'
AND d_chartitems.itemid = chartevents.itemid
AND value1num <= 9
GROUP BY CenturyICUstay;

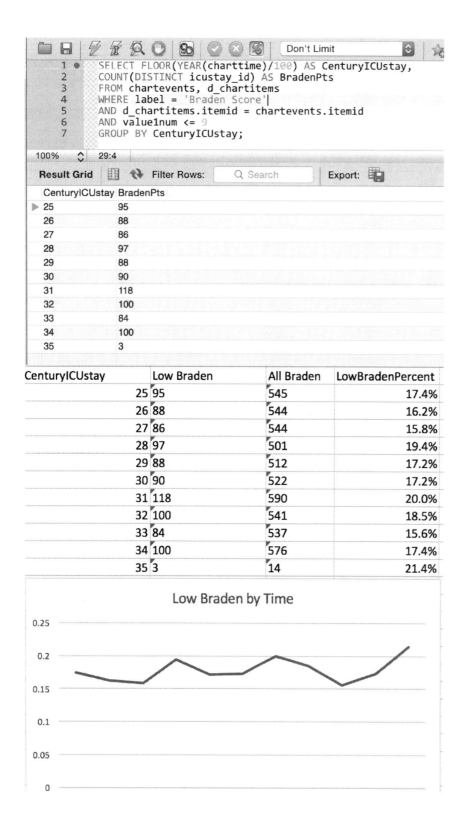

Answer 78

```sql
(SELECT icustay_id, charttime, category, label, 'ioevents' AS OrigTable
FROM ioevents, d_ioitems
WHERE ioevents.itemid = d_ioitems.itemid
AND subject_id = 4655)
UNION
(SELECT icustay_id, charttime, category, label, 'deliveries' AS OrigTable
FROM deliveries, d_ioitems
WHERE deliveries.ioitemid = d_ioitems.itemid
AND subject_id = 4655)
UNION
(SELECT icustay_id, charttime, category, label, 'totalbalevents' AS OrigTable
FROM totalbalevents, d_ioitems
WHERE totalbalevents.itemid = d_ioitems.itemid
AND subject_id = 4655)
UNION
(SELECT icustay_id, starttime, category, label, 'a_iodurations' AS OrigTable
FROM a_iodurations, d_ioitems
WHERE a_iodurations.itemid = d_ioitems.itemid
AND subject_id = 4655)
UNION
(SELECT icustay_id, charttime, category, label, 'additives' AS OrigTable
FROM additives, d_ioitems
WHERE additives.ioitemid = d_ioitems.itemid
AND subject_id = 4655)
ORDER BY charttime, OrigTable, category;
```

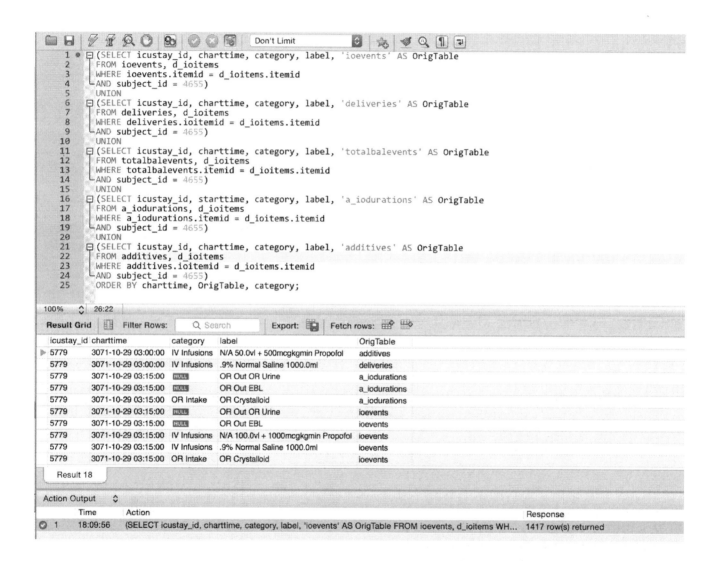

Answer 79

SELECT icustay_id, charttime, ROUND(cumvolume) AS Volume, label
FROM totalbalevents, d_ioitems
WHERE totalbalevents.itemid = d_ioitems.itemid
AND d_ioitems.label = 'Net Hourly Balance'
AND subject_id = 12613
ORDER BY charttime;

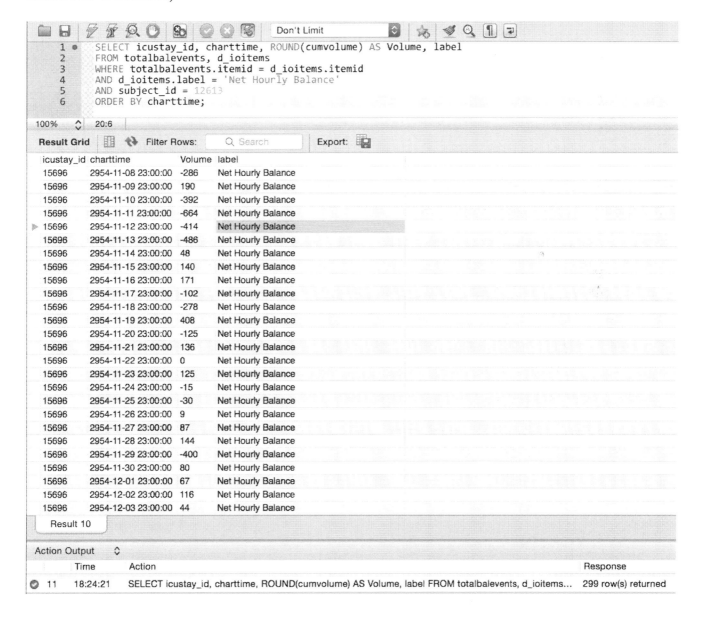

Answer 80

sofa_min	All Pts	Died	Mortality
0	789	140	17.7%
1	1066	179	16.8%
2	786	122	15.5%
3	697	163	23.4%
4	644	229	35.6%
5	483	231	47.8%
6	252	121	48.0%
7	162	97	59.9%
8	129	97	75.2%
9	80	67	83.8%
10	56	44	78.6%
11	50	48	96.0%
12	48	44	91.7%
13	36	34	94.4%
14	32	30	93.8%
15	17	17	100.0%
16	16	16	100.0%
17	13	13	100.0%
18	11	11	100.0%
19	6	6	100.0%
20	4	4	100.0%
21	5	5	100.0%
22	2	2	100.0%

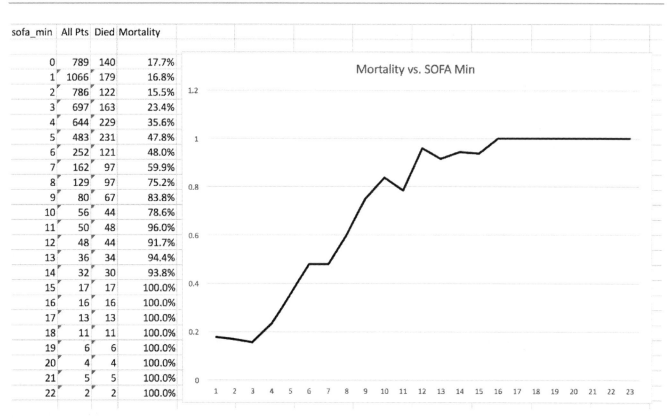

sofa_max	All Pts	Died	Mortality
0	285	84	29.5%
1	231	18	7.8%
2	303	21	6.9%
3	364	38	10.4%
4	504	63	12.5%
5	503	112	22.3%
6	425	86	20.2%
7	433	108	24.9%
8	425	177	41.6%
9	372	139	37.4%
10	271	100	36.9%
11	254	110	43.3%
12	221	99	44.8%
13	183	105	57.4%
14	157	95	60.5%
15	109	67	61.5%
16	91	69	75.8%
17	71	62	87.3%
18	45	42	93.3%
19	48	41	85.4%
20	37	34	91.9%
21	19	18	94.7%
22	21	20	95.2%
23	8	8	100.0%
24	4	4	100.0%

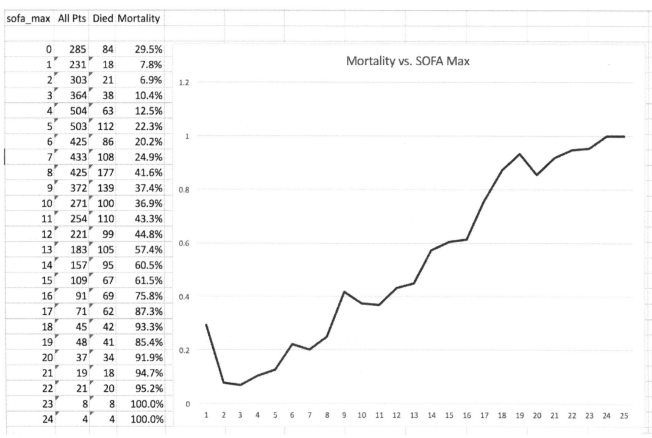

INDEX

1

1:1	7, 8
1:M	6, 8, 64, 79, 80, 201, 203, 356

60

60 seconds limit	20

A

Admission	143
Age	83, 84, 95, 102, 111, 142, 149, 175, 187
Aggregate	48
Alias	21, 28
Average	48, 51, 52, 54, 57, 94, 175, 187, 217, 225, 299, 300

B

Balance	379
Beth Israel Deaconess Medical Center	i, 10
Blood	214, 271, 272, 273
BMI	94, 102, 117, 118, 125, 134, 139, 142, 143, 320
BookGuests	14, 15, 16, 17, 19
Braden	259, 266, 275, 375

C

Calculate	111, 117, 130, 135, 141, 142, 143, 152, 162, 163, 164, 166, 189, 195, 198, 208, 216, 225, 232, 266
Care giver	248, 249
Chart	239
Client	20
Clinical query	91, 95
Cloud	2, 3, 10, 13
Column	129
Conceptual model	91, 92
Connect	12, 16, 17
Connection method	20
Cons	89
Consistent	100
Correct	99
Count	62, 70, 98, 208, 225, 257, 258

D

Date / Time	21, 43, 95
De-identification	9, 10
Description	84, 85, 308, 309
Discharge	239, 245

Disconnect	12, 18
Distribution	94
Domain	93, 385
Dose	220, 227
DRG	78, 81, 82, 83, 84, 94, 95, 154, 155, 161, 162, 163, 168, 169, 170, 171, 173, 199
Drug	217, 220

E

EHR	ii, iii, 2, 3, 92, 104, 385
Electronic Health Record	ii, 93
Entity	76, 77
ERD	47, 76, 77, 78, 79, 80, 82, 84, 85, 89, 90, 96, 98, 99, 103, 110, 111, 113, 115, 154, 161, 172, 201, 218, 219, 231, 232, 240, 242, 249, 250, 251, 255, 262, 267, 268, 269, 270
Ethnicity	28, 94, 102, 119

F

Failed connection	12, 19
Female	94, 130, 324
Filter	212
FK	6, 7, 74, 79, 83, 84, 90, 98, 103, 104, 219, 270, 310
Fluid	267
Foreign Key	6, 79

G

GCS	275, 276
Gender	95, 102, 109, 142, 147, 174, 175, 184
Grid	22, 23

H

Height	117, 118, 134
Hemoglobin	267, 271
HIPAA	10
Hostname	12, 14, 16, 19, 20
Hypoglycemia	200, 208, 212

I

ICD	154
ICU stay	239, 243, 248, 256, 257, 258, 265, 266, 272, 273, 278
Identifier	6
Imaging	175
Index	5, 134, 381
Information schema	76
Inner join	63
IV	39, 44, 217, 218, 220, 221, 222, 226, 295

L

Left join	63
Limit	44

LOINC	206
LOS	ii, iii, 51, 94, 95, 122, 139, 140, 141, 142, 143, 144, 153, 162, 163, 174, 175, 195, 230, 236, 274, 281
Lost connection	12, 18, 241

M

M N	7, 8, 94
Male	94, 130, 324
Many to Many	7
Map	91, 96
Maximum	48, 94
Microbiology	201
MIMIC2 Demo	i, 10
Minimum	48, 50, 94, 111
Mortality	94, 95, 106, 125, 126, 129, 130, 131, 134, 135, 136, 153, 157, 161, 174, 175, 190, 191, 230, 234
MRSA	200, 205
MySQL Community Server	10, 13
MySQL Workbench	10, 12, 13, 16, 17, 18, 19, 20, 22, 23, 24, 25, 78

N

Name	16
Nitroprusside	217, 226
NoSQL	3
Nursing	245, 246, 259, 275

O

One to one	7

P

Password	17, 20
Patient	6, 94, 95, 102, 103, 105, 204, 205, 239, 240, 353
Physician	6
Physionet	i, 10
PK	4, 5, 6, 7, 74, 78, 79, 83, 84, 90, 98, 103, 104, 106, 219, 270, 310
PK / FK	74, 83, 84, 90, 98, 104, 270
Port	16, 20
Prescription	6
Primary Key	4, 6, 78, 80
Procedure	230
Profile	95, 174, 175
Pros	89

R

RDBMS	2, 4, 5, 8, 10, 34, 90
Readmission	95, 146, 153, 168, 175, 196
Relationship	76, 77
Restraints utilization	259, 264
Reverse engineering	76, 90
Right join	63
Route	220

S

SAPS-I	275, 276, 277
Score	266, 274, 275, 276, 375
Self-join	63, 165
Sepsis	174, 175, 177, 185, 186, 188, 191, 192, 346, 347, 348
SOFA	44, 274, 275, 276, 277, 278, 279, 280, 281, 282, 284
SQLi	ii, iii, 1, 2, 3, 8, 10, 13, 20, 21, 22, 23, 24, 26, 28, 30, 31, 32, 34, 38, 39, 44, 47, 49, 56, 60, 65, 66, 73, 74, 75, 85, 86, 94, 99, 109, 158, 185, 186
Standard deviation	48, 51

T

Test	17, 91, 99

U

Unique	6
User guide	9, 11
Username	16, 20

V

Venn	65, 185, 186, 188
Volumes	95, 174, 175, 179, 230, 233

W

Weight	102, 117, 118, 134

ABOUT THE AUTHOR

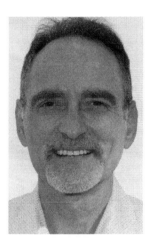

I am a physician board certified in Anesthesiology with a Bachelor's degree in computer sciences and a strong background in clinical informatics.

For more than two decades, I've worked with both vendors developing electronic health records and healthcare organizations implementing this technology, as a liaison between two highly educated groups of professionals— clinicians and information technologists — that unfortunately , rarely speak the same language.

This is my second book, trying to bridge this gap between medicine and informatics.
My first book being on the subject of Systems Analysis of the EHR Medications Domain.

You can contact me by sending a letter, preferably in Structured Query Language and with a well-behaved homing pigeon, to drscarlat at gmail dot com.

Made in the USA
Columbia, SC
27 March 2018

A SURPRISING COMPANIONSHIP

40 PSALM-PRAYERS IN CONTEMPLATIVE VOICE

A SURPRISING COMPANIONSHIP

40 PSALM-PRAYERS IN CONTEMPLATIVE VOICE

Jerry Webber

Director of The Center for Christian Spirituality

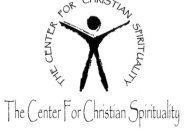

A ministry of Chapelwood United Methodist Church
11140 Greenbay Drive
Houston, Texas 77024
www.centerforchristianspirituality.org

A SURPRISING COMPANIONSHIP
40 PSALM-PRAYERS IN CONTEMPLATIVE VOICE

Copyright ©2014 Jerry Webber

ISBN: 978-0-692-32720-3

Published by The Center for Christian Spirituality
A ministry of Chapelwood United Methodist Church
11140 Greenbay
Houston, Texas 77024

713/465-3467 (phone)
713/365-2808 (fax)

www.centerforchristianspirituality.org
www.chapelwood.org

All rights reserved. No part of this book may be reproduced or transmitted in any form whatsoever without the written permission of Jerry Webber except in the case of brief excerpts or citations as part of articles or reviews. For further information, contact Jerry Webber or The Center for Christian Spirituality.

Cover, design and layout by Bobby Wooley

Printed in Houston, Texas, on
McCoy Silk Recycled Paper

Boasting 10% Post Consumer Waste, FSC Chain of Custody and SFI Fiber Sourcing certifications.
100% of the electricity used to manufacture McCoy was generated with Green-e certified renewable energy.

First Edition

*When Jacob woke up from sleep
he said to himself,
"Surely the Lord is in this place
and I wasn't even aware of it."*

*So he named that place Beth-El,
which means, "house of God."*
— **Genesis 28:16, 19**

For all those who help me
wake up from sleep
and realize that every time, person, and place
is Beth-El . . .

. . . especially
        Sr. Adeline, Kaye, and Janet

        Eric Deal, my friend and favorite altar-server

        Gregg Taylor

        Paul Ilecki . . .

God was here all along
        and I had not noticed

CONTENTS

INTRODUCTION AND ACKNOWLEDGMENTS i

DAY (**01**)	PSALM 19:1 – 4 PRAYER	A psalm of story-telling	1
DAY (**02**)	PSALM 107:4 – 9 PRAYER	A psalm of surprising companionship	2
DAY (**03**)	PSALM 42 PRAYER	A psalm of always-present connection	4
DAY (**04**)	PSALM 61 PRAYER	A psalm for stepping into the unknown	7
DAY (**05**)	PSALM 91 PRAYER	A psalm for burrowing into God	9
DAY (**06**)	PSALM 119:145 – 152 PRAYER	A psalm that barters with God	12
DAY (**07**)	PSALM 39 PRAYER	A psalm for bearing life	14
DAY (**08**)	PSALM 29 PRAYER	A psalm celebrating God's voice	16
DAY (**09**)	PSALM 79 PRAYER	A psalm of mercy	18
DAY (**10**)	PSALM 20 PRAYER	A blessing psalm	20
DAY (**11**)	PSALM 44 PRAYER	A psalm about worthiness	22
DAY (**12**)	PSALM 36:5 – 9 PRAYER	A psalm for finding God all-ways	25
DAY (**13**)	PSALM 119:113 – 120 PRAYER	A psalm of kinship	26
DAY (**14**)	PSALM 137 PRAYER	A psalm from a foreign land	28
DAY (**15**)	PSALM 51:7 PRAYER	A psalm in praise of unbounded love	30
DAY (**16**)	PSALM 93 PRAYER	A psalm acclaiming God's DNA	33
DAY (**17**)	PSALM 84 PRAYER	A psalm for being at home in God	34
DAY (**18**)	PSALM 119:105 – 112 PRAYER	A psalm extolling stillness	36
DAY (**19**)	PSALM 127 PRAYER	A psalm for a life of meaning	38
DAY (**20**)	PSALM 62 PRAYER	A psalm of waiting	40

DAY (**21**)	PSALM 122 PRAYER	A psalm of *shalom*	42
DAY (**22**)	PSALM 129 PRAYER	A psalm for when life presses down	44
DAY (**23**)	PSALM 30 PRAYER	A psalm of being pulled from darkness	46
DAY (**24**)	PSALM 142 PRAYER	A psalm of help and rescue	48
DAY (**25**)	PSALM 133 PRAYER	A psalm of healing balm	50
DAY (**26**)	PSALM 38 PRAYER	A psalm to heal toxic shame	52
DAY (**27**)	PSALM 16:1 – 5 PRAYER	A psalm for waking up	55
DAY (**28**)	PSALM 119:65 – 72 PRAYER	A psalm for blossoming delight	56
DAY (**29**)	PSALM 75 PRAYER	A psalm advocating mercy	58
DAY (**30**)	PSALM 119:1 – 8 PRAYER	A psalm for exploration	60
DAY (**31**)	PSALM 40:1 – 14 PRAYER	A psalm for carrying weights	62
DAY (**32**)	PSALM 131 PRAYER	An honest psalm of restlessness	65
DAY (**33**)	PSALM 90 PRAYER	A psalm for living fully our days	66
DAY (**34**)	PSALM 144:13 – 16 PRAYER	A psalm of real-life faithfulness	68
DAY (**35**)	PSALM 24 PRAYER	A psalm of the One who comes	70
DAY (**36**)	PSALM 33:1 – 11 PRAYER	A psalm for acclaiming God	72
DAY (**37**)	PSALM 76 PRAYER	A psalm for an alternative vision	74
DAY (**38**)	PSALM 82 PRAYER	A psalm for hearing God's voice	76
DAY (**39**)	PSALM 22 PRAYER	A psalm to the unbridled God	78
DAY (**40**)	PSALM 100 PRAYER	A psalm of God's Oneness	81

INTRODUCTION

A Surprising Companionship. . . . The words floated upon me fresh as I prayed one of the psalms included in this collection. That phrase, "surprising companionship," immediately stirred my heart. The image spoke to me of times I felt lost or still-lost, only to discover that I was companioned in unanticipated ways. Sometimes that companionship took the form of a person who stood with me through a painful experience. Sometimes my companion was a whispered prayer, connecting me resiliently to hope when all I could feel was despair. Sometimes my tangible companion came toward me on four, furry legs, sitting at my feet as if she knew the difficulty of the moment. And sometimes the companion was a simple trust that held me through the dark hours, a faithful buoy for my soul that would not allow me to drown.

Hindsight reveals a constant thread in these varied experiences. In each situation, somehow and in some way, there was God . . . God's unanticipated presence throughout all of life. That presence may be manifested in various ways and may feel like a "surprising companionship," but it is steady throughout every season of life.

In the Christian context, the word "gospel" signifies good news. The good news is that God comes, God companions, God gives, God accompanies. God does not stand far off, does not forsake, does not turn a deaf ear.

This companionship is frequently surprising because we continually uncover it in places we didn't think to look, in people with whom we don't anticipate God's embodiment, and in situations through which we never imagined God could be seen.

God's surprising companionship is not limited to certain pious people, to "holy" places, or to special times. God doesn't merely show up here or there, on a whim or as a fate. Rather, God is always and everywhere, ever-present in time and place.

To be honest, I usually notice God's companionship in hindsight. I am a slow learner. I tend to sleepwalk through life, not always awake and alert to God's always-everywhere presence. Frankly, in darker and more strenuous days, I tend to see more quickly this companionship already within and around me.

Through these psalm-prayers, I hope you experience God's surprising companionship wherever you are. Whether you find yourself in joyful celebration, or deep inside darkness, pressed down like a vein of ore squeezed through rock, God is in that place within you and around you. I hope these words help you pray honestly from that place.

ON SPIRITUALITY AND PRAYER, PSALMS AND CONTEMPLATIVE VOICE

Spirituality has to do with being consciously connected to God in a way that shapes our lives in relationship with God, self, others, and the created world. This connection transforms us inwardly, so that our lives make a difference in the world. Transformed people transform the world. The goal of spirituality is not greater piety, self-righteousness, or escape from reality, but rather a grounded and intimate connection with God that allows for deeper engagement with life-as-it-is.

One manifestation of this conscious connection is prayer. Prayer gives us a listening and speaking language for our life with God. Prayer invites us to a posture of receptivity that allows for a more full-bodied communion with God. Immersed in this communion, we find a lens of mercy and compassion through which to view the world.

There is no single way to pray. Prayer takes many forms. Just as we can never exhaust or get to the end of our relationship with God, so it is with prayer. To pray is to enter a vast and unending terrain that invites us to exploration. Parts of the landscape may feel familiar and cozy, and the temptation is to find one part of the terrain – or one way to pray – and to settle there, as if one expression of our life in God could be the totality of prayer.

Years ago I decided to enter through the gate, to explore the landscape of prayer and conscious connection with God. I began my exploration in the Psalms of the Old Testament. I prayed these ancient prayer-poems daily, learning from them a vocabulary for prayer. These prayers permitted me to bring every aspect of life into my prayer. I found the psalms to be honest about life. They were raw, unedited speech, not shouted at neighbor or foe, but aimed at God. From the Hebrew Psalms, I slowly learned that prayer hinges on bringing real life – not life as it should be, ought to be, or might be – to God.

Thus, some psalms are shaped by thankfulness and praise, while others are sparked by situations of animosity or trouble. Some are meant to be prayed personally, and others are meant as corporate expressions of faith. Some celebrate life as well-ordered, and some lament life as fragmented and chaotic. Some are parochial and nationalistic, while others are global and inclusive.

So in my beginnings, I explored this corner of the prayer-landscape with psalms. I have continued to pray psalms these many years later. But my exploration of prayer did not end there. At some point in the journey, I found a part of prayer's geography called "contemplative prayer." Modern use of the word suggests that "contemplative" indicates something we think about or contemplate, but that is a narrow misconception. Sometimes called "the prayer of quiet listening" or "the prayer of the heart," contemplative prayer practices gently lead to openness and receptivity. They are ways of prayer that mold our hearts, quietly shaping us inwardly. They enable us to listen for the still, small voice of God. They are the practices that dispose us toward the gentle winds of God's Spirit.

As I explored contemplative prayer – while still praying in many different ways – I found my outlook changing. Opening to God and listening to God altered my awareness. It shaped the way I viewed other persons. It slowly shifted the way I perceived events and life situations. Contemplative prayer became more than just another way to pray. It became a stance or a posture for seeing God, myself, others, and the created world . . . a stance rooted in quietness and peace, in mercy and compassion.

Further, contemplative prayer shaped every other devotional practice, including my prayer with psalms. For example, I found myself unable to demand that God give victory to my family, my team, my race, or my nation, as many of the Hebrew Psalms so honestly implore. I prayed less for vengeance and retribution, and more for healing and mercy. I prayed less that walls would separate us from strangers or foreigners, and more for the common desires that live within all humans. I prayed less about my enemies in the outer world, and more about the enemies that live within me and hinder my capacity to be God's reconciling person in the world. I found myself with fewer answers and with more questions. Less and less did I believe that the way I saw and experienced life was "the way it is." More and more I opened myself to the vantage-point of others, especially those very different from me.

This book comes as a result of my own exploration. The prayers are rooted in the Hebrew Psalms, but they are offered in my own "contemplative voice," the melding of my own engagement with psalms from the perspective of a listening heart. In that sense, these prayers entwine two aspects of a vast landscape. But they are not exhaustive. They represent only a small part of prayer's expansiveness.

GOD-LANGUAGE

The prayers of scripture offer many images for God (Shepherd, King, Provider, and so on). None of the metaphors exhaust God, yet each speaks to some aspect of God in relationship to humans. As my own prayer has evolved, I've experimented with contemporary equivalents for these biblical images. Some of those metaphors find their way into this collection.

For example, the word "Lord" in the Old Testament often translates the Hebrew word, "Yahweh." The word, from the Hebrew verb "to be," is almost unutterable and beyond knowing. Generally, it is translated "I Am Who I Am." In the ancient world, most all deities were identified by function . . . god of war, goddess of hearth, god of fertility, goddess of the moon, and so on. But at the burning bush, for instance, God is revealed to Moses as Yahweh, "I Am Who I Am" (Ex. 3). God is being, Essence. In other words, God is. Period. God is more than a job description. God is deeper than a function. God is named by the vastness and mystery of being.

Thus, in some psalm-prayers, I have found it sufficient simply to affirm that "God is" or that "God is to me." In that is-ness I sense a depth that no words can completely mine or exhaust.

I also experience God to be "One." The Shema clearly declares, "Hear, O Israel, the Lord is one, and you shall love the Lord with all your heart, soul, and strength," (Dt. 6:4 – 5). Even in the mystery of Trinity, there is unity. Within this wholeness resides God's impulse to bring all things into union. God's movement toward reconciliation speaks to the one-ing of fragmented parts. This oneness is the essence of Jesus' prayer for us in John 17. For centuries, the saints and mystics have written that our spiritual destination is what they called, "divine union," that is, knowing ourselves intimately connected to God in oneness. Thus, I have often called God "the One" in these prayers.

In these prayers, I affirm that God acts generously without limits. In gracious generosity, God gives to the world, yet never exhausts what it means to be God. Thus, in other psalm-prayers I refer to God as "Source."

You will also see psalm-prayers which refer to the "Magnetic Center." I often use that phrase, as well as "True Pole," to translate the Hebrew notion of Mount Zion. Mount Zion was literally the centralized worship place to which all persons went to praise and offer sacrifice. People traveled from the entire known world in order to worship at this "center." In these psalm-prayers, I use "Magnetic Center" and "True Pole" to suggest a dynamic, modern-day equivalent.

Finally, I frequently lean into the idea that God is "always" (in time) and "everywhere" (in space). I find that most of us are frequent atheists, living as if God is present from time to time, but also as if God is absent much of the time. Our great challenge in prayer, Teresa of Avila wrote 400 years ago, is that we often pray as if God were absent. In my psalm-prayers, I affirm that God is "always and everywhere." It reminds me that God's companionship is constant, not occasional or conditional.

FORMAT AND LAYOUT

You will notice that I have used little punctuation in my prayers, and almost no periods. We are never finished with prayer and prayer is never finished with us. We may begin to pray with set times and parameters, but prayer actually involves all of life. From my Benedictine brothers and sisters, for instance, I learn that when I pray, I am doing work. By the same measure, when I am doing my work, I am at prayer. In other words, all of life is prayer, holy interaction, and divine communion.

When I have resisted putting a period at the end of a line or the end of a prayer, I mean to suggest that prayer carries on. It doesn't stop. We don't cease praying because of a dot at the end of a sentence.

By giving attention to layout – and not merely to word choice – I hope to imply that prayer is more than words. Sometimes prayer cascades as a visual image and sometimes it becomes stopped up. Perhaps a time or two in these pages, you will find yourself not so drawn to the words themselves as to the movement of lines, words, and phrases across the page.

I have used capitalization and spacing to suggest sentence structure. Even so, there are times when the lack of punctuation allows for a line to be read both as completing a previous thought and as introducing a new thought.

USING THIS RESOURCE

In two previous collections of psalm-prayers, *Sometimes an Unknown Path* and *Fingerprints on Every Moment*, I offered numerous suggestions for using the books. I will not repeat those prompts here.

I compiled these prayers for use during Advent and Christmas, though they are appropriate for any time of year. The phrase " Surprising Companionship" naturally expresses Christ's incarnation and God's willingness to take up residence in our world within humans. Jesus is born among us and his name "Immanuel" means, "God with us." His birth takes place in the midst of real-life issues . . . the infertility of faithful couples, taxes to be collected, rigorous work schedules, unforeseen pregnancies, make-shift maternity wards, dictators who act madly, and wise elders who have clung tenaciously to hope for decades. Into th challenging world of struggle and ordinariness, Christ comes.

Thus, in his Christmas carol "O Little Town of Bethlehem," Phillips Brooks could write,

> *Yet in thy dark streets shineth*
> *the everlasting light;*
> *the hopes and fears of all the years*
> *are met in thee tonight.*

Bethlehem's setting becomes a metaphor for our lives. The one born at Christmas meets us in the fullness of our hopes and ou fears. Born in humility, he comes as our surprising companion.

These prayers also may be useful during the Lenten and Easter seasons. The Risen Christ is proclaimed alive in the world, among us always and everywhere. The message of Easter reaffirms this experience of presence. After Jesus' crucifixion and resurrection, a group of disciples walking the road to Emmaus found themselves companioned by a stranger. They had not expected God alive in the world, but to their surprise, found that Jesus himself walked with them and then shared their table. So it is with the Risen Christ.

Most of all, my desire is that you would take a step into the Hebrew Psalms for yourself. You might find it helpful, for examp to read these psalm-prayers with a traditional Bible translation in one hand and these prayers in the other. You will note how I prayed the words of the actual psalm. More importantly, you might consider how you would pray those same words. What voice arises from your own soul to express the words of the psalmist? And if that practice led you to write a few psalm-prayer in your own voice, I would be delighted.

Psalms are not the end of the landscape of prayer, but they are a part of it. I hope you will explore them for yourself. Don't solely trust me as your guide. Pray them in your own idiom. Find your own vocabulary for prayer. Psalms comprise an important part of prayer's terrain.

ACKNOWLEDGEMENTS AND GRATITUDE

I am thankful for the scores of persons who have shaped me through words, kindnesses, prayer, welcome, and lived witness. I cannot name each of you, though your presence has beamed light into the world.

I am grateful for numerous opportunities to be with spiritual seekers in settings of the Academy for Spiritual Formation (The Upper Room Ministries) around the country. Friends like John Lockhart, Annette Breazeale, Brenda Anderson-Baker, Lindsay Churchman, Allison Boone, Carmen Gaud, Jane Vennard, Jerry Haas, and Johnny Sears have provided opportunities to be with Academy sojourners in ways that have shaped each of us.

I am indebted to the people and staff of Chapelwood United Methodist Church in Houston, Texas, where I have served for 14 years. They support a ministry of prayer, spiritual formation, and contemplative life in numerous ways. I am grateful for retired Senior Pastor Jim Jackson, current Senior Pastor John Stephens, and Executive Pastor Bob Johnson. They provide encouragement as we explore the terrain of prayer and contemplative life.

Many persons in Southeast Texas participate in the ministry of The Center for Christian Spirituality. Through worship, classes, and on retreats, they have prayed many of these psalm-prayers with me. They form a life-giving community of embodied grace, contemplative prayer, and surprising companionship. They are friends who make a difference in the world.

Each week, a Chapel-full of people gather for Contemplative Worship at Chapelwood. Partners in ministry lead that service along with me: Lori Anderson, Melissa Maher, Peter Johns, and Wick Stuckey. We explore and create, we laugh together and weep together. These companions are soul-friends to whom I owe much.

Kristin Lewis and Nancy Sterling assist me in daily ministry. Kristin handles countless ministry details that I am either too old or too unwilling to learn. I'm glad to be able to lean on her. Nancy cares for many ministry concerns that arise daily, serving with a compassionate heart. She also gives her editor's eyes to manuscripts like this one, suggesting ways to make it clearer.

Karen Firenza and the Communication's Ministry at Chapelwood have shepherded this project to completion. I am indebted to Bobby Wooley, a colleague and friend, who has masterfully laid out these pages and made my often-unintelligible work accessible for others. His spirit is imprinted on these pages in ways you will notice, though his name is scarcely seen. The layout and design of this book is the fruit of his artistry.

Finally, I cannot think about "a surprising companionship" without remembering my dear friend, Paul Ilecki. Paul and I eased into a quick and deep friendship several years ago. In fact, the word "friendship" seems far too trite for the depth of life we shared together over a relatively short time. He was a quiet, gentle, wise presence. If he were still alive to say it to me, he would resist any way I could describe him . . . so I won't try. I have grieved through these months since his sudden death, but have also sensed his companionship in a way I cannot explain, in a way that transcends long-distance internet chats. In that spirit, I remember Paul with this book.

Please forgive the shortcomings on these pages. They are mine and mine alone.

JERRY WEBBER
All Saints, 2014

DAY ONE

PSALM 19:1 – 4 Prayer
A psalm of story-telling

The ducks and stars
    oaks and rabbits
        still ponds and night-cereus
            all tell Your story
                and display Your artisanship

Light speaks to light
Darkness teaches the next darkness

They have no words
    but their silence is a shout

They speak the language of being

Their testimony spreads far

Their message of the God-life
    told day after day
        night after night

I, too, have a story to tell
    with my lips
    with my life

Here it is . . .

For reflection: What is your story? What story does your day-by-day life tell? Make this the material of your prayer.

DAY TWO

PSALM 107:4 – 9 Prayer
A psalm of surprising companionship

Lost in a wasteland
    I wandered

        No landmarks to lead me home
        No discernible path to a dwelling place

Driven on by hunger, thirst
    desiring more
        the inner fire flickering within

Crying out in my lostness
    seeking help in the darkness

And then . . .
    . . . an unexpected presence!
    . . . a surprising companionship!

The way did not come clear
    but I felt myself accompanied

I saw just one next step
    of the path
        appear before me
    not knowing where it led
        yet trusting it
            to carry me home

So met by mercy
    I offer You thanks
A receiver of compassion
    I am grateful

Lost in a wasteland
    You uncovered a path onward
Blind in the darkness
    You beamed a glimmer of light
Hungry for more
    You wafted the faintest aroma of peace

Lip-praise
And life-praise
    to You
        my Surprising Companion

For reflection: As you reflect on this psalm-prayer, ask the Holy Spirit to remind you over the next 24 hours of God's companionship with you. Be prepared to notice God's companionship in surprising, unexpected places.

03 DAY THREE

PSALM 42 Prayer
A psalm of always-present connection

The deer, the bear, the mountain lion
    gather at the river in Pecos for nourishment
        drawn by thirsty cravings

So my body craves air and water
    with a determined longing

So my soul cannot be other than You
    entwined with You
    united with You
    linked with You
So I don't need to go anywhere to find You
    no holy place
    no beautiful reserve
    no inspiring overlook
    no awe-full experience
    no temple of the outer world

So why the separation I feel?
    Why have I convinced myself
        You are not here?
    Others say, "Go here to meet God"
        or "God showed up then"
        or "God was in this place"
    And I, too, live out of that false assumption
        that You are basically absent
            except for periodic appearances
                the moments I catch a glimpse
                    or lose my breath

I remember my beginnings . . .
    inviting You to "show up"
    encouraging congregants to "meet You" in worship

    I spent my energy trying to lead people
        to meet numinous You
            in a moment of luminosity
        to lead people to You
            in the sacred place
        to discover Your presence,
            then take people there
        to catch You – Genie-God –
            in a bottle and have You for always

How dull
    How confused
You were within all along
    woven into my being

My soul's heaviness
    does not equate
        to Your absence

My deeps open to You
    touching Your deeps
I am a sponge in the depths of the ocean
    full of the ocean's water
    and surrounded by the ocean's water
You have covered me
    filled me
    consumed me

DAY THREE (Cont)

So that by day
       Your merciful kindness is the ground I walk on
And by night
       Your love and peace are the air I breathe

Thus, the situations of my life are not indicators
       of Your presence or absence
As if difficulties were a sign of Your
       rejection and abandonment
             when I feel overwhelmed
                broken
                confused
As if Your connection to my soul
       was fleeting
       and conditional
       and tied to my response
              toward these life-situations

The day-to-day happenings of my world may seem dire
       but none of them change the interior connection
       none of them dissuade You from presence

Trust God, then, my soul
       but also
Trust your own interior connection
       with God
Trust what you have
       what is real
Trust the truth

For reflection: Where are the geographical places where you feel most closely connected to God? Can you believe that God is no more present to you in those settings than in the ordinary, mundane places of your life? Bring this awareness into your prayer.

DAY FOUR

PSALM 61 Prayer
A psalm for stepping into the unknown

I show up, it seems,
    with a list in my hands
        of troubles and holes
    the traps into which I have fallen

Always waiting for rescue
    the turning of the wind
    the lifting of the weight
    the liberating of the heart

Awaiting the dawn when You set me
    above the fray
        beyond the tree-line
            looking down on the clouds
As if Your job were to keep me clean
    to brush the dust from my shirt
    and wash the mud from my knees
        a brilliant sparkle to my being

This is a messy life
    and the path leads downward
        through the muck
The shelter I seek is not immunity
    from the difficulty
    but with-ness for the journey
        not the fore-seeing that knows
            what is ahead
    but the faithfulness that steps
        into the "I-know-not-what"

DAY **FOUR** *(Cont)*

The sum of my days is unknown to me
    – dare I pray for more of them
        from my darkened corner? –

Somehow give me the grace to live my hours
    in a way that reflects Your original design
        woven into my heart
Let me step into the unknown future with a spirit
    of mercy, graciousness, and openness
Let me never stop becoming
    through every happening
        in me
        and around me
That my becoming
    would be Your praise
        and fulfill Your dream
            for me

For reflection: Is there a part of this prayer that comforts you or gives you a sense of peace? Take that part of the prayer into your own conversation with God.

DAY FIVE

PSALM 91 Prayer
A psalm for burrowing into God

When I burrow into You
    my sight clears
I find myself

I see others as my sisters
    and brothers
I take on Your way
    of being in the world

I say to You
    "I want to be here forever
    I want to experience this fullness of life always
    Please don't ever lose me
        from Your heart"

Even when I'm burrowed into You
    terrible things still happen
My life in Your heart is not a hiding
        not a safety
        not protective insulation

    It is a seeing
        a loving
        a mercy-ing
    so that my stance toward those terrible things
        is altered
    so that I'm changed from the inside-out
    so that my perspective shifts

I'm no longer afraid of the fearsome midnight
    the dark pit of despair
    the daily upsets and tumults
        of life in this world
The cancers that threaten to decimate me
    no longer offer the last word

DAY FIVE *(Cont)*

I cannot coerce others
        into dwelling here with me
Only open the door
        and invite them in

Some will fall aside
        seeking to go it alone
                to weather the storm in their own resources

As for me
        I must find a home in You
                a moment-by-moment connection
                      that animates my being

Life still crumbles and falls
Evil still erupts
        – sometimes within *me* –
But it need not shake me
        need not bring me to final harm

Unseen messengers flood the world
        angelic guardians
        the wavelengths of prayer
        the peace of those who share good will
They care for me in ways mostly unnoticed

One day, the curtain will be pulled back
        we will see

This I hear You say:

> "Don't live in an anxious mess
> Root yourself in My love
> Walk trust-fully step-by-step
>   without worry or fear
> Use My name
> Let Me be your anchor
>   when the winds blow
>   and the storm rushes in
> I am that near
>   closer than your breath
> In fact, think of your breath
>   as a prayer
>   constantly breathing in
>   breathing out
>   My name
>   My being
>   'Yah-weh . . . Yah-weh'
>
> Thus, there will never be a time
>   when you are without Me
> There will never be a place
>   where you are separated from Me
>
> Peace now, my lovely one
> Peace always"

For reflection: Traditionally, Psalm 91 is a night-prayer of comfort and shelter. If you find a line or stanza in this prayer that resonates with you, let your prayer today begin there. You might want to offer the prayer at the end of your day.

06 DAY SIX

PSALM 119:145 – 152 Prayer
A psalm that barters with God

Whole-hearted
Half-hearted
Some other-hearted

When I call to You
    I plead with the only heart
        I have

This heart that is mostly concerned for me
    wants to deal and barter:
"If You'll answer as I desire
    I can more surely keep Your commands"

"If You would rescue me
    in my distress
        I would be faithful to You"

My life and faith
    full of these conditions
        these responses to You
            that are predicated
                on how life is going for me

Early each morning
    I rehearse the pleas
    I trust Your word –
        to the extent it gets me
            what I want –

I lay awake at night
    Perhaps more vigil
        through the dark hours
        will convince You of my earnestness
            my righteousness

Maybe my loud shouts
    will catch Your ear
    and You will give me
        what I long for

I am terminally special
    uniquely unique

Unlike others
    who are mindless
        heedless
            no doubt
        far from You

You must be near to me
    so near
        You can hear

I have taken this stance with You so long
    I'm ready for my reward

Sigh . . .

For reflection: What "deals" have you made with God? In what ways do you live today under the influence of past bargains you've made with God? You may want to reflect on your images of God, recognizing that God does not deal with you on the basis of merit or what you deserve. Our efforts at earning God's favor by our work or our "rightness" only put God under our control. A loving relationship with God is difficult when we continually try to barter with God or earn God's favor.

DAY SEVEN

PSALM 39 Prayer
A psalm for bearing life

Silence is my home
    Stillness is the language
        of my First Love
In quieting my mind
    I do not trash my neighbor
In guarding my tongue
    I honor the other

At times, I have lived in this posture
    speaking little
        listening much
        refusing to spew my angry vomit
            on those around me

In some ways, this did not diminish my pain
    but intensified it
Holding my anger
    the venom turned inward
        on myself
    a flame threatening
        to consume my interior

There are days, God, when I only want the burning
    to be over
I want to be free of the pain
    the poison
    even death is preferable
        to the sharp stab of my conflicted self-interest
    my existence
        just a cloud blown by the breeze
        a shadowed darkness
        a vain accumulation of objects

Hope . . .
    what is it?
Hope . . .
    who is it?

I could recite a creed,
        but it would not be mine
I want my life to write
        my own creed
                its own expression of:
                        "This I believe . . ."

I pray that Your mercy and love
        will absorb all my missteps
                the ways I've brought harm
                        into the world
Give me the grace to bear my life
        with a quiet heart
Give me the grace to bear afflictions
        with hope and peace
Give me the grace to live among others
        as a healing presence

When the night turns dark
        and You slowly remove from me
                what I have not the strength
                        to give You
        find me open and willing
                to live in the darkness
                        and disorientation

This is my prayer
        my heart's cry
For I wander through life
        seeking a way
                allowing the way to emerge
        with You as companion

Don't forget me
        God

For reflection: If there is pain or some difficulty you are bearing right now, find a line or two in this psalm-prayer that you could offer as your own prayer for bearing up through these days.

DAY EIGHT

PSALM 29 Prayer
A psalm celebrating God's voice

All you demi-gods
    you semi-gods
        you arrogant and self-sufficient
            mini-gods
You who take yourself to be the center
    a weak and pathetic play
        sham of life
Step into the center
    say it loud
        with your breath
    sing it loud
        with your life
    bring your mess and imperfection
        your knee bent
        your tongue loosened

The waters, Lord, voice Your love
    the downhill-moving stream
        in symphony with the smooth stones
The skies cracking open
    in brilliant flashes
        Your rumble rolling in from the north
The waves relentlessly shouting
    coming, calling
    each swallowing the last
        swell and crash and tumult

How mighty Your voice!
    How relentless Your speech!
        How glorious Your words!

As oaks give voice to the mighty wind
    as even the strong oaks
        the long oaks
    crack under the weight
        of the pressing storm
    Your speech presses into every corner of the cosmos

At Your cue
    the peoples dance like the newborn foal
    the mountains come alive like a calf finding his legs
When You speak
    the world moves

Your word goes out
    like tongues of flame
        lapping the night air
    like quaking earth
        from which there is nowhere to hide

Elm and cypress tremble
    Black forests fall bare
and across the planet
    all created things call out,
        "Yes!"

You are All
    in All
    All now
    All forever

Giving Your All
    to people
        like me
        like us
    calling, shouting
    whispering, silencing
        "Peace
            be well
            be whole
        Be"

For reflection: Offer to God your intention to hear God's voice as you go through the next few days. As often as needed, renew your desire to be attentive to God's voice. Then listen . . . to others . . . to sounds found in the created world. What do you hear?

09 DAY NINE

PSALM 79 Prayer
A psalm of mercy

Not once, God,
    have I stepped into the worship place
   that it hasn't been filled
      with an odd mix
         of the holy and the profane
The heathen keep company with the saints
    Which is which?
    Who is who?
       I can't keep track
          even with a scorecard

The same mis-matched company that comprises the people of God
    the same spirit of self-interest
       that threatens
         our corporate life
    lives within me
       feeding on rumor
       puffed up in indignation
       plying a façade of saintliness
       cutting off those who seem less
         or behind

That part of me – so real
      so familiar –
  cuts and sheds blood
  blazes and flames fire

And You?
    I would, if in Your shoes
      in my disgust
      throw down stones
        of fire upon
          such small-mindedness
     begging Your destruction
        upon the vile and destructive elements
         in me
           and
         in the world

Eye for eye
Tooth for tooth
  God-justice

Mercy me, Generous One
Heal me, Gracious One
Compassion me, Heartful One
  that I – and we –
    may not be overwhelmed
      by our petty self-interest
      by our faults
      by our insecurities

  that we not harm ourselves
    – or others –
  beyond the point of healing

Free us from our prison
    of retribution
  our impulse
    to destroy

Free us for compassion
  and healing

That I – and we –
  would be like You

Your mercy and compassion
  in the world
    first
      with ourselves

For reflection: The brokenness of the world also lives within me, you, and each of us. We may come in touch with our brokenness, but it does not have to overwhelm us. We also may touch and abide in God's mercy and compassion.

DAY TEN

PSALM 20 Prayer
A blessing psalm

May you cry when life hurts
    and know that you are heard
May you discover your name
    in the Nameless One

May you know the help of
    the Always-Everywhere One
May your most secret center
    know strength

May all your letting go's
    practice you for life-giving surrender
May you make a habit of opening your hands
    in sacrifice

May you know yourself
    and your innermost desires
May you live fully into the original purpose
    for which you were created

Bless us, God, with the grace to celebrate
    Your work
    Your Name
    Your boundlessness

You answer prayer
          surely
     not according to my desires
          but according to Your design
               for all people

So 'tis folly to bow before power and influence
          to trust size and initiative
          to believe only in knowledge and strategy

In wisdom we call upon You

There is no future in human scheming
     it collapses
          without fail

But those who trust Your
     always-everywhereness
         stand

In love and trust
     now
     and ever

For reflection: Consider someone you know who needs blessing today. Write a series of life-affirming blessings for them: "May you . . . ." You don't have to share the list with them, though you may. Most importantly, bless them in your prayer.

DAY ELEVEN

PSALM 44 Prayer
A psalm about worthiness

We have read the stories of scripture and saints
   Your deliverance at the water's edge
      in the dark cave
   How You cleared a path
      how You brought angel-armies to fight
      how You came alongside those who had no resources

They did not overcome by their might or their wiles
   they were not more worthy or holy
      than their adversaries

In an act of grace
   You came for them
      opened a way for them
         delivered them from narrowness to expansiveness

And so with me
   my strengths and abilities
      do not commend me to You
   I don't find the open terrain of expansive living
      by bull-rushing my way through the obstacles

I look to You
   I intend to participate with You
      in Your larger project for the world

Yet, I sit here alone
   confined
      in the rags and bones of my life
   as if someone had plundered my energy
      stolen the treasures that were hidden inside
         my inner vaults

These difficulties devour me
          I'm scattered, unable to touch the Center
     as if my very soul had been sold
          at someone's profit
    a cheap trinket scorned by those who know me
          derided as of little value
               humiliated
               ashamed
               mocked

This is my lot
     And my well-developed system
          of rewards and punishments
          tells me that
          I don't deserve this darkness
    I haven't been knowingly destructive
    I haven't spoken ill of You
          It seems as if I haven't been rewarded
               for my behavior
                    – I kept the rules
                         I adopted the code –

If I do right, I should be rewarded
If I do wrong, You have an obligation to zap me

This is my framework
    my adolescent faith

My current misery – according to that template –
     means I've mis-stepped
          displeased You
          forgotten You

DAY ELEVEN *(Cont)*

In fact, this suffering feels like it comes
    from Your hand

And You sleep
    You reject me
    You hide Your face
    You forget I exist

        all while I sink into shame
          fall into guilt
        become dust

There is something wrong here . . .
    either with You . . .
        or with my system

For reflection Many persons commonly believe that with God, they get what they deserve. Grace, mercy, and love all claim that we don't get what we deserve or what we feel worthy of receiving. Instead, we get God.

DAY TWELVE

PSALM 36:5 – 9 Prayer
A psalm for finding God all-ways

Love loves beyond reach

Faithfulness faiths even when belief is dry

Righteousness rights no matter the opinion polls

Justice justs without measuring conventional wisdom

Salvation saves indiscriminately

Your love cannot be bought
        only received
                freely, no cost

You protect us from nothing
        You abide with us
                in all things

In Your house is fullness
        and emptiness

In Your river is delight
        and difficulty

You are the Light by which we see
        You are the Darkness in which we are birthed

For You are all of life –
        nothing excluded –
    Alpha and Omega

For reflection: God is never locked into one way of being in the world . . . or one way of being with you. Reflect on some of the various ways you have experienced God. For instance, consider how you have experienced God in both light **and** darkness. Or remember how you have experienced God in fullness **and** emptiness.

DAY THIRTEEN

PSALM 119:113 – 120 Prayer
A psalm of kinship

Divided hearts
    divide the world
Divided hearts
    parse the world
        into insiders and outsiders
            us and them
            good and bad
            moral and immoral
            conservatives and liberals
            Palestinian and Israeli
            rebels and loyalists
            documented and undocumented
            Christians, Muslims, Jews, Buddhists, or Hindus

    So that all life
        becomes over-against
  and the stance of over-against-ness
        leaves no room
            for love

You, God, are the undivided Center
    the Magnetic Core
        to whom all are drawn

Save me from the easy demonizing
    and blaming
        that divides
        and makes a villain
            of the other

Hold me, God, in the tension
      of this otherness
Let my discomfort melt
      into kinship

Hold me, God, in Your undivided heart
      where I know my connection
           to the other

For none of us are pure
      none of us completely spurn deceitfulness
      none of us can claim a moral high-path
           that has earned the right to judge
                another

In the fire of Your love
      we all melt into Your heart
When I sink into silence
      I see others through the lens of love

Dread and fear are lame masters
      they gateway paranoia
           guilt and shame

Love, kinship, compassion
      these unlock
           every door

For reflection: The notion of kinship invites us to notice our commonality with other persons, rather than creating walls based on our differences. Kinship doesn't divide, but draws together. Ask God to help you notice your kinship with others you meet over the next few days. Try to be conscious of your kinship with everyone you meet.

DAY FOURTEEN

PSALM 137 Prayer
A psalm from a foreign land

I sat in a foreign land and wept
    among those of strange tongue
    among those who hated me
    among those who wanted me gone
I remembered You
    remembered the thought of You

My songs and instruments
    hung in a closet
        stored away
            no longer needed or useful
  I was
    who they said
        I was

The dialogue ended
        no more give-and-take
  now there was one way
    their way
  the tone of taunt in every exchange:
    "Why can't you sing your song?
        We'll play the music . . .
            you just sing along"

The song You've given
buried deep inside me
    I don't want to sing their song
        I'll do anything to keep from singing
            a pseudo-song

God, don't ever let me be too far away
        to forget Your song
    burn it upon my heart
    weave it into my soul

And for them, these pretenders
        who take their delight in my despair
                who have won the struggle
                        to steer the ship
        who said,
                "Damn you! Damn you!"

Oh, the warrior in me wants to fight to the death,
        to take them down
        and stand over their plot

And the introvert in me wants to run far
        to get out of their sight
                and reach
        and make a new life somewhere else

And the poet in me – at this moment –
        just wants to sing my song
        to spill out the verse from within
                no vengeance or vindication
                      just song

so that the cycle stops
        and all the little ones
                saved

For reflection: Remember a time when you felt great opposition, when it felt as if you lived "in a foreign land." Does this prayer reflect your experience in that land? Does it give voice to your own experience? Allow these memories to lead you into prayer . . . perhaps prayer for others involved in the situation you are remembering, or prayer for healing (yourself or the others).

DAY FIFTEEN

PSALM 51:7 Prayer
A psalm in praise of unbounded love

"You love those centered in truth" (Ps. 51:7)

"You love those centered in truth,"
    the Book says
A witness only to part of the truth

But I say more
    and besides . . .

You love.
    Period.
Love loves what is
    as it is

You love those centered in truth
    and You love those far away from truth
    and You love those who have fallen over the map-edge looking for truth

You love those who grow in attentiveness
    and You love those who cannot see straight

You love those who see You for who You are
    and You love those who see only illusions

You love those moving inward toward stillness
    and You love those whose lives are consumed with busyness

You love those who have lost inertia
    and You love those in the pits of despair
    and You love those floating amidst the clouds of delight

You love those who cultivate the inner life
    and You love those who move toward the world mending the broken

You love those who are aware of Your nearness
    and You love those who have never given You a thought

You love those who daily call Your name
    and You love those who have never before heard Your name

You love those drowning in depression
    and You love those laughing with friends

You love those who look like success
    and You love those who experience failure after failure

You love those who have nobody near
    and You love those surrounded by a supportive host

You love the hard-charging workaholic
    and You love the quiet Sister given to prayer

You love the kindergartener on her first day of school
    and You love the juvenile spending his days in lock-up

You love those who offer themselves for others
    and You love those who lazily sit, moving neither inward nor outward

You love those who love You
    and You love those who hate You
    and You love those who don't care one way or another

DAY FIFTEEN *(Cont)*

You love those whose lives have fallen apart
        and You love those who believe they are all put-together

You love those who regularly and intentionally nourish the soul
        and You love those who only want to make more money

You love addicts – all of us –
        and You love sojourners – all of us –

You love those moving toward the Center
        and You love those living on the periphery

Let my Book say:
You love what is
        as it is

You love.
        Period.

For reflection: Write two or three of your own couplets about love. "You love . . . and You love . . ."

DAY SIXTEEN

PSALM 93 Prayer
A psalm acclaiming God's DNA

The created world is Your domain, God
    and You wear it well
Your being deep within every created thing
    – *inscape*, Father Hopkins called it –
    Every cloud and leaf
        squirrel and sandstone
    Your fine clothing
        and You wear it well

You are the steady Presence at the center of everything
    the sure love of all things

Causing beginnings
Sustaining through time
Holding into the boundless future

Even the waters tell Your story
    alive with Your DNA
        every flowing mountain stream
            gathered lake
            salty sea
    acclaiming You in its own way

And You are more, still
    beyond ocean waves
    and mighty tsunamis
    and the continent-spanning rivers
Always more

Our witness to You
    like the waters
    is small and never enough
Inadequate praise is what we offer
    for You are right and good and true

And You are always

For reflection: The psalm-prayer follows Psalm 93, which affirms that even water tells the story of God. What is water's voice in its many expressions? How does the image of water illumine your own life in connection to God and to others?

DAY SEVENTEEN

PSALM 84 Prayer
A psalm for being at home in God

You Who Are
    You flame in unburned bushes
        the "I AM" who is the Essence of Everything
    at home in the vastness of the created world
    at home in the interior of the human heart

I am restless with longing for You
    my soul shaped to live in union with You
        to make my home where You dwell within me
        and to find my home in the unpredictable creation

Like the cardinal nesting in the low-shrub,
    so my soul comes home to myself
    and finds her connection to You there

Contented are those at home in You
        in self
          in the world
    They find grace to live praise

Blessed are those content in their weakness
        willing to let You make weakness strength
    for they will know the peace to discover secret trails
        that lead to You
        written on their hearts

Not even bitterness and desolation
    can turn them aside
In crisis, even, they know You
    as their well-spring

Their walking in weakness is a journey of strength,
    for they don't need fair weather
        to travel on
They see You, notice You
    at every turn

So I offer my life, You-Who-Are,
    as my prayer
Hear me with Your God-ears
Look upon me with Your God-eyes

For one moment in the interior of Your castle
    is better than a lifetime in any other room
Even waiting at the doorway of Your home
    is preferable to the comforts of deceit and self-centeredness

For You, God of Everything, are a sure guide
    You generously spend grace
        and shining brightness
    You dole out goodness
        to any who open themselves to You

YOU ARE
I AM
    God of Everything
        content is my heart
            as I dwell in You

For reflection: One of the many images found in Psalm 84 is the image of making a home in God. What does it mean for you to be "at home" in God? What images or pictures illustrate for you what it means to make a home in God?

DAY EIGHTEEN

PSALM 119:105 – 112 Prayer
A psalm extolling stillness

Your first language is silence

Your language illumines my life
Your silence gives me space
          to truly hear
Stillness clears the clutter
    and helps me to see

By keeping my silence
    and attending to Yours
I am able to discern
        truly
    the path that opens
        before me

When I am troubled
    I sit still before You
My stillness becomes my prayer
    My tears plead my cause

Let this, my God
    be the prayer that transforms me
        whether the words I speak
        or the silences I keep
  my ears
  my heart
      a listening
      a receiving

I have grasped tightly my life
    holding my very being in hand
Yet, I hear Your invitation
    to open my hands
        to let go of my closed-in life

Even when the extremes of daily living
    hem me in –
        the crazy-making medications
        the shaming directives
        the aging, aching body
        the stinging chemotherapies
        the narrowing parameters of job
My desire is faithfulness
    to lean into You
    to be still with You
    to allow You to fortify my heart
        in unseen
            unspoken ways

I give myself, with intention
    to press my head into Your chest
    to rest in Your heart
    to be at One with You

Now
    and always.

For reflection: Pray today in silence. Repeat a single word (Abba, love, peace, mercy, etc.) slowly and quietly for several minutes. Be aware, as you do, of God's life in you, nearer than your next breath.

DAY NINETEEN

PSALM 127 Prayer
A psalm for a life of meaning

You build to last
    lay foundations
    post beams
    nail up frames
    span trusses

Every other house
    is built on illusions
        glue and duct tape
        smoke and mirrors
    nothing lasts, nothing stands
    structures of my own ego
        erected with a mind to power and control
            my own pleasure
            my own wobbly sense of self

You watch always
    provide sentry
    round-the-clock care
    guard the vulnerable places
    shore up the weaknesses

Every other watch-post
    is built on fantasy
        the deluded dream
        I have for my life
    You stand over
        like an ever-vigilant guard-dog
        protecting the light and life
            within
                the way You've shaped a life
                so that nothing is lost

A vain stranglehold
    I have on my life
    that I would be so anxiously vigilant
        as to choke life
            controlling through the daylight hours
                and keeping watch of my own treasure
                    through night

You watch
You guard
> You give
>> to my weary body
>>> sleep
>>> rest
>>>> ahhhh . . .
>>>>> sweet rest

There are others who inherit
> the promise from us
What do I have to give them?
>> my anxiety about the future?
>> my tight hold on life?
>> my worry about government or economics?
>> my narrow vision of life?
>> my *shoulds*, *musts*, and *oughts*?

Happy and blessed and wise
> the man or woman
>> who shares the promise with others
>> who does not hoard light
>> who does not accumulate a storehouse of life
>> who gives generously of who they are
>>> and what they have

> They spend themselves
>> for future generations

> Their spending
>> You replenish
>>> always

For reflection: Choose one of the images from this psalm-prayer (building a house or a sentry keeping watch) and reflect on how that image shapes your life. In what ways does it illumine your connection to God? How does that image encourage you to invite others into your story?

DAY TWENTY

PSALM 62 Prayer
A psalm of waiting

I wait
    hungry
    silent
I wait for You
My soul waits
    through the rush and scurry of life
My insecure self
    clawing, clamoring
        for more
My soul patient
    still
        till all else recedes
        and there is only You
            the Center
            the Solid Ground

The windy bustle threatens my house
    shakes and shimmies the tiles
    but cannot touch the Center

Your agenda is not to stop the wind
        or fortify the roof
    but to draw me into the Center
        the secure Center of Your heart

There I wait
    hungry
    silent
I wait for You
My soul waits
    patient
    still
        till all else recedes
        and there is only You
            the Center
            the Solid Ground

You, my Illumination
      my Safety
      the Heart of my heart

My mortal life is bounded
          finite
      in time
      and space
one day I will be no more
      will have no weight

All the gains of this life will evaporate
      they won't last
          whether contrived dishonestly
          or attained with integrity
      How hard it is to accumulate much
          – of anything –
      and not trust the "muchness"

In gratuity, You scatter strength and love
          in the world
      generously spreading Your life
          like seed thrown wide
You scatter blindly
      with no thought of merit
You scatter indiscriminately
      to those deserving or not

This is my hope in life, God
      to catch a seed
          or two
      as they fall
          at my feet

For reflection: Let your prayer be silent. Sit still for a few minutes. You don't have to do anything or think anything. Just sit with God. Wait . . . hungry . . . silent.

DAY TWENTY-ONE

PSALM 122 Prayer
A psalm of shalom

My soul warmed within me
    when I heard the Voice say
        "Hide yourself in the Center
            make your home in My heart"

This, I know, is the place of *shalom*
    Your heart is my home

This is the place with thousands
        of gates
    the home with millions
        of entryways
    the address to which all
        are invited
    the dwelling in which all
        find a room

Somehow it is written on our hearts
    the yearning for this Home
    the longing to come into the Center
Here we find ourselves
    and here we see others
        through mercy's lens

Here the foundation prayer is
    "Peace" for all
    the wholeness of *shalom*
        for every corner of creation
    the divine union
        that reconciles every division
    the oneness
        that holds together every fragment

Here, love reigns
    love for family and friends
    love for strangers
    love for those who seem separate from us

"*Shalom*, my friends"

"The wholeness of God fill you
    my sisters and brothers"

And you, too, my readers
    sojourners with me
        into this spacious God-heart

In love
    I pray for your well-being
In mercy
    I pray for your wholeness

Shalom

For reflection: Shalom is more than peace. It means bringing together that which is separated and fragmented. It is wholeness and completeness. Offer your prayer for people and situations that are fragmented and broken apart.

DAY TWENTY-TWO

PSALM 129 Prayer
A psalm for when life presses down

Life presses in on me

Life has pressed in on me since my youth
        – it's the truth –

Life has pressed in on me
        but it has not squeezed me to death

As if I had been hit by a pick-up truck
        and left for dead in the road
            smashed
            run over
                    time after time after time
                    one small death after another

Yet You have not let the life be pressed out of me
        each death has led to more life
        each narrow space has opened up into spaciousness

You have not let those things intended for harm
        have final sway over me
            the quenchers
            the defeaters
            the life-robbers

In the end, they will have no voice
                no power
        their dominion lasts only a short while
            then it is gone
        they have no final say over You

Like weeds in a spring wind
        their seed is blown away
            scattered far
        their impact diminished

So they no longer lay claim to my life
        they no longer poison my becoming
        they no longer pacify me with weary clichés
            as they draw knives from their scabbards:
            "Bless your heart, dear brother
                    trust God
                          and it will go well with you"

For reflection: Every person has experienced their share of being "pressed down" by life. Allow God to suggest to you one or two times in your life when you were pressed down beyond your capacity to bear up under the weight. In hindsight, can you see how God was present in that situation, even if you didn't notice God at the time? Usually, our clearest sight comes at some moment after the incident, when we see the situation with fresh clarity of vision.

DAY TWENTY-THREE

PSALM 30 Prayer
A psalm of being pulled from darkness

Some mornings I sit lifeless, exhausted
    my own near-death experience
  Hope is distant
    no sense of Your within-ness
All is cloud and shadow
    a miserable, sinking depression
      wrestling with absence as I long for presence

Sometimes – not always – sometimes
    I am lifted out of that deep darkness
  For reasons unknown to me
    the weight becomes lighter
    the way clearer
    the sky bluer
    the dreams more vivid

No accident
  this is You
    Your right hand stretched into my life
      reaching into the cloudy soup
        to pull me – if only
          for the moment –
      out of the stranglehold
    You give me breath again
    Your light penetrates the diseased cells
      heals the marrow
    Your energy seeps into the pores
      animates the muscles of my being

It is my own resurrection
    or at least
        with Lazarus
    a resuscitation
        pulling me from the tomb
        a momentary unbinding
            of the grave clothes

The gift of another day
    to see and feel and be
        in the world
And so my heart sings God-songs
    sings in harmony with my soul
        and body
          and tired mind
    a four-part hymn of praise
        to You who have rescued
        You who have given respite
            from the creeping despair
                and hidden loneliness

Sing songs
    my soul
Sing with heart
Join, O mind and body
    the praise
        God-songs
    the Mystery Presence

For reflection: Remember a time in your own experience when you were unexpectedly brought out of a season of "cloud and shadow." Remember what that experience of deliverance was like. Offer your thanks to God.

DAY TWENTY-FOUR

PSALM 142 Prayer
A psalm of help and rescue

I cry out to You
    my voice
    my heart
    my hands
    my being
        loud supplications
        loud petitions
I complain and moan
    I empty the troubles out of my pockets

My spirit is weakened
    I'm hungry – angry – lonely – tired
        vulnerable in my weakness
    Unable to withstand the advances
        of adversaries
            the thoughts and feelings
            that dive me into swirled despair

O Path-Maker, Path-Keeper
    show me the traps
    awaken me to the pitfalls
        along this way I walk

I would flee if I could – my first instinct
        to run far away –
    to run toward those who don't know me
    to a place where I do not stand out

But I have nowhere to go
    I have no one in whom to hide

So I open myself to You, hopeful
    that You would be a refuge
    that You would be my Meal
        of sustenance in this land

Listen as I cry out for help
    I am poor
    I have nothing
        Yet many clamor after me
            clawing for a piece of me

Save me
    the grief, the despair, the emptiness
        that pursues me
    is too strong for me

Throw wide the prison door
        – I already have the key! –
    that I may live freely in fullness

    I give thanks to Your Name

For You are generous
        endlessly
    and the plenty in Your hand
        is more than enough

For reflection: This psalm invites us to cry out for help and rescue. It is something like "Prayer 101": "Help me, God. Save me." If that kind of prayer is appropriate for where you are right now, offer the prayer for yourself. If you are not in a place where you need help or rescue, then pray this prayer on behalf of someone you know who does need it.

DAY TWENTY-FIVE

PSALM 133 Prayer
A psalm of healing balm

This is the way
    life was intended to be . . .
This is what humans
    are made for . . .

To live without walls
    no borders
    no categories
    no jurisdictions

To know ourselves
    in harmony
        with every other living being
To delight in our common humanity
    to celebrate with those who laugh
    and to weep with those who suffer

To drop judgments
    and egocentric posturing
To peer through
    the foggy illusion
        of our separateness
To see the blue skies
    of each other
rather than to judge
    the cloudy storms

Such seeing
    knowing
        living
            is healing balm
                for our world
            anointed oil
                running down the face
                    even of those who intend harm

Our world is suffocating
    for lack of this air

Our world perpetuates brokenness
    for lack of this balm

For You smile at this harmony

Your heart delights

And those who step into this alternative vision
    become Your balm
        for the world

For reflection: As a point of reference, you might want to refer to a traditional version of Psalm 133. Notice the ways this psalm-prayer takes those original lines and makes prayer from them. Then notice the lines or phrases in the prayer that resonate most with you. Pluck them out and let them lead you into your own prayer.

DAY TWENTY-SIX

PSALM 38 Prayer
A psalm to heal toxic shame

My history says, God
    that You steam in anger
    that Your punishment is steered
        toward those who stir Your wrath
    that You shoot arrows of disgust
        toward wrong-doers
    that Your hand presses hard
        upon "sinners"

So I sit in my sickness
        in my soul's despair
        in my body's dis-ease
and can only believe
        that I've brought this crushing weight upon myself
reaping what I have sown
inviting a burden by my bad behavior
        festering wounds borne of my foolishness and folly

Shame . . . my only response
    I am laid low
        in my own badness
this pain what I must bear
        the fruit of my mis-sown life
without feeling
    spirit crushed
    body disabled
    heart-less

This is my narrative
        the script from which I live
                telling the story of my fallen humanity
                      my weak will
                      my faulty heart
                      my failing strength
                      my nearsighted vision

And because the narrative is common
        to those closest to me
No one draws near
        I am anathema
                forsaken
                accursed

You, alone
You, only
        see me
                as I am . . .
You alone
        know this narrative
                is a sham
                a shameful projection
                      of a fractured life
                that has forgotten its Source
                      and has grown disconnected
                            from its Truth

DAY **TWENTY-SIX** *(Cont)*

From this toxic shame, God, heal me
    more than the body's pain
    or the heart's despair
    or the blood's cancer

    From this narrative
        deliver me
  connect me to You
        in a way that imparts life
  and heals the toxins
        that reside deeper than my bone's marrow

Do not leave me in this cesspool
    of shame
        in the rotted corpse
            of these dead frameworks

Heal me
    here
Make haste to help me

For reflection: As an interior toxin, shame convinces us that we are bad and unworthy at our core. Many of us have built lives on foundations of shame. Convinced we are bad, we are also convinced that God sees us as flawed and failed. How does this psalm-prayer invite you to bring your shame to God?

DAY TWENTY-SEVEN

PSALM 16:1 – 5 Prayer
A psalm for waking up

Take me into Your heart, O God
      as I make my home in You

This is my praise:
      You are
      and You are to me
      and You are Source of all good and truth and right

My heart delights in those who seek You
      whose hearts are waking up to You
      who swim upstream courageously
           to find life with You

Those who step unseeing and unconscious into the day
      stir trouble and bring harm upon themselves
           and others
They live heedlessly
      without concern
      without consideration

Once awake, though,
      we cannot turn back to sleep
Once seeing
      we see everywhere

I do not want to live in the dullness
      that is blindness of heart
      nor sleepwalk through my shortened days

For You, God, are my daily Bread
      the Cup I drink
      the bounteous Land in which I live

For reflection: In your own prayer, think about your praise. How would you complete this phrase: "This is my praise . . . ."?

DAY TWENTY-EIGHT

PSALM 119:65 – 72 Prayer
A psalm for blossoming delight

Everywhere
                and
Always
        You give Your Self away
                generously
            as the Book promises

So shape my heart
        to follow You in the same abundant flow
            giving my own self away

Some of life
        I have borne
            as a weight or a burden
                that has pressed me
                further down into my self

But Your creative word
        frees me from self-interest
            bestows the grace of self-giving

You are Good
        and good in the world
            is a sign unto You

Let me notice the good
        and life-giving
            when I see it

Self-centeredness makes false
        perpetuates illusions
God-centeredness orients me
        to fullness of life
One makes stubborn and mean
        the other, wise and self-forgetful

Darkness has been good for me
        the shaping of night
            stumbling forward in blindness
                that I would trust You

Slowly, I learn Your ways
        Your life is becoming within me

Delight blossoms

For reflection: God is generously and endlessly Self-giving. Like a sower scattering seed indiscriminately, God scatters goodness, beauty, and life upon the world. A part of what it means for humans to be created in the "image and likeness of God" is that we, too, are invited to self-giving, giving ourselves away for the good of the world in God's name. This self-giving does not diminish us; rather, when we spend our lives for God's sake, delight blossoms.

DAY TWENTY-NINE

PSALM 75 Prayer
A psalm advocating mercy

We come with thanksgiving
    our God
We come with thanksgiving
    to praise Your Name
    and speak aloud
        the wonders we have seen

This I hear You say:

"Time is in My hands
    all time is
and thus,
    I am always
And always
    My judgments look like mercy

Even when you experience the world
    as tenuous
        and crumbling
I hold all things
    in being
I set all thing
    upon Rock

Empty talk
    and posturing
        does not impress Me
Neither does the proud power
    of the overlords

You who are self-defenders
You who hold power
    stop making a show
        of your position
        of your sway

Look at Me
       Watch how I hold the universe
           in My hands
      I hold the cosmos
          in mercy."

Indeed, God,
    Your judgments
        look like mercy
   a mercy that cannot
       come from the harsh terrain
          or the untamed wilderness

You take no delight in the pain and suffering
    of humans
        even those who act in malice
You do not react vengefully
      tit-for-tat
    to the skewed self-centeredness
      of our tribe
You have no interest in punitive justice
          retribution
   as if punishment – or
      the fear of punishment –
would awaken us

Only love unlocks
    every door
Only mercy cracks
    the heart
Only compassion softens
    the jagged edges

Thus, I sing
    and rejoice
And we together
    long for Your healing redemption
        Your saving of our race

For reflection: Make "mercy" your prayer for others today. Imagine the face of someone for whom you want to pray, then simply whisper, "Mercy," upon them. Next, bring another person to mind, and pray mercy for them, as well. Pray in this way for all the persons you carry on your heart.

DAY THIRTY

PSALM 119:1 – 8 Prayer
A psalm for exploration

Heart-content are they who walk a mindful path
    who travel a becoming road
    whose self evolves as they explore
Heart-content are they who are unafraid of failure
    who risk getting lost
        for the sake of the great soul-treasure

Who fall and get up
    resiliently
    time after time
Who press toward You
    as a vein of ore
        squeezes through stone
Who know the bitter edge of failure
    but not the final failure
        of stopping
            stalling out
                in a safe place

You invite us to exploration
    to find ourselves in You
    and in relationship to others
        in love

This, O God, is Your command
    that we would live in love's light
        and with love's light
            for our good
            and the good of the world

So many days I wish it were more clear-cut
    that the way would be more obvious
    that I could know beyond doubt
        if I was getting the steps right

But that would only make me proud
    more self-full

And so I live in the foggy gray of not-knowing
    trusting alone

Thank You for the light You share
    the illuminations of heart
        that enliven the path

I am bound to You in love
    but not as deeply as
        You are bound
            to me

For reflection: Think of exploration as a spiritual practice. In what ways have you explored the terrain of your own soul? What have you discovered? What practices assist you in the day-by-day exploration of your soul?

DAY THIRTY-ONE

PSALM 40:1 – 14 Prayer
A psalm for carrying weights

I stood under this weight
    bearing the heaviness of the days
You would not allow me to be crushed
    You became to me the "Weight-Bearer"

The weight did not disappear
    nor did the heaviness dissipate
But You led me on
    I walked ahead
        one step at a time

My spirit sang as I walked
    sang a song of thanks and praise
I do not walk this way for attention
    to draw the notice of others
I simply intend to live the only life I have
    to live with You at the center of it

Those who find their life in You are at peace
    They trust the Source
        rather than their own twisted self-interest
            which distorts good and evil
    They do not resort to cruelty in order to satisfy
        their own desires
    And they do not turn to cultural icons
        for fulfillment

    They recognize the Source,
        that from Your heart flows goodness
        from Your heart flows beauty
        from Your heart works a Oneness within all creation

It happens everywhere around me
                – the world is saturated with Your wonders –
        but my dim eyes miss so much

In the end, though, what You really desire is that I see
        that I see and participate in this one-ing
                which originates in Your heart
You aren't interested in piddling sacrifice
              – for the things that seem so huge to me
                      are really so microscopic to You –

To see
To participate
To bring my life into Your wholeness
        so I can walk with others into their wholeness
                and thus participate in the wholeness of the planet –
This is what You have asked

What does Your book say of me?
        "My image is woven into his soul
                Though he is broken
                      and bears the weight
                day after day I uncover my likeness in him"

What, then, shall I do with this uncovering?
        I tell what I know
                what I have seen
                what I have experienced
        When the time is right
                I speak my truth
                      to those who will listen

DAY **THIRTY-ONE** *(Cont)*

I have no magic formulas
        or secret potions
Only my own slow-roasted life
        and my willingness to open up to others
I have spoken my truth
        told my story
                as much as possible
                      in the larger community

I cannot pray for safety as I move forward
        I won't pray for a lighter weight
        I pray this:
                to know the abundance of Your mercy and compassion
                to be deeply connected to Your love and unending generosity
These will be enough to hold me in being
                forever

For the weight is heavy
        the challenges non-stop
                – ever more opportunities to find my faithfulness
                in You –
at any moment I could be overwhelmed
                overtaken
                driven into the dust
                      by this leaden, crushing rock

In Your pleasure
        I will stand
In Your pleasure
        I will not be driven to dust

For reflection: Bring to this psalm-prayer any weights or sadness you carry. Perhaps you could borrow two or three lines from this prayer to help you carry those weights.

DAY THIRTY-TWO

PSALM 131 Prayer
An honest psalm of restlessness

O Lord, I *am* proud
    I *do* have haughty looks

I make small matters great
    and occupy my mind with the trivial
I run from simplicity
    and complicate the mundane

My body is not still
    and my mind is not quiet
I *am* restless with pent-up energy
    even in my weariness

I *am* like a child on mother's breast
    an uneasy, squirming, bawling child
        who wants to escape
            mother's imprisoning embrace
        and run away
            independent of ties and nurture and help

And yet
    my soul remains quiet through this craziness
        waiting
            waiting
                waiting
                      for the racing to stop
                          to come home
                          to rest into You

So it is

So here am I

For reflection: Sit still for a few moments. Consciously open yourself to God, ready to receive whatever God gives. Perhaps your posture (opening your hands or spreading wide your arms) would reflect your openness. No words are necessary. Receive.

DAY THIRTY-THREE

PSALM 90 Prayer
A psalm for living fully our days

Day after day, our God
        time after time
                through every season of life
You are our Source

Beyond all You do – every act
        of creating, sustaining, healing –
You are

The I AM
        Essence of all things
        Being-ness

And we humans are, too

Only for a shortened span of days
        do we live our lives
Yet, forever is our I AM connected to You

You are in time and outside time
        You do not count the days

Yet in our mortality, our bodies wear out
        we are born for vitality
            and live in exuberance
        we get old
        we die
We are not gods
        but humans – weak and limited –

You know our frailty
        familiar with our weaknesses and limitations
            better than we are
        what we consider a secret
            You hold in plain sight
                nothing hidden from You

When our time is over
        we breathe our last
Some at a young age
        and some older

Some after struggle and diminishment
    and some by sudden tragedy

Not always do we see our end coming

So give us sobriety about life
    a heart to live fully each moment
        in self-giving
We have no days to "waste"
    no time that is not priceless

Our days are not commodities we can
    cheaply discard

Give us the grace, God
    to live in Your mercy and generosity

In You I find my morning satisfaction
    I hope to live all my days in contentment of soul

Many days I have experienced my afflictions
    For years I have faced adversities

I hope these afflictions and adversities
    dig a deep well within me
    push me to find my Source in You
    drive me deeper into Your heart

For I would find You in the depths
    I would live in Your generous graciousness
    I would make Your heart my home

    I want to be rich in You
        prosperous in Your love
        wealthy in Your peace
        extravagant in Your mercy

For reflection: At the burning bush (Exod. 3), God is revealed to Moses as YAHWEH. The English translation of that name might be something like I AM WHO I AM or I WILL BE HOWEVER I WILL BE. This self-revelation is important, because it suggests that God is identified more by essence and being than by function. So, too, are humans much more than function, roles, or deeds. We bear the image of the One who is I AM.

DAY **THIRTY-FOUR**

PSALM 144:13 – 16 Prayer
A psalm of real-life faithfulness

Even when our sons disappoint
    and our daughters rebel . . .
Even when none of our children dare
    call out Your name . . .

Even when our barns are empty
    and drought has scorched the crops
        leaving only brown, shriveled
            shards of death . . .

Even when our flocks find no nourishment
    and are ravaged by disease . . .

Even when we have run out of job prospects
    the mortgage is due
    the checking account dry . . .

Even when our work environment is toxic
    and our co-workers hostile . . .

Even when our relationships are strained
    and bleed us of energy . . .

Even when darkness spirals us downward
    and we wallow in despair . . .

Even when we drink to medicate
    and shop to medicate
    and run to porn to medicate
    and use to medicate . . .

Even when our walls have crumbled
        and enemies are rushing us from every side . . .

Even when we are exiled
        away from home
        among those very different from us . . .

Even when our wailing
        is the only prayer we have . . .

Yet, will we trust in You

Happy and blessed
        . . . not the ones who have life turn out
              with ease and comfort
              and a fortified ego-self

        . . . but who are faithful
              and know they are held
              even from the pit

        . . . who trust You and open themselves to You
              even when they cannot see the end
                  from where they stand

This is fullness of life
        This is the essence of life with You

For reflection: Write your own series of expressions that begin, "Even when . . ." How have you experienced God's love and mercy, "even when . . ."? Let that remembrance lead you into prayer.

DAY THIRTY-FIVE

PSALM 24 Prayer
A psalm of the One who comes

Always and everywhere
    You are
Every time is Yours
    and every place
Earth, world, universe
People, every race and tribe
Four-footed beasts, winged fowl, fish
Mountains and marshes
    oceans and plains
Always and everywhere
    You are

So who is the one aware of Your presence?
Who acknowledges You in the world?
    The one with open hands and a quiet heart
    The one humbly rooted in the ground of their truth
    The one who practices Your presence, even when washing dishes
        and unafraid when You seem absent
    The one who can hear You in utter silence
        and does not run from the darkness
    The one who lays aside self-interest
        and does not perpetuate conventional wisdom
            that dollars rule
            that bigger is better
            that success is measurable
            that others exist to serve me

    Such a person lives in fullness of life
        they bless others
            and bless the world

Open wide, you door of my heart
Swing wide, you long-closed gates
    Your Heart-lover
    Your Soul-shaper
        lays siege to you
            silently awaiting an opening to enter

    Who is this Heart-lover
    Who is this Soul-shaper
        besieging me?
    The Glorious One
        my Beloved
        my Friend

Open wide, you door of my heart
Swing wide, you long-closed gates
    Your Heart-lover
    Your Soul-shaper
        lays siege to you
            silently awaiting an opening to enter

    Who is this Heart-lover
    Who is this Soul-shaper
        besieging me?

Ahhh, my Beloved
    my Friend
        it's You
            You at last

Come in

For reflection: This psalm-prayer contains several images. As you read it again, notice the one image that seems to draw you most, then linger with that image quietly in your prayer.

DAY THIRTY-SIX

PSALM 33:1 – 11 Prayer
A psalm for acclaiming God

Find your joy in God, all you who are righteous
    you who would like to do right
    you who haven't given a thought to doing right
    you who make yourself righteous
    you who are repulsed by self-righteousness
  It is good to find your life outside your self
    to discover your Center in God

Heart-acclaim to the One
  use all your instruments
    all your tools
  find your voice hidden in psalms
    write your own song of acclaim

Sing to God the song of your life
  your one and only life
    in all its treble and blast
    through all its delight and passion
    with all its glorious galaxies
      and humble dust

For God is straight
  the true Center-Pole around which we circle
And what God does
  makes whole

Your heart, O God, is ever-inclined
        to what is receptive and ready
        to what is impoverished and open
        to what is marred and cast aside
    So "Mercy" is Your nickname
        and Your generosity saturates everything

Your speech ordered the cosmos in its place
    and Your breath sustains all You have made

The waters of river, lake, and sea
    the deep places, the high places
Stir the hearts of us all
    to awe You
    to wonder You

Your speech continues to shape us
    Your ongoing word to animate our living

So while we assume to master our destinies
        to plot and plan for our futures
    our designs together come to a small speck

Your design, though, exists from forever
    and invites us to openness and participation
        the praise of lives formed for You

For reflection: For this pray-er, God's name is "Mercy." What is your personal name for God? In quiet prayer, take a few minutes to follow where that personal name takes you.

DAY THIRTY-SEVEN

PSALM 76 Prayer
A psalm for an alternative vision

Are there any who know You?
        Are there any who live into Your name?
Are there any who will let You be
        simply and profoundly
        THE ONE WHO IS?
    Dwelling in every place
        and every time?

Former generations named You in victories
        located You in battles won
            among swords and tanks
                profits and margins
                bountiful harvests and sleek livestock
                promotions and salaries
    We, too, assume You must be predisposed
                to winners
                to acclaim
                to prosperity

How splendid, how brilliant
        Your being
    shining brilliance beyond the brightest star

So all the heroes we've trusted
        have come to nothing
    their exploits are puny
    they have no power to transform
    they cannot stand shoulder to shoulder with You

You alone are God
You alone are
You alone
You

Not from afar do You send anonymous pronouncements
Not from a distance do You hurl lightning bolts of judgment
        to pin humans against their sin

No, Your intimate presence in our hearts
        surprises us
We find ourselves in company with You
        in the unexpected ones
        in the foreigner
        in the little and the least
        in those of every race and tribe –
                how surprised we were to find You there!?!?

You invite every human person
        to turn their intention toward You
        to make of their lives an offering

You are no respecter of our attainment
                our fought-after position and rank
        no respecter of what we hold in our hands
                our addiction to much-ness and many-ness

You see only the state of our hearts

                thankfully

For reflection: For a few moments rest in knowing that God sees all the way through you, to your heart. God doesn't see all the exterior trappings of your life. "People look at the outward appearance, but the Lord looks at the heart," (1 Sam. 16:7). How do you feel about that?

DAY THIRTY-EIGHT

PSALM 82 Prayer
A psalm for hearing God's voice

You stand, God, waist-deep
  in the muck of all the tiny things
    we make into gods
all the small idols
  to which we bend a knee

  the fears and insecurities
  the self-interest and divisiveness
  the successes and failures
  the lust for power and control
  our ongoing comparison and competition

"Listen up:

How long will you live small?
  How long will you content yourself
    in mindless living?
  How long will you wear names
    not your own?

Go where I go
Do what I do
  meet both the weak and the strong
    the power-less and the power-full
  be a voice for the voiceless
  give a voice to the voiceless
Live in kinship and community with those
  who are different from you
Be in solidarity with the have-nots
  – everyone, I remind you, is a have-not in some way –

Give yourself
        – time, energy, resources –
    on behalf of others
Visit the dark places in this world
    crawl into the holes in which people live
        be with those who hide in the shadows
            hold their hands
            mercy them
        so that even the darkness
            becomes light

This I say to you:
    Your destiny is divine
    I have created you in My own image
    Your being is stamped with My likeness
        You and I are forever connected
            soul-to-soul
        with a cord that can never be severed

        so that even when your days on earth
            run out
        we are still connected
                you and I
            eternally linked"

Grow strong in me, God
    and in us
    and in our world

And open our eyes
    to see it happen

Amen

For reflection: Have a conversation with God today in which you both speak and listen. What does God say to you? What do you say to God? You might write out the conversation on paper or in a journal. Pay special attention to what you sense God saying to you.

DAY THIRTY-NINE

PSALM 22 Prayer
A psalm to the unbridled God

My Love, my Mercy
      why have You turned away?
Why are You at a distance
      beyond the reach of my cries?
Why are You outside
      looking in
            on my trouble?

Why?
Why?
Why?

If I knew the answer
      would I find relief?
Would a satisfied understanding
      relieve the pain?
Could the chaos evaporate
      simply by knowing the "why"?

I confess my smallness
      my limitation
           my inability to see and know
                  the wider scope of life
                  the intricate Divine design
                      of the universe

All I know – here and now –
      is this wretched pain
      this searing heat
           that erupts from within
                  a lone voice echoing through hollow halls
                  a solitary figure wilting in the noonday sun

Who are You, anyway?
And where are You enthroned?

Have I totally missed You?
                misrepresented You?

In days past
        others have nailed You down
                in images easy to bear
        fixed You in ways that could be grasped
                by those who seek
They held the key to who You are
                to what You do
They used the key
        they got what they were after
        they spoke of You as their personal god
                and national deity
And so it was for me at one time
        so I experienced You in former days

But I know You that way no more
        I find my way in darkness
The only shouts I hear are silent
        I feel no need of convincing myself
                that You are Someone
                      Something
                      Somewhere
                              You are not

I can only speak as a man
        not a saint
        not an angel
        not a god
I see what I see
I know what I know
I hear what I hear

DAY THIRTY-NINE *(Cont)*

I make no claims of "better-than"
    or "farther-than"
I am who I am
I am where I am
    all any human can say

I so want to give myself to You in love
I so want to entrust my being to You
    even in confusion of cloud
        and
    in the unknowing of darkness

I no longer want to lie about You
    make up tales that pretend to smooth
        all the rough edges
    apart from my experience of You

Today, I'm willing to let You be who You are
    to unbridle You freely in my life
        wherever and whatever

I don't need to fit You into a tidy frame that adorns my life
    I don't need You to be this or that

I only need You
    to Be
    and to help me come into who I am
        the "me" You created me to be

This is the great life-work
    to which I give myself
This is Your beauty and glory
    toward which I walk

For reflection: Most of all, spirituality involves seeing truly . . . seeing God as God is . . . seeing myself as I am . . . seeing others as they are. Perhaps your prayer today is for eyes to notice, a heart that sees.

DAY FORTY

PSALM 100 Prayer
A psalm of God's Oneness

Loud voices to God, all you people
Loud lives for God
Loud silences with God
      listen
      stillness
      ssshhhhhh!

Let your song be prayer, O people
          – pray twice! –
     the silent, chanted converse
         of a soul connected with God
Let your life be divine dance, you lands
     offer to God your light and darkness
     live as if every moment
         you were in the presence of God

     Because you are

This is what we experience:
     You, God, are One
         We are created in Oneness
              for Oneness
          our destiny is divine
        Together we embody the One
          the walking, talking,
          moving around,
          graciously living
              incarnation of the One
     You mark us with Your Oneness
     We bear Your image within us
         Your likeness upon us
            We belong to You

DAY **FORTY** *(Cont)*

Enter God's heart gratefully
    Rest in God's heart peacefully
    Come and go offering thanks
In God's house
    let the ambience of the Host
        be your breath
        fill your pores
        feed you Bread
        serve you Cup

For You, my One
    are good and generous
You are durable kindness and faithful love
    mercy and compassion
        flow out from You
    and You are solid
        rock solid
            always
                and everywhere

For reflection: In John 17:11, 22, Jesus' prayer affirmed his oneness with the Father. He prayed that we would be one with God and one with each other as he was one with God. That oneness is not a dream for you, but a current reality. In what ways do you experience oneness with God and with others in your daily experience?